EVIDENCE-BASED TREATMENTS FOR EATING DISORDERS: CHILDREN, ADOLESCENTS AND ADULTS

EVIDENCE-BASED TREATMENTS FOR EATING DISORDERS: CHILDREN, ADOLESCENTS AND ADULTS

IDA F. DANCYGER AND
VICTOR M. FORNARI
EDITORS

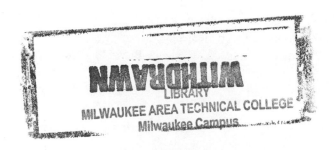
Nova Science Publishers, Inc.
New York

Library of Congress Cataloging-in-Publication Data

Evidence-based treatment for eating disorders : children, adolescents, and adults / Ida F. Dancyger, Victor M. Fornari (editors).   p. ; cm.
 Includes bibliographical references and index.
 ISBN 978-1-60692-310-8 (hardcover : alk. paper)
 1. Eating disorders. 2. Evidence-based medicine. I. Dancyger, Ida F. II. Fornari, Victor M.
 [DNLM: 1. Eating Disorders--therapy. 2. Evidence-Based Medicine. WM 175 E93 2009]
 RC552.E18E95 2009
 616.85'26--dc22   2008041221

Published by Nova Science Publishers, Inc. ✛ *New York*

Contents

A Book Reflecting the Kaleidoscopic Nature of the Treatment of Eating Disorders

Walter Vandereycken

Symptoms associated with food avoidance or overeating varied considerably over time. In view of this historical variability, eating disorders apparently belong to those disorders whose features show a remarkable susceptibility over the span of centuries to prevailing economic and sociocultural conditions as well as to developing medical knowledge. The current constellations of symptoms comprising anorexia nervosa and bulimia nervosa are to be considered the latest – and conceivably not the last – variants in an ever-existing, but constantly changing pattern of disordered eating behavior. Preoccupations with weight and shape and the use of weight control strategies like dieting and self-induced vomiting, have acquired popular and medical attention relatively recently and predominantly in Western or westernized countries. Hence, in medicine, the specific syndromes of anorexia nervosa and bulimia nervosa appear to be relatively "modern" clinical entities. Our diet-culture started more than a century ago and it is going to be with us for many years to come, probably together with eating disorders, "old" or "new" ones...

More than a century after the first systematic clinical observations, eating disorders still induce quite opposite reactions in clinicians: their "therapeutic appetite" may be either stimulated or suppressed. A considerable number of health care professionals do not want to treat patients with eating disorders, mainly because of feelings of frustration and lack of empathy with these patients. Others devote their entire professional career to the research and/or treatment of eating disordered patients. Why are these disorders so fascinating for some and so frustrating for others?

An ever-recurring pitfall in writings about one particular diagnostic category is the "uniformity myth", i.e. the assumption of homogeneity. Such a myth can easily be detected when one asks a clinician to briefly describe the major characteristics of anorexia nervosa. We all have a prototype in our mind, a kind of typical model which has been imprinted in our memory when first hearing or learning of the disorder. A common anorectic prototype is the "skinny teenage girl refusing to eat". If that picture becomes the leading image in our perception, we are likely not only to miss the diagnosis in several cases, but to mistreat many patients. Regardless of its diagnostic simplification into a DSM code, each person with an eating disorder reflects a complexity of biopsychosocial issues. This book bears witness to that kaleidoscopic picture. An impressive list of leading international experts presents a comprehensive review of the evidence supporting the best practices in the field.

Nowhere in a medical discipline is the plurality of opinion as great as in psychiatry. Does this diversity reflect the appealing richness of the discipline or is it symptomatic for a hybrid professional identity? This colorful picture is even more striking in the management of eating disordered patients, including the whole spectrum of professionals and the most diverse therapeutic arsenal in health care. But what treatment,by whom is the best for which patient? A book like this can be compared to a global positioning system tracing a variety of roads – the easiest, the fastest, and the most scenic – toward the desired goal. But for navigation in daily clinical practice, can science be the only reliable and useful guide?

Treatment for serious eating disorders can last many years and still its long-term outcome remains difficult to predict. So, how long should one go on with treatment trials? When does the disorder become chronic or "recalcitrant"? And what should we do for those patients who have "chosen" a life as an abstainer or a bulimic? Challenged by the reality of health care costs, be it in varying degrees depending on the health care system of the country involved, therapists dealing with seriously ill patients have to face some difficult decisions, both clinically and ethically, for which no clear-cut evidence-based guidelines exist.

Evidence-based medicine, in general, uses the double blind randomized controlled trial as the gold standard for judging the effectiveness of an intervention. The outcome of this type of research is then translated in algorithmic guidelines and manual-based treatments. For an increasing number of clinicians, only this approach can guarantee the scientific status of their work and safeguard the quality of care for a diversity of patients. For others, this scientific mainstreaming is experienced as the ultimate straitjacket squeezing their professional creativity into some form of pre-programmed practice. In recent years, the most challenging task in health care appears to be the fruitful merging of an evidence-based and an experienced-based approach. As in general medicine, this is the case in the field of eating disorders. Indeed, daily practice of working with eating disorder patients is not summarizable to some simple "do's and don'ts". Therefore, a book like this cannot offer easy-to-use recipes. However, *Evidence Based Treatments of Eating Disorders: Children, Adolescents and Adults* proposes a rich variety of methods and ingredients for the creative clinician who faces the challenges of caring for these individuals, and wants to be able to integrate the best current knowledge available.

Walter Vandereycken

Preface

This book represents the opportunity to bring together the currently available evidence for the best practices in the treatment of the eating disorders (EDs). We feel privileged that we have been able to assemble such a distinguished international group of experts in the field of eating disorders research and treatment. We will be gratified if clinicians across the wide range of disciplines treating individuals with eating disorders find the chapters in this book helpful to them in their work with patients, whether in treatment facilities, in the community, or in private practice. The chapters describe evidence-based or evidence-informed practices for the full range of eating disorders- including anorexia nervosa, bulimia nervosa, binge eating disorder, and obesity, and cover the full range of individuals with EDs seen across the life cycle: from childhood through adolescence and into adulthood, including a special section on males as well.

The topics are organized into four sections: (I) Overview of the evidence on the underpinnings of anorexia nervosa, bulimia nervosa, binge eating disorder, and obesity, as well as the tension in the field between research and clinical practice (Chapters 1-4); (II) Intensive treatments of eating disorders, including particular attention to treatment resistance (Chapters 5-10); (III) Evidence based and informed approaches to the psychotherapy of eating disorders, including cognitive behavioral, interpersonal, dialectical behavioral, family-based, and integrative cognitive-affective therapies (Chapters 11-17); and (IV) Pharmacological therapies for anorexia and bulimia nervosa (Chapter 18 and 19). Authors share with the reader their vast clinical experience and provide clinical vignettes in order to highlight important treatment considerations.

The book begins with Federici and Kaplan in Chapter 1 providing an informative overview of the bio-psycho-social risk factors underlying anorexia nervosa (AN). This chapter reviews the breadth of empirical evidence regarding neuro-biological, socio-cultural, familial, and psychological variables.

Brewerton in Chapter 2 presents the underpinnings of bulimia nervosa (BN) as it results from the dynamic interplay between biological, psychological, and social dimensions that operate along a developmental continuum. The research evidence is comprehensively examined as it relates to predisposing, precipitating, and perpetuating factors underlying BN, as there is no single etiology.

Cuzzularo and Vetrone in Chapter 3 provide an overview of the evidence for the underpinnings of binge eating disorder (BED) and obesity. BED is the most distinct subgroup in the eating disorder not otherwise specified (EDNOS) category. An account of the current knowledge on the epidemiology of BED and obesity is given along with the nosological status of this possible new diagnostic category.

Banker and Klump in Chapter 4 offer the reader an exciting review of the dynamic tension in the eating disorder field between research and clinical practice. The "research practice gap" is evidenced by discrepancies between the rate at which research results are re-produced and the rate at which the results are utilized in practice. The factors underlying the gap are explored and the authors provide a "road map" for closing this gap.

The second section begins with Parikh, Bellace, and Halmi in Chapter 5 describing the inpatient psychiatric treatment of adolescents and adults with an eating disorder. There are no standardized, universally accepted, evidence based criteria for the inpatient treatment of patients with EDs, but the multidisciplinary team approach for the inpatient care of individuals with AN and BN is emphasized.

Together with Katz, in Chapter 6 we examine the emergence of day treatment in the spectrum of care for AN. The evidence for its utility is reviewed, including the unique challenges and pitfalls with the different care options.

Fisher in Chapter 7 clearly summarizes the four key areas in the medical and nutritional care of children, adolescents, and young adults with EDs. This includes several consensus statements from professional associations describing a team approach as well as the clinical experience of the author.

Chapter 8 by Madden focuses on the challenge of the care of children with EDs where the evidence base for treatment remains weak. Developmental issues and their impact on treatment provide a framework to clinicians for identifying and managing the care of these young children.

An increasing incidence of males with EDs has been observed in recent years, specifically BN and EDNOS as described by Fernandez-Aranda and Jimenez-Murcia in Chapter 9. Therapy for males with EDs has received relatively little attention in the literature to date; however, description of a specific therapy program for males is fully presented.

Guarda and Coughlin in Chapter 10 discuss the critically important issue of ambivalence towards treatment and treatment resistance, both characteristics of patients with EDs, particularly AN. The matters of persuasion, perceived coercion, and treatment refusal, including competency and capacity to give or refuse consent, are among the many challenges facing clinicians and are thoroughly examined.

Section three begins with Pike and Yamano's up-to-date description of cognitive behavioral therapy (CBT) for AN in Chapter 11. There is an emerging data base that CBT has the potential to be an effective psychotherapy, particularly for individuals with weight-restored AN.

Chapter 12 by Braun offers a detailed overview of the impressive data on CBT in treating BN, with a brief description of underlying related brain functioning.

Brownley, Shapiro, and Bulik in Chapter 13 review current evidence-based treatment for obesity and BED. Topics include novel therapies that have shown promise in limited clinical studies, available pharmacological treatments, and effective behavioral therapies.

Interpersonal psychotherapy to treat patients with EDs is described by Murphy, Straebler, Cooper, and Fairburn in Chapter 14. The authors provide a detailed rationale for how helping patients identify and resolve current interpersonal difficulties can lead to recovery from deviant eating behaviors.

Chapter 15 by Wisniewski, Bhatnagar, and Warren presents a promising model for Dialectical Behavioral Therapy (DBT) enhanced CBT for the treatment of EDs. This chapter describes DBT, reviews relevant literature, and offers a novel approach for fusing principles of CBT with those of DBT.

Lock offers clinicians the latest advancements in an evidence based approach to family treatment for AN and BN in Chapter 16. An evaluation of existing research on family-based treatments, as well as skills necessary to implement this model, is provided.

Empirical research on emotions and EDs, the neurobiology of emotion, and a new treatment for BN called Integrative Cognitive-Affective Therapy (ICAT) are discussed in Chapter 17 by Engel, Wadeson, Lystad, Simonich, and Wonderlich.

The concluding two chapters present the empirical evidence for pharmacological therapies for AN in Chapter 18 by Roerig, Steffen, Mitchell, and Crow and for BN in Chapter 19 by Brown, Kotler, and Walsh. Randomized, double-blind, placebo controlled trials are emphasized.

We are delighted that so many of the leading international experts in the field of eating disorders have provided in this volume a compendium of the best studied treatments currently available. This book is thus intended to serve as a framework to the clinician searching for guidance on how to proceed with treatment when caring for an individual with an eating disorder. We are grateful to the authors for their generosity in sharing their clinical expertise, insights, and wisdom. We hope that the reader will appreciate and benefit from these contributions. Ultimately, patient care relies on the artful therapist who can integrate the best available evidence to inform his or her practice while tailoring the treatment for each individual. We sincerely hope that readers will find this book a useful reference, whether they are beginning or seasoned clinicians.

Acknowledgments

We are particularly delighted to have the opportunity to co-edit this book together. We are very fortunate to have collaborated these past ten years in our clinical and academic work with children, adolescents and adults with an eating disorder. We dedicate this volume to the many individuals and families with whom we have had the privilege to work with, and who have taught us about the complexities of caring for those struggling with these challenging disorders.

It has been an immense honor to work with our outstanding group of contributors; the researchers, clinicians and scholars who have so generously contributed not only their knowledge, but also their passion to the treatment of those with eating disorders. Several of the authors have been not only our teachers, but also international leaders in this field.

This book would not have been possible without the administrative help, dedication, intelligence and commitment from Nicole Taylor at North Shore University Hospital, who helped with the early organization of the project; and Marie Stercula at Long Island Jewish Medical Center, who helped with the preparation of the manuscript.

Finally, we would like to thank our families, for their continued support and enthusiasm throughout this lengthy project. To my husband, Ken, an extremely gifted and prodigious writer, your constant belief in me and your loving input whenever requested made this dream of mine come true. To my wife Alice, for your continuous love and encouragement.

In memory of our parents, Mendel and Malka Flint and Ermanno and Alice Notrica Fornari.

List of Contributors

Judith D. Banker, MA, LLP, FAED
Center for Eating Disorders, Ann Arbor, Michigan

Dara Bellace, PhD
Eating Disorders Program, New York Presbyterian Hospital-Payne Whitney Westchester
Department of Psychiatry, Cornell Weill School of Medicine, White Plains, New York

Kelly Bhatnagar, MA
The Cleveland Center for Eating Disorders and Case Western Reserve University,
Cleveland, Ohio

Devra Lynn Braun, MD
Weill Cornell Medical College, New York, New York
Integrative Medicine and Psychotherapy of Greenwich, LLC, Connecticut

Timothy D. Brewerton, MD, DFAPA, FAED
Department of Psychiatry and Behavioral Sciences,
Medical University of South Carolina, Charleston, South Carolina

Amanda Joelle Brown, BA
The New York State Psychiatric Institute, New York, New York

Kimberly A. Brownley, PhD
Department of Psychiatry, University of North Carolina at Chapel Hill, North Carolina

Cynthia M. Bulik, PhD
Departments of Psychiatry and Nutrition,
University of North Carolina at Chapel Hill, North Carolina

Zafra Cooper, DPhil, DipPsych
Department of Psychiatry, University of Oxford, United Kingdom

Janelle W. Coughlin, PhD
Department of Psychiatry and Behavioral Sciences, The Johns Hopkins School of Medicine,
Baltimore, Maryland

Scott J. Crow, MD
Department of Psychiatry, University of Minnesota Medical School, Minneapolis, Minnesota

Massimo Cuzzolaro, MD
Eating and Weight Disorders Unit, Department of Medical Physiopathology,
University of Rome, Sapienza, Roma, Italy

Ida F. Dancyger, PhD
Department of Psychiatry, The Zucker Hillside Hospital,
North Shore-Long Island Jewish Health System, Glen Oaks, New York
Clinical Associate Professor of Psychology in Psychiatry,
New York University School of Medicine, New York, New York

Scott G. Engel, PhD
Neuropsychiatric Research Institute, Fargo, North Dakota
University of North Dakota, Grand Forks, North Dakota

Christopher G. Fairburn, DM, FMedSci, FRCPsych
Department of Psychiatry, University of Oxford, United Kingdom

Anita Federici, MSc
Department of Psychology, York University, Toronto, Ontario, Canada

Fernando Fernández-Aranda, PhD, FAED
Eating Disorder Unit and Research Group
Department of Psychiatry, University Hospital of Bellvitge and
CIBER Fisiopatología de la Obesidad y Nutrición (CIBEROBN),
Instituto Carlos III, Barcelona, Spain

Martin Fisher, MD
Division of Adolescent Medicine, Schneider Children's Hospital,
North Shore-Long Island Jewish Health System, New Hyde Park, New York
New York University School of Medicine, New York, New York

Kathleen Kara Fitzpatrick, PhD
Department of Psychiatry, Stanford University School of Medicine, Stanford, California

Victor M. Fornari, MD
Director, Division of Child and Adolescent Psychiatry, Department of Psychiatry,
The Zucker Hillside Hospital, North Shore-Long Island Jewish Health System,
Glen Oaks, New York
Professor of Psychiatry, New York University School of Medicine, New York, New York

Angela S. Guarda, MD
Department of Psychiatry and Behavioral Sciences, The Johns Hopkins School of Medicine,
Baltimore, Maryland

Katherine Halmi, MD
New York Presbyterian Hospital-Payne Whitney Westchester
Cornell Weill School of Medicine, White Plains, New York

Susana Jiménez-Murcia, PhD
Department of Psychiatry, University Hospital of Bellvitge and CIBER Fisiopatología de la
Obesidad y Nutrición (CIBEROBN), Instituto Carlos III, Barcelona, Spain

Allan S. Kaplan, MD FRCP(C)
Eating Disorders, Toronto General Hospital
Department of Psychiatry, University of Toronto, Ontario, Canada

Jack L. Katz, MD
Department of Psychiatry, The Zucker Hillside Hospital,
North Shore-Long Island Jewish Health System, Glen Oaks, New York
New York University School of Medicine, New York, New York

Lisa A. Kotler, MD
The New York State Psychiatric Institute, New York, New York
Columbia University College of Physicians and Surgeons, New York, New York

Kelly L. Klump, PhD, FAED
Department of Psychology, Michigan State University, East Lansing, Michigan

James Lock, MD, PhD
Division of Child Psychiatry and Pediatrics, Department of Psychiatry and
Behavioral Sciences, Stanford University School of Medicine, Stanford, California

Chad M. Lystad, MS
Neuropsychiatric Research Institute, Fargo, North Dakota

Sloane Madden, MB BS (Hons) FRANZCP
Child and Adolescent Eating Disorder Program, Psychiatry,
The Children's Hospital at Westmead, Sydney, Australia

James E. Mitchell, MD
Department of Clinical Neuroscience, University of North
Dakota School of Medicine and Health Sciences, Fargo, North Dakota
Neuropsychiatric Research Institute, Fargo, North Dakota

Rebecca Murphy, DClinPsych
Department of Psychiatry, University of Oxford, United Kingdom

Parinda Parikh, MD
Child and Adolescent Eating Disorder Program,
New York Presbyterian Hospital-Payne Whitney Westchester
Cornell Weill School of Medicine, White Plains, New York

Kathleen M. Pike, PhD
Temple University, Japan

James D. Roerig, PharmD, BCPP
Department of Clinical Neuroscience, University of North Dakota School of Medicine and
Health Sciences, Fargo, North Dakota

Jennifer Shapiro, PhD
Department of Psychiatry, University of North Carolina at Chapel Hill, North Carolina

Heather K. Simonich, MA
Neuropsychiatric Research Institute, Fargo, North Dakota

Kristine Steffen, PharmD
Neuropsychiatric Research Institute, Fargo, North Dakota

Suzanne Straebler, APRN-Psychiatry, MSN
Department of Psychiatry, University of Oxford, United Kingdom

Walter Vandereycken, MD, PhD
Department of Psychiatry, Catholic University Leuven, Belgium

Giuseppe Vetrone, MD
Department of Philosophical Research, University of Rome Tor Vergata, Roma, Italy

Andrea Wadeson, BA
Neuropsychiatric Research Institute, Fargo, North Dakota
North Dakota State University, Fargo, North Dakota

B. Timothy Walsh, MD
The New York State Psychiatric Institute, New York, New York
Columbia University College of Physicians and Surgeons, New York, New York

Mark Warren, MD, MPH
The Cleveland Center for Eating Disorders and Case Western Reserve University,
Cleveland, Ohio

Lucene Wisniewski, PhD, FAED
The Cleveland Center for Eating Disorders and Case Western Reserve University,
Cleveland, Ohio

Steve A. Wonderlich, PhD
Neuropsychiatric Research Institute, Fargo, North Dakota
University of North Dakota, Grand Forks, North Dakota

Marisa A. Yamano, BA
Temple University, Japan

In: Evidence-Based Treatments for Eating Disorders
Author: Ida F. Dancyger and Victor M. Fornari

ISBN 978-1-60692-310-8
© 2009 Nova Science Publishers, Inc.

Chapter I

Overview of the Biopsychosocial Risk Factors Underlying Anorexia Nervosa

Anita Federici[1] and Allan S. Kaplan[2]
[1]York University, Toronto, Ontario, Canada
[2]University of Toronto, Ontario, Canada

Abstract

Historically, anorexia nervosa has been a poorly understood and difficult to treat psychiatric illness. With the advent of more sophisticated medical technology, enhanced research methodology, and widespread international interest, current conceptualizations of the disorder have become increasingly more refined and advanced. The goal of this chapter is to review the breadth of empirical evidence regarding risk factors for the development of anorexia nervosa, spanning neuro-biological, sociocultural, familial, and psychological domains.

Introduction

Developing an evidence based theory regarding the etiological underpinnings of anorexia nervosa (AN) is an important yet challenging task. Many variables have been hypothesized to be risk factors for AN, however, their relative contribution and specificity to the development of the disorder is unknown (Fairburn, Cooper, Doll, and Welch, 1999; Pike, 1998). In addition, there are relatively few longitudinal studies with adequate cohort sizes to allow proper examination and identification of potential risk factors in AN. Nevertheless, there is evidence in the published literature that certain biological, personality, and familial variables appear to contribute to the development of AN. We will attempt to comprehensively review these risk factors in this chapter.

Phenomenologically, AN is characterized by a refusal to maintain a body weight at or above what is considered a minimal normal weight for age and height. Individuals with AN exhibit intense fears of becoming fat despite being underweight and display severe disturbances in the way their bodies are perceived and experienced (DSM -IV, American Psychiatric Association (APA), 2000). The presence of amenorrhea is also part of the current diagnostic criteria, although the necessity of this feature is currently under review (Garfinkel et al., 1996). Depending on symptom presentation, the illness may be further nosologically characterized as a restricting subtype (e.g., absence of any binging or purging behaviour during the course of the illness) or a binge-purge subtype (e.g., regular occurrence of binge eating and/or purging behaviours). AN is prevalent in approximately 0.5 % of the female population and the long-term prognosis of the disorder is poor (APA, 2000; Steinhausen, 2002). In comparison to other psychiatric conditions, AN is considered to be one of the most severe and life-threatening as it confers a standardized mortality rate that is 12 times higher than the general population of females aged 15-24 (Sullivan, 1995). Mortality rates as high as 22% have been reported (Lowe, Zipfel, Dupont, Reas and Herzog, 2001; Birmingham, Su, Hlynsky, Goldner, and Gao, 2005). Identifying and elucidating the factors that contribute to the development and maintenance of AN are paramount to our ability to effectively treat the disorder.

While early descriptions of the origins of AN typically focused on discreet causal factors (e.g., maturational fears, familial difficulties, repressed sexual conflicts), modern theoretical accounts are predominately multifactorial in nature. Most theorists agree that a single etiological cause of AN does not sufficiently address the complexities of the illness (Garfinkel and Garner, 1982). AN is best understood using a more sophisticated, multidimensional model. From this perspective, the disorder is likely a manifestation of biological, psychological and sociocultural risk factors (Anderson, Bowers and Evans, 1997; Jacobi, Hayward, de Zwaan, Kraemer, Agras, 2004).

I. Biological Factors

There is increasing evidence for the importance of neurobiological factors in potentiating the vulnerability to anorexia nervosa. These include genetic factors, changes in brain structure/blood flow, neurotransmitter/ neuropeptides, and pre- and perinatal factors.

Genetic Factors

Family and twin studies have shown that genes contribute substantially more than 50% of the risk for AN (Klump, Kaye, and Strober, 2001). Over the past decade, a number of association and linkage studies have identified specific genetic diatheses contributing to the development of AN. Association studies have examined genes responsible for the regulation of various neurotransmitter systems. The most well studied is the serotonin system. A meta-analysis of the studies examining the 5HT2a receptor gene found a very significant association between AN and the AA genotype, suggesting a role for the 5HT2a receptor in the genetic risk for AN (Gorwood, Kipman, and Foulon, 2003). Other neurotransmitter and neuropetide systems have been examined, including the opioid, dopamine, neuropeptide Y, leptin and agouti related protein genes, with largely negative results, possibly related to inadequate sample sizes (Klump and Gobrogge, 2005.) Linkage studies emanating from a large multi-site consortium have shown modest evidence of linkage on chromosomes 1, 4 11, 13 and 165 and much stronger linkage on chromosome 1 when only restrictor anorexics were included in the analyses (Grice et al., 2002). Candidate genes such as the delta opioid receptor (OPRD1) and serotonin 1 D receptor (5HTR1D) genes were also associated with AN in this cohort (Bergen et al., 2003). These studies point to significant genetic effects in the risk for AN but require replication.

Changes in Brain Structure/Cerebral Blood Flow

Structural neuroimaging studies have demonstrated enlarged ventricles and loss of gray matter in underweight subjects with AN, changes which are thought to be related to the state of emaciation and starvation and to reverse with refeeding and weight gain. (Wagner et al., 2006). However, more recent studies suggest that these changes may persist in the recovered state (Mühlau et al., 2007). Regional blood flow changes utilizing SPECT (single photon emission computed tomography) have been reported in adolescents with AN (Lask et al., 2005). These studies have found unilateral reduction in blood flow in the temporal lobe in about 75% of subjects studied. There was no association between this reduced blood flow and nutritional state, length of illness, associated comorbidity, or eating disorder psychopathology, suggesting a primary phenomenon independent of starvation. This reduced blood flow was associated with impaired visual processing and memory and enhanced information processing, suggesting altered cognitive functioning in AN. These findings are intriguing and require further research.

Neurotransmitter/Neuropeptide Systems

Many changes in monamines described in the past among individuals with AN are virtually all due to either the starvation state or emaciation and correct with nutritional rehabilitation and weight gain (Kaplan, 1990). Recent functional neuroimaging studies have implicated several of the neurotransmitters and neuropeptides in the etiology of AN. These studies have found that recovered subjects with AN had reduced 5HT2a receptor activity in the cingulate and other cortical areas and normal 5HT1A activity (Frank et al., 2002). Observed abnormalities in serotonergic functioning could contribute to the symptoms seen in AN, such as changes in appetitive behaviors, and increased anxiety and obsessionality (Kaye, Frank, Bailer, and Henry, 2005). In addition, abnormalities of the dopaminergic system found in recovered restricting anorexics could contribute to other symptoms seen in AN such as hyperactive motor behavior and abnormalities in reward and behavioral inhibition (Kaye, Frank, and McConaha, 1999).

some researchers speculating that the two disorders are etiologically related (for a review see Serpell et al., 2002).

Other identified personality traits include neuroticism, negative emotionality, harm avoidance, compulsivity, social inhibition, emotional restraint, compliance, and low self-esteem (Geller, Cockell, Hewitt, Goldner, and Flett, 2000; Vervaet, van Heeringen, and Audenaert, 2004; Vitousek and Manke, 1994; Zaitsoff, Geller, Srikameswaran, 2002). Problems with identity formation, issues with autonomy, maturity fears, and negative self-evaluation are also common in AN sufferers (de Groot and Rodin, 1994; Fairburn et al., 1999; Stein and Nyguist, 2001).

There is also some empirical support for characterological differences between AN subtypes. For example, individuals with the binge-purge subtype are more likely to score higher on measures of impulsivity and sensation-seeking (Claes, Vandereycken, and Vertommen, 2005; Lacey and Evans; 1986; Rossier, Bolognini, Plancherel, and Halfan, 2000; Vervaet et al., 2004). In contrast, individuals with the restricting type of AN are more likely to be compulsive, constricted, and neurotic (Wonderlich, Lilenfeld, Riso, Engel, and Mitchell, 2005).

With regard to specific Axis II pathology, Cluster C disorders, particularly obsessive compulsive and avoidant personality disorder, are more commonly observed among the restricting subtype of AN while Cluster B pathologies are more frequently associated with patients who engage in binging and purging behaviours (Bornstein, 2001; Cassin and von Ranson, 2005; Rastam, 1992). Borderline personality disorder (BPD) is considered to be the most common Axis II disorder among this latter population (Dennis and Sansone, 1997). Data from epidemiological studies consistently show that a significant subgroup of ED patients meet criteria for BPD (Skodol et al., 1993; Vitousek and Manke, 1994). Sansone, Levitt, and Sansone (2005) reported that BPD was prevalent in 35% of patients with AN (25% with the binge/purge subtype and 10% with the restricting subtype). Individuals with comorbid AN and BPD have significantly greater difficulty regulating internal emotional states and are more likely to engage in self-injurious behaviours, substance abuse, and other impulsive and reckless acts; thus, they represent a more challenging and complex patient population. Impulsivity has been associated with a more protracted course of illness, poor treatment outcome, premature dropout, and higher rates of relapse (Agras et al., 2000; Johnson-Sabine, Reiss, and Dayson, 1992; Finfgeld, 2002; Sansone, Sansone, and Levitt, 2004).

Emotion Dysregulation

Deficits in the ability to recognize, integrate, and express emotion are hypothesized to play a central role in the development and maintenance of AN (Bruch, 1978). As early as the 1960s, conceptualization of AN included a pervasive inability to identify and describe internal emotional states and many researchers have since described eating disorder symptoms (e.g., self-starvation, binging, vomiting) as maladaptive attempts to regulate intense negative emotions (Bruch, 1988). Certainly, it is not uncommon for individuals with AN to report feeling disconnected from their feelings or to feel confused and overwhelmed by emotion. Numerous studies have shown that the most commonly cited trigger for symptomatic behaviours is stress or negative affect. Eating disorder patients have consistently reported that symptoms provide relief from emotions that are perceived as threatening, overwhelming, or that exceed their existing coping abilities (Cockell, Zaitsoff, and Geller, 2004). Identifying, tolerating, and expressing negative affect has also been identified as an essential component in the recovery process (Federici and Kaplan, 2007).

Some researchers have speculated that alexithymia (referring to the inability to identify and describe feelings, difficulty discriminating between physical sensations and emotions, and a concrete, externalized orientation) may be an important predisposing factor in the development of AN (Schmidt, Jiwany, and Treasure, 1993; Zonnevijlle-Bendek, van Goozen, Cohen-Kettenis, van Elburg, and van Engeland, 2002). Studies using the Toronto Alexithymia Scale (TAS) provide consistent evidence that alexithymia is, in fact, more prevalent in eating disorder populations (Bydlowski et al., 2005; Schmidt et al., 1993). Compared to control groups, where the prevalence of alexithymia ranged from 6.7% to 26%, Bourke, Taylor, Parker, and Bagby (1992) reported prevalence rates as high as 77% in female AN patients, 56% in patients with BN, and 64% in patients with BED. Zonnevijlle-Bendek et al. (2002) demonstrated that, compared to a control group, patients with AN and BN have greater difficulty recognizing and labelling affective states. In addition, Bydlowski et al. (2005) demonstrated lower levels of emotional awareness among individuals with AN compared to those with BN, highlighting a more pronounced deficit in the ability to recognize and accurately label affective states. It is not uncommon for patients with AN to report that the onset of their symptoms were preceded by a pervasive sense of ineffectiveness, feelings of shame or worthlessness, a feeling of being internally flawed, and strong fears of criticism and rejection. One of the identified functions of severe food restriction and binge eating or purging behaviours, is to regulate, dismiss, or reduce aversive mood states. Similarly, a significant subgroup of patients with AN engage in recurrent episodes of self-harm and self-mutilation, often in an attempt to regulate intense negative affect. In a meta-analysis of studies conducted between 1986 and 2000 examining self harm and suicidal acts in patients with an ED, Sansone and Levitt (2004) found that 11% of outpatients with AN reported a history of attempted suicide and 22% of outpatients with AN reported engaging in self injurious behaviours.

The significant and pervasive problems with affect observed in those with AN has prompted clinicians to incorporate emotion regulation strategies into existing treatment protocols (Corstorphine, 2006; Fairburn, Cooper, and Shafran, 2003). In addition, alternative treatment approaches that focus on the processing of emotional experience (e.g., Emotion Focused Therapy) and teaching specific affect regulation skills (e.g., Dialectical Behaviour Therapy) are currently being adapted for use in clients with eating disorders (Telch, 1997; Telch, Agras, and Linehan, 2001).

Cognitive Factors

Cognitive models have been particularly influential in providing a theoretical framework for the conceptualization of disordered eating. Such models posit that eating disorders are the result of core disturbances in thinking, perception, and memory. Individuals with AN demonstrate maladaptive, rigid, and idiosyncratic schemas involving food, weight, and shape which directly influence their thoughts, feelings, and subsequent behaviours (Green, McKenna, and De Silva, 1994; Sackville, Schotte, Touyz, Griffiths, and Beaumont, 1998; Vitousek and Hollon, 1990). Obsessive thoughts about eating and body weight, overly rigid, dichotomous, and perfectionist styles of thinking, and body size overestimation are all well documented phenomena in the literature on AN. In addition, investigators have recently found evidence to support the presence of thought-action fusion (TAF) or thought-shape fusion (TSF) in patients with AN (Shafran, Teachman, Kerry, and Rachman, 1999). Typically used to describe a cognitive distortion common among patients with OCD, TAF refers to the belief that a thought about something aversive occurring can increase the likelihood of a negative event happening and/or is equivalent to having actually carried out the negative event. Radomsky, de Silva, Todd, Treasure and Murphy (2002) found that the act of writing an aversive sentence (e.g., "I am eating cake") significantly increased anxiety, depression, guilt, and increased subjective ratings of fatness among individuals with AN. Notably, 75% of the sample chose to act on urges to neutralize or correct the statement (e.g., crossed out/modified/covered the sentence). The presence of such ingrained and dysfunctional cognitive patterns serves to direct, organize, and classify incoming information in such a way as to reinforce the core assumptions and beliefs.

In their seminal paper exploring the role of schematic processing in eating disordered individuals, Vitousek and Hollon (1990) argued that eating disorders are maintained and intensified by particular attentional biases to weight and body-related stimuli. People with eating disorders are expected to detect food and weight-based cues more quickly, and to attach greater meaning and be more attentive to schema-related information in their environment. Vitousek and Hollon (1990) further proposed that anorexic and bulimic sufferers would exhibit selective memory for schema-consistent information, be resistant to details perceived as schema-inconsistent, and perceive ambivalent stimuli as weight, shape, or food-related, thus differentiating them from non-eating disordered individuals.

There is some empirical evidence for the presence of specific memory and attentional biases for food and weight-related stimuli in AN. Hermans, Pieters and Eelen (1998) reported that patients with AN showed a pattern of selective recall of anorexia-related words on a task of explicit memory compared to a control group. Modified versions of the Stroop colouring naming task have demonstrated that individuals with AN and BN are slower to colour-name the ink in which food or body-related words are

written (Fairburn, Cooper, Cooper, McKenna, and Anastasiades, 1991; Cooper, Anastasiades, and Fairburn, 1992). Using the dot probe visual detection task, Rieger et al. (1998) found that, compared to unrestrained eaters (e.g., non-dieters) individuals with AN and BN detected target probes faster when they appeared in the same location as negative body shape/weight words (e.g. fat). Differences in response patterns have also been detected between patients with AN and BN, with the former group having greater difficulty colour naming food–related words and the latter group responding more slowly to body shape and weight words (Ben-Tovim and Walker, 1991; Channon, Hemsley, and de Silva, 1988; Cooper and Todd, 1997). Observed colour-naming latencies and interference effects are thought to be the result of difficulties attending to emotionally salient and highly evocative stimuli. These data provide compelling evidence that patients with AN selectively attend to, and prioritize, schema-congruent stimuli. It is unclear, however, whether these cognitive patterns are etiological in nature or a by-product of chronic hunger and starvation. Some data have shown that hunger alone is not sufficient to account for these observed effects. For example, Placanica, Faunce, and Job (2002) examined the effect of hunger on attention in a sample of female undergraduate students. While fasting increased the detection of high-calorie food words across the entire sample, individuals with elevated drive for thinness and body dissatisfaction scores processed food words significantly faster than participants with low scores. More research is needed to further understand the nature of the relationship between cognitive biases and the development of AN.

Sociocultural Factors

While the association between disordered eating and socio-cultural influences are commonly acknowledged in the literature, the degree to which such factors play a causal role in AN is widely debated (Keel and Klump, 2003; Striegel-Moore and Smolak, 2002). Feminist and sociological theories of the etiology of AN have long proposed that cultural ideals of beauty, sex-role stereotypes, and the increasing demands on women to occupy multiple roles have oppressed women and presented them with conflicting messages about their bodies and their relationships with food (Szmukler and Patton, 1995; Stice, 2002).

Given the disproportionately greater prevalence of AN among Caucasian women in Westernized societies, many have suggested that the emphasis and value placed on slenderness in modern society (and the concurrent hostility toward overweight body types) facilitate and reinforce the internalization of a "thinness ideal", particularly among women (Harrison and Cantor, 1997; Mills, Polivy, Herman, and Tiggerman, 2002). Internalization of the thinness ideal occurs when an individual accepts and integrates societal norms and expectations about body weight and shape into her developing self concept. As a result, self-esteem and self-worth become dependent upon one's perceived ability to approximate and successfully achieve such standards. The inherent paradox, however, (i.e., that cultural standards for weight and shape are virtually unattainable and unrealistic for the majority of women) tends to foster body dissatisfaction, cultivate a drive for thinness, and promote dieting behaviour; factors that have each been identified as prominent risk factors for the development of disordered eating.

In lab settings, with both clinical and non-clinical populations, exposure to thin media images is associated with greater negative affect and body dissatisfaction. Yamamiya, Cash, Melnyk, Posavac and Posavac (2005) found that degree of internalization moderated the effect on mood and body shape concerns among a sample of 123 college females exposed to a five-minute display of thin fashion models. The impact of the messages espoused by industrialized countries on non-industrialized societies has also been studied. Investigations evaluating the influence of television exposure among a sample of female adolescents from Fiji found that exposure to Western media was related to an increased desire to reshape the body, identification with female television characters as role models, and greater eating disordered attitudes and behaviours (Becker, 2004; Becker, Burwell, Gilman, Herzog, and

Hamburg, 2002). Similarly, the degree to which one's peer group ascribes to culturally sanctioned weight ideals is correlated with a greater likelihood of body dissatisfaction and low self-esteem. For example, Mills and Miller (2007) reported that restrained eaters (i.e, chronic dieters) were more likely to rate themselves as heavier, less attractive, and more depressed when a same-sex peer (e.g., a fellow undergraduate student), compared to a same-sex non-peer (e.g., a PhD student), guessed their weight to be 15 pounds heavier than their actual weight. Peer influences appear to play an important role in the promotion of body dissatisfaction, social comparison, and dieting behaviours (Grigg, Bowman, and Redman, 1996; Schutz, Paxton, and Wertheim, 2002; Stice, Maxfield, and Wells, 2003). Individuals suffering from AN have identified weight and shape-based teasing and pressures to be thin by female peers as contributory factors in the development of their disorder (Nilsson Abrahamsson, Torbiornsson, and Hagglof, 2007; Tozzi, Sullivan, Fear, McKenzie, and Bulik, 2002).

While these findings paint a compelling picture of the detrimental effects of sociocultural ideas linking beauty and success with thinness, these particular influences alone fail to account for the relatively low base rate of AN in the general population. In contrast to the increasing incidence rates of BN over the past several decades, rates of AN have remained relatively stable over time (Willi, Giacometti, and Limacher, 1990) . Given the pervasiveness of the media and the fact that significant numbers of adolescents (McVey, Tweed, and Blackmore, 2004) and adult women are dieting at any one point in time, one would expect to observe a much greater prevalence of AN in Westernized societies. In contrast, only a small proportion of individuals exposed to the noxious influence of the media go on to develop the disorder. It is best to conceptualize societal pressures and cultural influences as environmental risk factors that promote dieting behaviours and poor body image and interact with genetic factors in biologically vulnerable individuals to produce the illness; i.e., gene-environment correlation (Bulik et al., 2005). It is important to clearly distinguish the severe psychiatric illness of AN which has genetic and psychopathological determinants from the type of body dissatisfaction and aberrant eating beahviour which is ubiquitous among young women in most Westernized societies.

Furthermore, there is increasing evidence that AN exists in non-industrialized societies where the influence of Western culture is either unlikely or non-existent. In their review of the literature, Keel and Klump (2003) identified cases of AN in India, Malaysia, Nigeria, Hong Kong, and Pakistan. Documented cases of self-starvation, sometimes leading to death, also date back to the 12th century, and possibly earlier (Lacey 1982). Such evidence calls into question the notion that modern Westernized views of the female body are necessary for the development of AN. In addition, there are important historical and cross-cultural variations of the illness which suggest that dominant cultural norms tend to shape and influence the outward expression of the syndrome as opposed to directly causing the disorder. For example, the current conceptualization of AN considers weight and shape concerns to be a defining feature of the illness and a necessary diagnostic criterion. Such concerns, however, are endorsed with far less frequency in historical writings and in non-industrialized societies among individuals who otherwise meet diagnostic criteria (e.g., Hong Kong; Lee, Ho, and Hsu, 1993). It appears as though the presentation of AN and the specific motivations for food refusal (e.g., religious devotion, gastric discomfort) is culturally dependent but that the disorder itself is not culture-bound.

Family Systems and Environmental Risk Factors

Family dysfunction and negative childhood experiences have consistently been implicated as significant contributory factors (Beresin, Gordon, and Herzog, 1989; Button and Warren, 2001; Tozzi et al., 2002). Much has been written over the decades regarding the role of family dynamics as a contributory factor in the development of AN (Bruch, 1978; Minuchin, Rosman, Baker, and Lester, 1978). Hilde Bruch (1978) proposed that several characteristic traits of the disorder (e.g. emotional distress, low self-esteem, a sense of ineffectiveness) were partially the result of insufficiently met needs in childhood and inadequate maternal validation. Individuals with AN consistently describe their early home environments as controlling and emotionally invalidating. In their qualitative study exploring causes of AN, Tozzi et al. (2002) reported that the most frequently cited etiological factor was a dysfunctional family environment. Families are often described as intrusive, enmeshed, overbearing, and adverse to the emotional and psychological needs of the developing child (Beresin et al., 1989; Garfinkel and Garner, 1982; Polivy and Herman, 2002). Research has also demonstrated that AN families have more difficulty resolving conflict and are less communicative with one another (Lattimore, Wagner and Gowers, 2000). Less secure, and more avoidant /anxious attachment styles have also been implicated as salient predisposing factors (Latzer, Hochdorf, Bacher and Canetti, 2002; Ward and Gowers, 2003). Marital discord, high parental expectations, expressed value on thinness, and chronic dieting behaviours in the home have also been hypothesized to exacerbate body dissatisfaction and disordered eating. Given that AN typically develops during adolescence, these data underscore the importance of understanding the relative contribution that dysfunctional family dynamics play in the pathogenesis the illness. Having said this, much of the disturbance in family dynamics seen in the families of individuals with AN is more likely the result of having a child who is tenaciously pursuing thinness and engaged in self starvation rather than being directly causative of the disorder.

Recent research has also identified that having a mother with either an active eating disorder or a past history of one is an environmental risk factor for AN (Mazzeo, Zucker, Gerke, Mitchell, and Bulik, 2005). Disturbed feeding practices (Russell, Treasure, and Eisler, 1998), disturbed attitudes towards feeding and weight (Stice, Agras, Hammer, 1999), conflictual mealtime interactions (Stein, Woolley, Cooper, and Fairburn, 1994) interference with parenting and meeting the child's needs (Stein and Woolley, 1996), and difficulties with interpersonally relating to their children (Franzen and Gerlinghoff, 1997) have all been reported to contribute to this risk.

Patients with AN have also reported an association between symptom onset and stressful life transitions. Advancing from high school to university, moving to a new home, losing a close friend, or experiencing difficulties in intimate relationships have frequently been identified as precipitating factors (Beresin et al., 1989; Nilsson et al., 2007; Tozzi et al., 2003). Childhood sexual abuse has also been implicated as a risk factor for the development of AN. While trauma histories are not uncommon among individuals with AN and continue to be an important focus of research and treatment, the empirical evidence to date does not support a direct, causal link between trauma exposure and the development of the illness (Brewerton, 2005; Wonderlich, Brewerton, Jocic, Dansky, and Abbott, 1997). At this time, there is a stronger association between sexual abuse and the development of BN rather than AN (see Fallon and Wonderlich, 1997 and Brewerton, 2005 for review).

Conclusion

Notable advances have been made in recent years with respect to our understanding of the risk factors that contribute to the development of AN. The goal of this chapter was to provide a comprehensive overview of the etiological factors that have been empirically identified to date. While the precise mechanisms and associations between these risk factors are yet to be determined, the data presented in this chapter highlight that AN is a distinct and multi-determined serious clinical disorder. The precise interactional effects between predisposing biological, social, and psychological determinants is unique to each individual and understanding these interactions is key to our ability to effectively treat this complex and debilitating illness.

References

Agras, W. S., Crow, S. J., Halmi, K. A., Mitchell, J. E., Wilson, G. T., and Kraemer, H. C. (2000). Outcome predictors for the cognitive behaviour treatment of bulimia nervosa: Data from a multi-site study. *American Journal of Psychiatry, 157,* 1302-1308.

American Psychiatric Association. (2000). *Diagnostic and Statistical Manual of Mental Disorders,* fourth edition, text revised (DSM-IV-TR). Washington, DC: American Psychiatric Press.

Anderluh A. B., Tchanturia, K., Rabe-Hesketh, S., and Treasure, J. (2003). Childhood obsessive-compulsive personality traits in adult women with EDs: Defining a broader ED phenotype. *American Journal of Psychiatry, 160,* 242-247.

Anderson, A. E., Bowers, W., and Evans, K. (1997). Inpatient treatment of anorexia nervosa. In D. M. Garner and P. E. Garfinkel (Eds.) *Handbook of treatment for eating disorders* (2nd ed.). *(*pp. 327-348). New York, NY: The Guilford Press.

Bastiani, A. M., Rao, R., Weltzin, T., and Kaye, W. H. (1995). Perfectionism in anorexia nervosa. *International Journal of Eating Disorders, 17,* 147-152,

Becker, A. (2004). Television, disordered eating, and young women in Fiji: Negotiating body image and identity during rapid social change. *Culture, Medicine and Psychiatry, 28,* 533-559.

Becker, A. E., Burwell, R. A., Gilman, S. E., Herzog, D. B., and Hamburg, P. (2002). Eating behaviours and attitudes following prolonged exposure to television among ethic Fijian adolescent girls. *British Journal of Psychiatry, 180,* 509-514.

Ben-Tovim, D. I., and Walker, M. K. (1991). Further evidence for the stroop test as a quantitative measure of psychopathology in eating disorders. *International Journal of Eating Disorders, 10*, 609-613.

Beresin, E. V., Gordon, C., and Herzog, D. B. (1989). The process of recovering from anorexia nervosa. *Journal of the American Academy of Psychoanalysis, 17*, 103-130.

Bergen, A. W., van den Bree, M. B. M., Yeager, M., Welch, R., Ganjei, J. K., Haque, K., et al. (2003). Candidate genes for anorexia nervosa in the 1p33 linkage region: serotonin 1D and delta opioid receptor loci exhibit significant association to anorexia nervosa. *Molecular Psychiatry, 8*, 397-406.

Birmingham, C. L., Su, J., Hlynsky, J. A., Goldner, E. M., Gao, M. (2005) The mortality rate from anorexia nervosa. *International Journal of Eating Disorders, 38*, 143-146.

Bornstein, R. F. (2001). A meta-analysis of the dependency-eating-disorders relationship: Strength, specificity, and temporal stability. *Journal of Psychopathology and Behavioural Assessment, 23,* 151-162.

Bourke, M. P., Taylor, G. J., Parker, J. D., and Bagby, R. M. (1992). Alexithymia in women with anorexia nervosa. A preliminary investigation *The British Journal of Psychiatry, 161*, 240-243.

Brewerton, T. (2005). Psychological trauma and eating disorders. In S. Wonderlich, J. Mitchell, M. de Zwaan, and H. Steiger (Eds.), *Eating disorders review: Part I* (pp. 137-154). Oxford: Radcliffe Publishing.

Bruch, H. (1978). *The golden cage. The enigma of anorexia nervosa.* Cambridge, MA: Harvard University Press.

Bruch, H. (1988). *Conversations with Anorexics.* New York: Basic Books.

Bulik, C. M. (2002). Anxiety, depression and eating disorders. In C. G. Fairburn and K. D. Brownell (Eds.), *Eating Disorders and Obesity: A Comprehensive Handbook* (2nd ed.). (193-198). New York, NY: The Guilford Press.

Bulik, C. M. (2004). Genetic and biological risk factors. In J. K. Thompson (Ed.), *Handbook of eating disorders and obesity* (pp. 3-16). New Jersey: John Wiley and Sons Ltd.

Bulik, C., Reba, L., Siega-Riz, A. M., and Reichborn-Kjennerud, T. (2005). Anorexia nervosa: Definition, epidemiology, and cycle of risk. *International Journal of Eating Disorders, 37*, S2-S9.

Button, E. J., and Warren, R. L. (2001). Living with anorexia nervosa: The experience of a cohort of sufferers from anorexia nervosa 7.5 years after initial presentation to a specialized eating disorders service. *European Eating Disorders Review, 9*, 74-96.

Bydlowski, S., Corcos, M., Jeammet, P., Paterniti, S., Berthoz, S., Laurier, C., et al., (2005). Emotion-processing deficits in eating disorders. *International Journal of Eating Disorders, 37*, 321-329.

Casper, R. C. (1990). Personality features of women with good outcome from restricting anorexia nervosa. *Psychosomatic Medicine, 52,* 156-170.

Cassin, S. E., and von Ranson, K. M. (2005). Personality and eating disorders: a decade in review. *Clinical Psychology Review, 25*, 895-916.

Channon, S., Hemsley, D., and de Silva, P. (1988). Selective processing of food words in anorexia nervosa. *British Journal of Clinical Psychology, 28*, 329-340.

Claes, L., Vandereycken, W., and Vertommen, H. (2005). Impulsivity related traits in eating disorder patients. *Personality and Individual Differences, 39*, 739-749.

Cnattingius, S., Hultman, C., Dahl, M., and Sparén, P. (1999). Very preterm birth, birth trauma, and the risk of anorexia nervosa among girls. *Archives of General Psychiatry, 56*, 634-638.

Cockell, S. J., Zaitsoff, S, L., and Geller, J. (2004). Maintaining change following eating disorder treatment. *Professional Psychology: Research and Practice, 35*, 527-534.

Cooper, M. J., Anastasiades, P., and Fairburn, C. G. (1992). Selective processing of eating, shape, and weight-related words in persons with bulimia nervosa. *Journal of Abnormal Psychology, 101,* 352-355.

Cooper, M., and Todd, G. (1997). Selective processing of eating, weight and shape related words in patients with eating disorders and dieters. *British Journal of Clinical Psychology, 36*, 279-281.

Corstorphine, E. (2006). Cognitive-emotional-behavioural therapy for the eating disorders: Working with beliefs about emotions. *European Eating Disorders Review, 14*, 448-461.

de Groot, J. M., and Rodin, G. (1994). Eating disorders, female psychology, and the self. *Journal of the American Academy of Psychoanalysis, 22*, 299-317.

Dennis, A. B., and Sansone, R. A. (1997). Treatment of patients with personality disorders. In D. M Garner and P. E. Garfinkel (Eds.), *Handbook of treatment for eating disorders* (2nd ed.) (pp. 437-449). New York: The Guilford Press.

Fairburn, C. G., Cooper, P. J., Cooper, M. J., McKenna, F. P., and Anastasiades, P. (1991). Selective information processing in bulimia nervosa. *International Journal of Eating Disorders, 10*, 415-422.

Fairburn, C. G., Cooper, Z., and Shafran, R. (2003). Cognitive behaviour therapy for eating disorders: a "transdiagnostic" theory and treatment. *Behaviour Research and Therapy, 41*, 509-528.

Fairburn, C. G., Cooper, Z., Doll, H. A. and Welch, S. L. (1999). Risk factors for anorexia nervosa: Three integrated case-control studies. *Archives of General Psychiatry, 56*, 468-476.

Fallon, P., and Wonderlich, S. A. (1997). Sexual abuse and other forms of trauma. In D. M. Garner and P. E. Garfinkle (Eds.), *Handbook of treatment for eating disorders* (2nd ed.) (pp. 394-414). New York: The Guildford Press.

Faunce, G. J. (2002). Eating disorders and attentional bias: A review. *Eating Disorders, 10*, 125-139.

Federici, A. and Kaplan, A., S. (2007). The patients' account of relapse and recovery in anorexia nervosa: A qualitative study. *European Eating Disorders Review, 16,* 1-10.

Finfgeld, D. L. (2002). Anorexia nervosa: Analysis of long-term outcomes and clinical implications. *Archives of Psychiatric Nursing, 16*, 176-186.

Frank, G., K., Kaye, W. H., Meltzer, C. C., Price, J. C., Greer, P., McConaha, C. et al. (2002). Reduced 5HT2A receptor binding after recovery from anorexia nervosa. *Biological Psychiatry, 52,* 896-906.

Franzen, U., and Gerlinghoff, M. (1997). Parenting by patients with eating disorders: Experiences with a mother-child group. *Eating Disorders, 5*, 5–14.

Garfinkel, P. E., Lin, E., Goering, P., Spegg, C., Goldbloom, D., Kennedy, et al., (1996). Should amenorrhoea be necessary for the diagnosis of anorexia nervosa? Evidence from a Canadian community sample. *The British Journal of Psychiatry, 168*, 500-506.

Garfinkel, P. E., and Garner, D. M. (1982). *Anorexia nervosa: A multidimensional perspective*. New York, NY: Brunner/Mazel Publishers.

Geller, J., Cockell, S. J., Hewitt, P. L., Goldner, E. M., and Flett, G. L. (2000). Inhibited expression of negative emotions and interpersonal orientation in anorexia nervosa. *International Journal of Eating Disorders, 28*, 8-19.

Gorwood, P., Kipman, A., and Foulon, C. (2003). The human genetics of anorexia nervosa. *European Journal of Pharmacology, 480*, 163-170.

Grice, D., Halmi, K., Fichter, M. M., Strober, M., Woodside, D. B., Treasure, J. T., et al . (2002). Evidence for a susceptibility gene for anorexia nervosa on chromosome 1. *American Journal of Human Genetics, 70*, 787.

Grigg, M. Bowman, J., and Redman, S. (1996). Disordered eating and unhealthy weight reduction practices among adolescent females. *Preventive Medicine, 25*, 748-756.

Halmi, K. A., Sunday, S. R., Strober, M., Kaplan, A., Woodside, D. B., Fichter, M. (2000). Perfectionism in anorexia nervosa: Variation by clinical subtype, obsessionality, and pathological eating behaviour. *American Journal of Psychiatry, 157*, 1799-1805.

Halmi, K.A., Tozzi, F., Thornton, L.M., Crow, S., Fichter, M.M., Kaplan A.S., et al. (2005). The relation among perfectionism, obsessive-compulsive personality disorder and obsessive-compulsive disorder in individuals with eating disorders. *International Journal of Eating Disorders, 38*, 371-374.

Harrison, K. and Cantor, J. (1997). The relationship between media consumption and eating disorders. *The Journal of Communication, 47*, 40-67.

Hermans, D., Pieters, G., and Eelen, P. (1998). Implicit and explicit memory for shape, body weight, and food-related words in patients with anorexia nervosa and nondieting controls. *Journal of Abnormal Psychology, 107*, 193-202.

Jacobi, C., Hayward, C., de Zwaan, M., Kraemer, H. C., Agras, S. W. (2004). Coming to terms with risk factors for eating disorders: Application of risk terminology and suggestions for a general taxonomy. *Psychological Bulletin, 130*, 19-65.

Johnson-Sabine, E., Reiss, D., and Dayson, D. (1992). Bulimia nervosa: A 5-year follow-up study. *Psychological Medicine, 22*, 951-959.

Kaplan, A. S. (1990). Biomedical variables in the eating disorders. *Canadian Journal of Psychiatry, 35*, 745-753.

Kaye, W., Frank, G., Bailer, U., and Henry, S. (2005). Neurobiology of anorexia nervosa: Clinical implications of alterations of function of serotonin and other neuronal systems. *International Journal of Eating Disorders, 37*, S15-S19.

Kaye, W., Frank, G., McConaha, C. (1999). Altered dopamine activity after recovery from restrictor type anorexia nervosa . *Neuropsychopharmacology, 21*, 503-506.

Keel, P. K., and Klump, K. L. (2003). Are eating disorders culture-bound syndromes? Implications for conceptualizing their etiology. *Psychological Bulletin, 129,* 747-769.

Klump, K. L., Strober, M., Johnson, C., Thornton, L., Bulik, C. M., Devlin, B., et al. (2004). Personality characteristics of women before and after recovery from and eating disorder. *Psychological Medicine, 34*, 1407-1418.

Klump, K., and Gobrogge, K. (2005). A review and primer of molecular genetic studies of anorexia nervosa. *International Journal of Eating Disorders, 37*, S 43-S48.

Klump, K., Kaye, W., and Strober, M. (2001). The evolving genetic foundation of eating disorders. *Psychiatric Clinics of North America, 24*, 215-225.

Lacey, J. H. (1982). Anorexia nervosa and a bearded female saint. *British Medical Journal (Clinical Research Edition), 18*, 1816–1817.

Lacey, J. H., and Evans, C. D. H. (1986). The impulsivist: A multi-impulsive personality disorder. *British Journal of Addiction, 81*, 641-649.

Lask, B., Gordon, I., Christie, D., Frampton, I., Chowdhury, U., Watkins, B. (2005). Functional neuroimaging in early onset anorexia nervosa. *International Journal of Eating Disorders, 37*, S49-S51.

Lattimore, P. J., Wagner, H. L., and Gowers, S. (2000). Conflict avoidance in anorexia nervosa: An observational study of mothers and daughters. *European Eating Disorders Review, 8*, 355-368.

Latzer, Y., Hochdorf, Z., Bachar, E., and Canetti, L. (2002). Attachment style and family functioning as discriminating factors in eating disorders. *Contemporary Family Therapy, 24*, 581-599.

Lee, S., Ho, T., P., and Hsu, L. K., G. (1993). Fat phobic and non-fat phobic anorexia nervosa: a comparative study of 70 Chinese patients in Hong Kong. *Psychological Medicine, 23*, 999-1017.

Lindberg, L., and Hjern, A. (2003). Risk factors for anorexia nervosa: a national cohort study. *International Journal of Eating Disorders, 34*, 397-408.

Lowe, B., Zipfel, B. L., Buchholz, C., Dupont, Y., Reas, D. L., and Herzog, W. (2001). Long-term outcome of anorexia nervosa in a prospective 21-year follow-up study. *Psychological Medicine, 31*, 881-890.

Mazzeo, S. E., Zucker, N. L., Gerke, C. K., Mitchell, K. S., and Bulik, C. M. (2005). Parenting concerns of women with histories of eating disorders. *International Journal of Eating Disorders, 37*, S77-S79.

McVey, G., Tweed, S., and Blackmore, E. (2004). Dieting among preadolescent and young adolescent females. *Canadian Medical Association Journal, 170*, 1559-1561.

Mills, J. S., and Miller, J. L. (2007) Experimental effects of receiving negative weight-related feedback: A weight guessing study. *Body Image, 4*, 309-316.

Mills, J. S., Polivy, J., Herman, P. E., and Tiggerman, M. (2002) Effects of exposure to thin media images: Evidence of self-enhancement among restrained eaters. *Personality and Social Psychology Bulletin, 28*, 1687-1699.

Minuchin, S., Rosman, B. L., Baker, L. (1978). *Psychosomatic families: Anorexia nervosa in context*. Oxford, England: Harvard University Press.

Mühlau, M., Gaser, C., Ilg, R., Conrad, B., Leibl, C., Cebulla, M. H., et al. *(2007)*.Gray matter decrease of the anterior cingulate cortex in anorexia nervosa. *American Journal of Psychiatry, 164*, 1850-1857.

Nilsson, K., Abrahamsson, E., Torbiornsson, A., and Hagglof, B. (2007). Causes of adolescent onset anorexia nervosa: Patient perspectives. *Eating Disorders, 15*, 125-133.

Pike, K. M. (1998). Long-term course of anorexia nervosa: Response, relapse, remission and recovery. *Clinical Psychology Review, 18*, 447-475.

Placanica, J. L., Faunce, G. L., and Job, R. F. S. (2002). The effect of fasting on attentional biases for food and body shape/weight words in high and low eating disorder inventory scorers. *International Journal of Eating Disorders*, *32*, 79-90.

Polivy, J., and Herman, C. P. (2002). Causes of eating disorders. *Annual Review of Psychology, 53*, 187-213.

Procopio, M., and Marriott, P. (2007). Intrauterine hormonal environment and risk of developing anorexia nervosa. *Archives of General Psychiatry, 64*, 1402-1407.

Radomsky, R. S., de Silva, P., Todd, G., Treasure, J., and Murphy, T. (2002). Thought-shape fusion in anorexia nervosa: An experimental investigation. *Behaviour Research and Therapy, 40*, 1169-1177.

Rastam, M. (1992). Anorexia nervosa in 51 Swedish adolescents: Premorbid problems and comorbidity. *Academy of Child and Adolescent Psychiatry, 31*, 819-829.

Rieger, E., Schotte, D. E., Touyz, S. W., Beaumont, P. J. V., Griffiths, R., and Russell, J. (1998). Attentional biases in eating disorders: A visual probe detection procedure. *International Journal of Eating Disorders*, *23*, 199-205.

Rossier, B., Bolognini, M., Plancherel, B., and Halfan, O. (2000). Sensation seeking: A personality trait characteristic of adolescent girls and young women with eating disorders. *European Eating Disorders Review, 8*, 245-252.

Russell, G. F. M., Treasure, J., and Eisler, I. (1998). Mothers with anorexia nervosa who underfeed their children: Their recognition and management. *Psychological Medicine, 28*, 93-108.

Sackville, T., Scotte, D.E., Touyz, S.W., Griffiths,R., and Beaumont, P. J.V. (1998). Conscious and preconscious processing for food, body, weight and shape, and emotion-related words in women with anorexia nervosa. *International Journal of Eating Disorders, 23*, 77–82.

Sansone, R. A., Levitt, J. L. (2004). The prevalence of self-harm behaviour among those with eating disorders. In J. L. Levitt, R. A. Sansone, and L. Cohn (Eds.). *Self-harm behaviour and eating disorders: Dynamics, assessment, treatment* (pp. 3-14). New York, NY: Brunner-Routledge.

Sansone, R. A., Levitt, J. L., and Sansone, L. A. (2005). The prevalence of personality disorders among those with eating disorders. *Eating Disorders, 13*, 7-22.

Schmidt, U. (2003). Aetiology of eating disorders in the 21st century: New answers to old questions. *European Child and Adolescent Psychiatry* (Suppl 1), *12*, 30-37.

Schmidt, U., Jiwany, A., Treasure, J. (1993). A controlled study of alexithymia in eating disorders. *Comprehensive Psychiatry*, *34*, 54-58.

Schutz, H.K., Paxton, S.J., and Wertheim, E.H. (2002) Investigation of body comparison among adolescent girls. *Journal of Applied Social Psychology, 32*, 1906-1937.

Serpell, L., Livingstone, A., Neiderman, M., and Lask, B. (2002). Anorexia nervosa: Obsessive-compulsive disorder, obsessive-compulsive personality disorders, or neither? *Clinical Psychology Review, 22*, 647-669.

Shafran, R., Teachman, B., A., Kerry, S., and Rachman, S. (1999). A cognitive distortion associated with eating disorders: Thought-shape fusion. *British Journal of Clinical Psychology, 38*, 167-179.

Skodol, A. E., Oldham, J. M., Hyler, S. E., Kellman, H. D., Doidge, N., and Davies, M. (1993). Comorbidity of DSM-III-R eating disorders and personality disorders. *International Journal of Eating Disorders, 14*, 403-416.

Srinivasagam, N. M., Kaye, W. H., Plotnicov, K. H., Greeno, C., Weltzin, T. E., and Rao, R. (1995). Persistent perfectionism, symmetry, and exactness after long-term recovery from anorexia nervosa. *American Journal of Psychiatry, 152*, 1630-1634.

Stein, K. F., and Nyquist, L. (2001, January/February). Disturbance in the self: A source of eating disorders. Gurze Books: *Eating Disorders Review, 12*, 1.

Stein, A., Woolley, H., Cooper, S. D. and Fairburn, C. G. (1994). An observational study of mothers with eating disorders and their infants. *Journal of Child Psychology and Psychiatry, 35*, 733-748.

Stein, A. and Woolley, H. (1996). The influence of parental eating disorders on young children: Implications of recent research for some clinical interventions. *Eating Disorders: The Journal of Treatment and Prevention, 4*, 139-146.

Steinhausen, H. (2002). The outcome of anorexia nervosa in the 20th century. *American Journal of Psychiatry, 159*, 1284-1293.

Stice, E. (2002). Sociocultural influences on body image and eating disturbance. In C. G. Fairburn and K. B. Brownell (Eds.), *Eating disorders and obesity: A comprehensive handbook* (2nd ed.). (pp. 103 – 107). New York, NY: The Guilford Press.

Stice, E., Agras, W. S., Hammer, L. D. (1999). Risk factors for the emergence of childhood eating disturbances: A five-year prospective study. *International Journal of Eating Disorders, 25*, 375-387.

Stice, E., Maxfield, J., and Wells, T. (2003). Adverse effects of social pressure to be thin on young women: An experimental investigation of the effects of "fat talk." *International Journal of Eating Disorders, 34*, 108-117.

Striegel-Moore, R. H., and Smolak, L. (2002). Gender, ethnicity, and eating disorders. In C. G. Fairburn and K. B. Brownell (Eds.), *Eating disorders and obesity: A comprehensive handbook* (2nd ed.). (pp.251-255). New York, NY: The Guilford Press.

Sullivan, P. E. (1995). Mortality in anorexia nervosa. *American Journal of Psychiatry, 152*, 1073-1074.

Szmulker, G. I., and Patton, G. (1995). Sociocultural models of eating disorders. In G. I. Szmukler, C. Dare and J. Treasure (Eds.), *Handbook of eating disorders: Theory, treatment and research* (pp.177-192). West Sussex, England: John Wiley and Sons.

Tchanturia, K., Campbell, I. C., Morris, R., and Treasure, J. (2005). Neuropsychological studies in anorexia nervosa. *International Journal of Eating Disorders, 37*, S72-S76.

Telch, C. F. (1997). Skills training treatment for adaptive affect regulation in a woman with binge-eating disorder. *International Journal of Eating Disorders, 22*, 77-81.

Telch, C. F., Agras, W. S., and Linehan, M. M. (2001). Dialectical behaviour therapy for binge eating disorder. *Journal of Consulting and Clinical Psychology, 69*, 1061-1065.

Tozzi, F., Sullivan, P. F., Fear, J. L, McKenzie, J., and Bulik, C. M. (2002). Causes and recovery in anorexia nervosa: The patient's perspective. *International Journal of Eating Disorders, 33*, 143-154.

Vervaet, M., van Heeringen, C., and Audenaert, K. (2004). Personality-related characteristics in restricting versus binging and purging eating disordered patients. *Comprehensive Psychiatry, 45*, 37-43.

Vitousek, K. and Hollon, S. D. (1990). The investigation of schematic content and processing in eating disorders. *Cognitive Therapy and Research, 14*, 191-214.

Vitousek, K., and Manke, F. (1994). Personality variables and disorders in anorexia nervosa and bulimia nervosa. *Journal of Abnormal Psychology, 103*, 137-147.

Wagner, A., Greer, P., Bailer, U. F., Frank, G. K., Henry, S. E., Putnam, K., et al., (2006). Normal brain tissue volumes after long-term recovery in anorexia and bulimia nervosa. *Biological Psychiatry, 59,* 291-293.

Ward, A., and Gowers, S. (2003). Attachment and childhood development. In J. Treasure, U. Schmidt, and E. van Furth (Eds.). *Handbook of eating disorders* (2nd ed.). (pp. 103-120). West Sussex, England: John Wiley and Sons Ltd.

Willi, J., Giacometti, G., and Limacher, B. (1990). Update on the epidemiology of anorexia nervosa in a defined region of Switzerland. *American Journal of Psychiatry, 147*, 1514-1517.

Wonderlich S. A., Lilenfeld, L. R., Riso, L. P., Engel, S., and Mitchell, J. E. (2005). Personality and anorexia nervosa. *International Journal of Eating Disorders, 37*, S68-S71.

Wonderlich, S. A., Brewerton, T. D., Jocic, Z., Dansky, B. S., and Abbott, D. W. (1997). The relationship of childhood sexual abuse and eating disorders: A review. *Journal of the American Academy for Child and Adolescent Psychiatry, 36*, 1107-1115.

Yamamiya, Y., Cash, T. F., Melnyk, S., E., Posavac, H., D., and Posavac, S., S. (2005). Women's exposure to thin-and-beautiful media images: Body image effects of media-ideal internalization and impact-reduction interventions. *Body Image, 2*, 74-80.

Zaitsoff, S. L., Geller, J., K., and Srikameswaran, S. (2002). Silencing the self and suppressed anger: Relationship to eating disorder symptoms in adolescent females. *European Eating Disorders Review, 10*, 51-60.

Zonnevijlle-Bendek, M. J. S., van Goozen, S. H. M., Cohen-Kettenis, P. T., van Elburg, A., and van Engeland, H. (2002). Do adolescent anorexia nervosa patients have deficits in emotional functioning? *European Child and Adolescent Psychiatry, 11*, 38-42.

In: Evidence-Based Treatments for Eating Disorders   ISBN 978-1-60692-310-8
Author: Ida F. Dancyger and Victor M. Fornari   © 2009 Nova Science Publishers, Inc.

Chapter II

Overview of Evidence on the Underpinnings of Bulimia Nervosa

Timothy D. Brewerton
Medical University of South Carolina
Charleston, South Carolina, USA

Abstract

There is *no single etiology* or basis for any of the eating disorders, including bulimia nervosa, but similar to other mental disorders, bulimia results from the dynamic interplay between biological, psychological and social factors that operate along a developmental continuum. In this chapter these factors are further subdivided into predisposing, precipitating and perpetuating factors (the "3 P's), which creates nine categories of underpinnings from which to examine the evidence as it relates to bulimia nervosa. Latent vulnerability theory suggests strong genetic predisposing factors linked to anxiety, harm avoidance, obsessive-compulsiveness and drive for thinness, which are exposed, triggered and/or exacerbated by behaviors geared toward weight loss. Among a host of psychosocial factors, traumatic experiences often play important roles in predisposing, precipitating and perpetuating bulimic disorders, especially when there is psychiatric comorbidity.

Introduction

This chapter will review the underpinnings of bulimia nervosa (BN). In essence, underpinnings refer to the underlying foundations or bases of a condition. Such an understanding is a complex one that encompasses multiple levels or layers interacting over time. At the outset it is important to unequivocally state that there is *no single cause* or basis of any of the eating disorders (EDs), including BN. Nevertheless, one traditional approach to this etiological conundrum is to think of BN, like any other mental illness, as a result of a dynamic interplay between biological, psychological and social factors. Because these factors interact along a developmental continuum in which nature and nurture interact, for the sake of this discussion we can further subdivide these layers into the "3 P's," i.e., predisposing, precipitating and perpetuating factors. This creates nine categories of underpinnings from which to examine the evidence as it relates to BN. In the previous chapter the underpinnings of anorexia nervosa (AN) are reviewed, and in the following chapter those of binge eating disorder (BED) are reviewed. Many, but not all of these underpinnings, may also be relevant for BN. This chapter will seek to highlight those underpinnings that are more specific for BN (and to some extent the binge-purge type of AN).

Although Russell is often given credit for first reporting *BN*, which he described as "an ominous variant of anorexia nervosa" (1979), it was Boskind-Lodahl (1978) who described bingeing and purging in normal weight women first, a phenomenon she called *bulimarexia*. She perceived this condition as a Western culture-bound syndrome that developed from society's preoccupation with female thinness as well as its patriarchal oppressive restrictions of female gender roles. The Diagnostic and Statistical Manual of Mental Disorders (DSM) included *bulimia* for the first time in 1980 (American Psychiatric Association, 1980) and the term was changed to bulimia nervosa in DSM-III-R in 1987 (American Psychiatric Association, 1987).

Latent vulnerability theory provides an overarching, interactive perspective for understanding the underpinnings of BN. It goes a long way toward answering the question of why so many young women begin dieting but only a small minority of these go on to develop the illness of BN. In short, dieting, bingeing, purging and exercise all alter neurochemistry, which then expose a genetically mediated latent vulnerability. In other words, "genetics loads the gun and environment pulls the trigger." The remainder of this chapter will seek to illuminate these processes or underpinnings in more detail.

Predisposing Biological Underpinnings

Gender

Gender is an indisputable characteristic of BN. One of the most consistent findings in epidemiological studies is that BN occurs significantly more frequently in females than males. Depending on the study the ratio of females to males ranges from 10:1 (American Psychiatric Association, 2004; Hsu, 1996; Lewinsohn, Hops, Roberts, Seeley and Andrews, 1993; Neilsen, 1990; Schotte and Stunkard, 1987; Paton, Selzer, Coffey, Carlin and Wolfe, 1999; Vollrath, Koch and Angst, 1992; Whitaker, Johnson, Shaffer, et al., 1990) to 3:1 (Hudson, Hiripi, Pope, Kessler, 2007). Since gender is an unchangeable characteristic and uneven gender distributions have been found for several other mental disorders, female status appears to be a non-specific risk factor for BN.

Genetics

There is indisputable evidence from well-controlled twin and family studies that BN (like all EDs) runs in families. Twin studies with large sample sizes indicate that as much as 60% to 83% of bulimia's etiological variance is due to genetic factors (Bulik, Sullivan and Kendler, 1998). In a major family history study involving 504 probands and over 1800 relatives, the risk that a first degree relative of a bulimic proband also had BN was four times greater than a first degree relative of a non-bulimic proband (p < 0.05) (Strober, Freeman, Lampert, Diamond and Kaye, 2000). In summary, heritability estimates for BN have been reported to be on the order of 0.5-0.8 (Bulik, Sullivan, Wade and Kendler, 1998; Fichter and Noegel 1990; Holland, Hall, Murray, Russell and Crisp, 1984; Holland, Sicotte and Treasure, 1988; Hsu, et al 1990; Kendler et al 1991, 1995; Klump et al, 2002; Treasure and Holland 1990; Walters and Kendler, 1995).

One might ask what exactly is heritable. How is this genetic transmission accomplished? Studies indicate that not only are EDs inherited, but other related disorders that may predispose the individual to develop BN are also genetically mediated. These include anxiety and mood disorders as well as temperament and the personality traits of perfectionism, obsessionality, compulsivity, novelty seeking, sensation seeking and impulsivity. In addition, low self esteem, a trait quite common in BN and all eating disorders, been shown to be due in large part to genetic factors, a finding that is contrary to conventional social wisdom (Kendler, Gardner and Prescott, 1998).

In summary, AN, BN, EDNOS diagnoses and symptoms are transmitted in families. In addition, AN and BN are cross transmitted, and AN and BN are highly heritable. Family members have similar mood and temperament traits. Suspect genes have been identified. In particular, chromosome 10 has been implicated in BN (Bulik, Devlin, Bacanu, et al., 2003).

Trait-Related Biological Differences

Biological differences that appear to be related to specific personality traits linked to BN have been noted in the literature (Brewerton and Steiger, 2004). In comparison to healthy age matched controls, persistent alterations in serotonergic activity have been reported in women following long-term recovery from BN ($\geq$ 1 year), including increased cerebrospinal fluid (CSF) concentrations of 5-hydroxyindoleacetic acid (5-HIAA), the major metabolite of 5-hydroxytryptamine or serotonin (Kaye, Greeno, Moss, et al., 1998), reduced 5-HT_{2A} receptor activity on positron emission topography (PET) scanning (Kaye, Frank, Meltzer, et al., 2001), and reduced platelet [(3)H]paroxetine binding (Steiger, Richardson, Israel, et al., 2005). Furthermore, as in AN, these CSF 5-HIAA alterations have been found to correlate with obsessive-compulsive personality traits, perfectionism and behavioral inhibition, which are associated with a hypothetical tendency towards a hyper-serotonergic status. Given these results in recovered bulimic patients, it could be hypothesized that a disturbance of 5-HT activity may be part of the genetically determined biological vulnerability for the development of an ED including BN. However, whether these findings represent a true premorbid biological liability or a consequence of the ED itself cannot be definitively determined from these results. To tease out this issue studies of transmitter function in at-risk pre-morbid individuals as well as non-affected identical and fraternal twins, siblings, and other first-degree relatives of ED patients, could begin to confirm trait related disturbances (Brewerton and Steiger, 2004). To this end, Steiger, Gauvin, Joober, et al. (2006) studied paroxetine binding in the unaffected mothers and sisters of recovered patients with BN and found that they too had reduced platelet [(3)H]paroxetine binding compared to healthy controls and their mothers and sisters. Furthermore, there were significant within family correlations for Bmax, which indicates a heritable trait or endophenotype possibly linked to serotonin function and passed on by those with BN and their first degree relatives.

Age

In both clinical and population-based surveys, the peak incidence of EDs has been found in the age range from adolescence to early adulthood (Woodside and Garfinkel, 1992). BN typically begins later in life than AN, usually between the ages of 18 and 23 years, although onset may be variable. Clinical samples report earlier onset whereas representative and community samples report later onset (Dansky, Brewerton, O'Neal and Kilpatrick, 1997).

Ethnicity and Race

Eating disorders have been usually considered primarily Caucasian phenomena (Striegel-Moore and Smolak, 1996), but more recent literature has seriously challenged this notion. Results indicate that the ethnic distribution is much more complicated (Crago, Shisslak, and Estes, 1996; Smith and Krejci, 1991) with Native Americans reported as having higher rates of EDs than Caucasians, and Hispanics having comparable rates as Caucasians. Studies have indicated lower rates of BN among Asians (Chen, Wong, Lee, Chan-Ho, Lau and Fung, 1993; Ohzeki, Hanaki, Motozumi, et al., 1990), while other studies have indicated comparable rates of BN in Black women (Field, Colditz, and Peterson, 1997; Le Grange, Telch, and Tibbs, 1998; Pumariega, Gustavson, Gustavson, Motes, and Ayers, 1994). Still others report higher rates of laxative abuse, diuretic abuse, and/or self-induced vomiting in young Black women (Emmons, 1992; Field et al., 1997).

Pregnancy and Perinatal Complications

In a large population-based study by Foley, Thacker, Aggen Neale and Kendler (2001) complications of pregnancy were associated with a significantly increased risk for later developing BN. It was notable that these complications were not associated with the other psychiatric disorders but were specific for BN. Increased rates of perinatal complications have been reported in the histories of patients with both AN and BN (Favaro, Tenconi and Santonastaso, 2006). In this well-controlled study, patients with BN had significantly higher odds ratios for a number of complications, including hyporeactivity, low birth weight for gestational age, and early feeding problems. In addition, a highly significant odds ratio of 7.7 for developing BN was found for those patients with 2 or more complications (p < 0.001).

Seasonality of Birth

In a related area of research, Brewerton, Dansky, O'Neil, and Kilpatrick, (2007) reported significant alterations in the season of birth of individuals who later developed BN. Using results from the National Women's Study women with BN were more likely to be born in the fall and less likely to be born in the spring than women without BN. Similar seasonal findings have been fruitful in schizophrenia research in which an excess of winter births led to the identification of a relationship between intrauterine influenza and later onset of schizophrenia (neurodevelopmental aspects).

BMI and Obesity

Obesity during childhood has been reported to be an important risk factor for the subsequent development of BN and its symptoms. Fairburn, Welch, Doll, Davies and O'Connor (1997) reported that 40% of the bulimics vs. 13% of psychiatric controls and 15% of normal controls retrospectively reported childhood obesity. In addition, the bulimic subjects reported more parental obesity than subjects in either of the comparison groups. Childress, Brewerton, Hodges and Jarrell (1993) found that middle school children who reported bulimic symptoms such as vomiting to lose weight were heavier than those children without bulimic symptoms. Some longitudinal studies have also found that higher BMI or body fat is predictive of disordered eating (Killen, Taylor, Hayward, et al., 1994; Patton, Johnson-Sabine, Wood, Mann and Wakeling, 1990; Vollrath, Koch and Angst, 1992). However, this has not been true for all studies (Killen, Taylor, Hayward, et al., 1994; Patton, Selzer, Coffey, Carlin and Wolfe, 1999; Gowen, Hayward, Killen, Robinson and Taylor, 1999). Nevertheless, higher BMI appears to be an important risk factor for BN.

Pica and Early Digestive Problems

Marchi and Cohen (1990) found pica, early digestive problems, and weight reducing efforts to be related to later bulimic symptoms. The risk of BN was found to be almost seven times higher in those individuals with early childhood pica. However, this was not found in another longitudinal study (Kotter, Cohen, Davies, et al., 2001

Family History of Psychopathology

Many, many studies report elevated rates of an array of psychiatric disorders in first-degree relatives of patients with BN, including other EDs, anxiety disorders, mood disorders, substance use disorders and cluster B personality disorders (Jacobi, Hayward, de Zwaan, Kraemer, and Agras, 2004; Lilenfeld, 2004). Unfortunately, the temporal relationship of the psychiatric disorders of patients' family members in relationship to the onset of BN in the patients was not addressed in any of these studies. However, selected parental psychiatric disorders occurring prior to the onset of the child's BN were assessed retrospectively in a study by Fairburn, Welch, Doll, Davies and O`Connor (1997), who found that parental depression, parental alcoholism, and parental drug abuse predating the onset of the BN were significantly more frequent in patients compared to normal controls. Interestingly, parental alcoholism was even more frequent in the relatives of BN patients compared to those of psychiatric controls.

Predisposing Psychological Underpinnings

Perfectionism and Obsessive-Compulsive Personality Traits

In their retrospective assessment of reputed risk factors Fairburn, Welch, Doll, Davies and O`Connor (1997) found that premorbid perfectionism was elevated in bulimic patients when compared to healthy controls. However, measures in the BN group did not differ from psychiatric controls. More recently, Halmi, Tozzi, Thornton, Crow, Fichter et al., (2005) demonstrated that perfectionism and obsessionality are core features of EDs, regardless of diagnosis. In a large sample of ED subjects, they found no differences across diagnostic subtypes in the prevalence of obsessive-compulsive personality disorder (OCPD) and obsessive-compulsive disorder (OCD), or with the association between OCPD and OCD. Perfectionism was noted to be highest in individuals with OCPD with or without concomitant OCD. The authors emphasized that our developing understanding of the relationship between these traits and EDs may ultimately enhance our ability to identify pertinent behavioral endophenotypes for EDs, but the combination of perfectionism with OCPD may be a fundamental core behavioral feature underlying vulnerability to ED.

Establishing that perfectionism predates BN in longitudinal studies has been difficult. In one study (Killen, Taylor, Hayward, et al., 1994; 1996) measures of perfectionism at time one were not linked to subsequent disordered eating in multivariate analyses but did discriminate between symptomatic and asymptomatic girls at baseline in univariate comparisons (Killen, Taylor, Hayward, et al., 1994). In addition, studies by Leon, Fulkerson, Perry and Early-Zald (1995) and Leon, Fulkerson, Perry, Keel and Klump (1999) did not find perfectionism to be predictive in multivariate comparisons.

Low Self-esteem

The other side of perfectionism is low self-esteem. When one's actions can "never be good enough," then one always "falls short" and feels badly about oneself. Low self-esteem has been noted to be an important risk factor for the development of BN (Fairburn, Welch, Doll, Davies and O`Connor, 1997). Although this is typically thought of as a purely psychological phenomena twin studies show that self-esteem has a strong genetic component with as much as 50% of the variance being accounted for by genetic factors (Kendler, Gardner and Prescott, 1998). Patients with BN have consistently been found in the literature to possess lower self-esteem than healthy controls (Jacobi, Paul, de Zwaan, Nutzinger and Dahme, 2000). The retrospective assessment of self-concept and its temporal relation to onset of the BN has been considered in two cross-sectional studies. Fairburn, Welch, Doll, Davies and O`Connor (1997) found negative self-evaluation prior to onset of ED to be more common in BN subjects than in healthy and psychiatric controls. Low self-esteem was also reported by Raffi, Rondini, Grandi and Fava (2000) to be one of several prodromal symptoms of patients with BN as compared to controls. Kendler, MacLean, Neale, Kessler, Heath and Eaves (1991) also found that low self-esteem was a major risk factor for BN in a large group of twins.

Measures of self-concept have been included in four longitudinal studies. In the studies by Leon, Fulkerson, Perry, and Early-Zald (1995) and Calam and Waller (1998) they did not prove to be important predictors. On the other hand, low self-esteem predicted elevated Eating Attitudes Test (EAT) scores four years later in the study by Button, Sonuga-Barke, Davies, and Thompson (1996). Girls in the lowest self-esteem range had an eightfold increased risk for a high EAT score (≥ 20) compared to those with high self-esteem. Similarly, Ghaderi and Scott (2001) reported significantly lower self-esteem at time one for the group that developed an ED two years later.

Ineffectiveness

Early on Hilda Bruch noted a "profound sense of ineffectiveness" in patients with EDs (1973). This hypothesis as applied to BN and bulimic symptoms was tested using the Eating Disorder Inventory (EDI)-Ineffectiveness subscale in four longitudinal studies (Leon, Fulkerson, Perry, Early-Zald, 1995; Leon, Fulkerson, Perry, Keel Klump, 1999; Taylor, Hayward, Haydel, Wilson, et al., 1996). The EDI-Ineffectiveness scale score was found to be predictive of disturbed eating patterns or bulimic caseness in one study using multivariate analyses (Leon, Fulkerson, Perry, Keel Klump, 1999). Significant differences, however, were found in the univariate comparisons of the subsequent symptomatic and the asymptomatic groups (Killen, Taylor, Hayward, Wilson, Haydel, et al., 1994; Killen, Taylor, Hayward, Haydel, Wilson, et al., 1996).

Anxiety and Mood Disorders

Psychiatric disorders, particularly anxiety and mood disorders have long been hypothesized to play a primary role in the development of EDs, including BN. Bulik, Sullivan, Fear and Joyce (1997) compared prevalence and onset of co-morbid childhood anxiety disorders in anorexics, bulimics and clinical as well as healthy controls. They noted the prevalence of social phobia to be highest in the bulimic group, and overanxious disorder highest in both the bulimic and anorexic groups. In terms of chronology of onset, 94% of women with BN with lifetime anxiety disorders reported that their anxiety disorder predated the onset of their BN. Fornari et al (1992) reported anxiety disorders to be as prevalent as depressive disorders in individuals with an ED. Brewerton, Lydiard, Herzog, Brotman, O'Neil and Ballenger (1995) also reported high rates of anxiety disorders in a group of patients with BN and that the anxiety disorders predated the onset of BN in 70% of cases. Social phobia was the most common anxiety disorder noted in this sample. These and many other authors have also noted higher rates of mood disorders, particularly major depressive disorder, among subjects with BN (Brewerton, Lydiard, Herzog, Brotman, O'Neil and Ballenger, 1995; Dansky, Brewerton, O'Neil and Kilpatrick, 1997; Lilenfeld, 2004). In addition, in a large non-treatment seeking, representative sample of women in the United States, Dansky, Brewerton, O'Neil and Kilpatrick (1997) found higher rates of both lifetime and current posttraumatic stress disorder (PTSD) in subjects with BN as compared to non-bulimic subjects. (see trauma below)

Raffi, Rondini, Grandi and Fava (2000) explored mood- and anxiety-related prodromal symptoms of BN and found a number of symptoms to be significantly more common in BN patients than controls six months prior to onset. These specifically included depressed mood, anhedonia, low self-esteem, irritability, impaired work performance, generalized anxiety, reactivity, phobic avoidance, guilt, pessimism and strict dieting. However, to what extent these symptoms are a result of strict dieting was not addressed in this study. In a study of risk factors for BN in a large group of twins, Kendler, MacLean, Neale, Kessler, Heath and Eaves (1991) reported that an external locus of control and high levels of neuroticism were predictive of BN.

Negative emotionality has also been found to predict eating disturbances and disorders in a number of longitudinal studies (Attie and Brooks-Gunn, 1989; Graber, Brooks-Gunn, Paikoff and Warren, 1994; Killen, Taylor, Hayward, et al., 1996; Leon, Fulkerson, Perry and Early-Zald, 1995; Leon, Fulkerson, Perry, Keel and Klump, 1999; Patton, Johnson-Sabine, Wood, Mann and Wakeling, 1990; Patton, Selzer, Coffey, Carlin and Wolfe, 1999). For example, in the study by Patton et al. (1990) the change score in general psychiatric morbidity was found to be the lone predictor of bulimic caseness. Psychiatric morbidity also was found to predict the onset of EDs (apart from dieting status) in a subsequent study by Patton et al. (1999). Subjects in the highest psychiatric morbidity category revealed a nearly sevenfold increased risk of developing an ED. Leon et al. (1999) reported that negative affectivity was the only statistically significant predictor of ED risk assessed three to four years later. Finally, in the study by Killen et al. (1996), the temperament scales, distress and fear, discriminated symptomatic from asymptomatic girls

Novelty Seeking, Sensation Seeking, and Impulsivity

The personality traits of novelty seeking, sensation seeking, and impulsivity, which appear to be related to each other, have all been linked to BN by a variety of investigators (Bailer, Price, Meltzer, et al., 2004; Berg, Crosby, Wonderlich, and Hawley, 2000; Bloks, Hoek, Callewaert, van Furth, 2004; Brewerton, 1995; Brewerton et al., 1992; Brewerton, Paolone, Soefje, 2002; Bulik, Sullivan, Weltzin, Kaye, 1995; Bulik, Sullivan, McKee, Weltzin, and Kaye, 1994; Cassin and von Ranson, 2005; Fassino, Abbate-Daga, Amianto, Leombruni, Boggio, and Rovera, 2002; Fassino, Amianto, Gramaglia, Facchini, and Abbate Daga, 2004; Fernandez-Aranda, Jimenez-Murcia, Alvarez-Moya, Granero, Vallejo and Bulik, 2006; Kleifield, Sunday, Hurt, and Halmi, 1994; Klump, Strober, Bulik, et al. 2004; Mizushima, Ono and Asai, 1998; Mulder, Joyce, Sullivan, Bulik and Carter, 1999; Schmeck and Poustka, 2001; Steiger and Bruce, 2007; Tomotake and Ohmori, 2002; Vervaet and van Heeringen, Audenaert, 2004; Wade, Bulik, Prescott and Kendler, 2004). Many clinical researchers have conceptualized a number of bulimic symptoms and behaviors in terms of impulsivity, including bingeing, purging, substance abuse, stealing, self-injury, suicide, and sexual acting out. Lacey and Evans (1986) coined the phrase "multi-impulsive bulimia," which has been shown to carry a poor prognosis. In addition, Wonderlich, Crosby, Mitchell, and colleagues (2001) found that impulsivity mediated the effects of childhood trauma on the development of bulimic symptoms.

Girls who later turned out to be symptomatic in the study by Killen et al. (1994) showed elevations on subscales of Aggressive and Unpopular in a personality inventory when compared to asymptomatic girls. Girls who developed a partial syndrome in the study by Killen et al. (1996) had higher 30-day prevalence of alcohol consumption. High use of escape-avoidance coping as well as low perceived social support were found to be prospective risk factors for subsequent EDs, primarily BN and BED, in the study by Ghaderi and Scott (2001).

Trauma, Neglect and PTSD

Accumulating evidence indicates that BN, unlike restricting AN, is a trauma-related disorder (Brewerton, 2003; 2004; 2005; 2007; Wonderlich, Brewerton, Jocic, Dansky and Abbott, 1997). It is now well established that prior traumatic or victimization experiences are nonspecific yet significant risk factors for the development of BN, especially when in association with other comorbid psychopathology such as anxiety, mood, substance use and personality disorders. Many, many studies now confirm this relationship as shown in meta-analyses (Smolak and Murnen, 2002; Molinari, 2001) and major reviews (Jacobi, Hayward, de Zwaan, Kraemer and Agras, 2004). However, despite the plethora of studies indicating higher than expected rates of prior abuse experiences in BN patients, very few studies have also examined for the presence of current and lifetime PTSD, which is a more powerful predictor of BN than abuse per se (Brewerton, 2007; Dansky, Brewerton, O'Neil, and Kilpatrick, 1997).

The National Women's Study (NWS) remains the most comprehensive study of the relationship of trauma history and PTSD to EDs and related comorbidity. Detailed histories of crime victimization experiences (rape, molestation, attempted sexual assault, and aggravated assault), PTSD, major depressive disorder, EDs, and substance abuse/dependence were obtained using DSM-III-R and DSM-IV (BED) criteria (Dansky, Brewerton, O'Neil and Kilpatrick, 1997). Rape and molestation was reported to have occurred approximately twice as often in BN participants compared to non-bulimic participants, while aggravated assault was three times as common. In the great majority of cases the age of victimization occurred prior to the age of first binge. For example, the age of first rape occurred before the age of 1st binge in 84% of all BN rape cases. These results provide substantial validity to the notion that victimization is indeed a causative risk factor for BN, albeit a non-specific one. However, the subsequent development of PTSD following victimization appears to incur the greatest risk of developing BN. The age of first binge (in BN) was significantly earlier in cases of rape resulting in PTSD compared to those with rape not resulting in PTSD or no rape. In addition, prevalence rates for BN were significantly higher in subjects with rape histories with PTSD (10.4%) compared to those with rape histories without PTSD (2.0%) or those with no rape (2.0%). This strongly suggests that PTSD rather than prior abuse per se best predicts the development of BN. In both the National Comorbidity Study and the National Women's Study, psychiatric comorbidity was highly associated with a history of serious victimization and especially a lifetime history of PTSD (Kessler Sonnega, Bromet, Hughes, Nelson, 1995). The odds ratios for several major axis I disorders have been reported to be on the order of 2.4 to 4.5 in both the National Comorbidity Study and the National Women's Study in participants with PTSD compared to those without PTSD. In other words, PTSD itself is a strong predictor of psychopathology including BN.

Besides a lifetime history of PTSD, other specific features of childhood sexual abuse (CSA) have been found to be associated with the development of BN, including decreased social competence, a poor maternal relationship, unreliable parenting, and greater severity of CSA (Wonderlich, Brewerton, Jocic, Dansky and Abbott, 1997). Interestingly, most of these features are also predictive of PTSD in the face of trauma.

Johnson, Cohen, Kasen and Brook (2002) conducted the most comprehensive longitudinal study on childhood adversities (including CSA, physical abuse (PA), and neglect), and the subsequent development of eating- or weight-related problems, including EDs. The participants in this study included a large community-based sample of mothers and their offspring (n = 782) who were followed over an 18-year period. This study further established CSA as important predictor of BN and bulimic disorders. In addition, the role of physical neglect in forecasting disturbed eating behaviors was demonstrated.

Alexithymia

Alexithymia is the inability to put one's emotions into words, a psychological characteristic originally described in patients with a variety of psychosomatic disorders. In addition, alexithymia refers to a diminished fantasy life and confusion of physical sensations often associated with emotions. Measures of alexithymia have been reported to be common in individuals with EDs and/or related conditions, such as mood, anxiety, substance use and dissociative disorders. Specifically, a number of investigators have described high rates of alexithymia in patients with BN (Cochrane, Hodges, Brewerton, 1993; Jimerson, Wolfe, Franko, Covino, and Sifneos, 1994). Interestingly, Espina (2003) reported that the parents of daughters with EDs show higher scores on measures of alexithymia than the control parents. These data suggest that alexithymia may be a familial condition which predisposes to the development of eating and related disorders.

Predisposing Social Underpinnings

Cultural Pressures for Thinness

Notwithstanding the powerful biogenetic contributions to the development of EDs noted previously, it is evident from a number of sources that sociocultural factors also predispose toward the development of EDs, including BN. Cross-cultural studies indicate significant variations in the prevalence rates of EDs, which have led investigators to conclude that specific sociocultural factors are influential. Although EDs are found in all socioeconomic status (SES) groups, they do occur more frequently in cultures and subcultures that promote thinness and place a great deal of emphasis on the control of body shape and weight (Anderson-Fye and Becker, 2004). Such cultures are typically those that are said to be industrialized or "Westernized." In a study of risk factors for BN in a large group of twins in the U.S., Kendler, MacLean, Neale, Kessler, Heath and Eaves (1991) demonstrated that birth after 1960 and a slim ideal body image were significant risk factors for bulimia. In addition, to cultural ideals favoring thinness, other cultural factors that may predispose toward EDs include exposure to TV and print media, cultural and social transition (see acculturation), and modernization (Becker, Burwell, Gilman, Herzog, and Hamburg, 2002; Stice, Maxfield, and Wells, 2003). Specific subcultures have also been reported to have higher prevalence rates of EDs, such as homosexual men, and occupations or activities that place a high premium on thinness, weight loss, beauty and physical appearance, such as models, actresses, dancers, gymnasts, wrestlers, etc, or on food preparation (Hodges, Stellefson, Jarrell, Cochrane, and Brewerton, 1999).

Acculturation

Acculturation is the process of adopting the cultural traits or social patterns of another group. Several reports indicate a connection between the degree of acculturation within ethnic minorities and the occurrence of eating disorder symptoms, including those of BN (Davis and Katzman, 1999; Gowen, Hayward, Killen, Robinson and Taylor, 1999; Hooper and Garner, 1986).

High Achievement and Athletic Competition

In a comprehensive survey of 522 female elite athletes from six different sport disciplines (Sundgot-Borgen, 1994), 8% of the surveyed athletes met DSM-III-R criteria for BN. Slightly more conservative results were obtained in a recent national survey by Johnson, Powers and Dick (1999), in which 1.1% of the female and none of the male athletes met DSM-IV criteria for BN, while 9.2% of the female and 0.005% of the male athletes were reported as having subclinical bulimia

Family Dysfunction

In the majority of the cross-sectional studies on family interaction, functioning or attachment style, bulimic patients describe various aspects of their family interaction as more problematic or dysfunctional than healthy controls. Characterizations of "bulimic families: have included being "less expressive, less cohesive, and experiencing more conflicts than normal control families" (Hodges, Cochrane, and Brewerton, 1998; Johnson and Flach, 1985; Laliberte, Boland, Leichner, 1999). In one study families of BN patients were reported to exhibit significantly more lack of care, indifference, discord, and overall adversity than AN patients and normal controls, but they did not differ from psychiatric patients with major depression (Webster and Palmer, 2000). In the community-based study by Fairburn, Welch, Doll, Davies and O`Connor (1997) parental variables such as low contact, high expectations, and critical comments about body shape and weight by family members were reported to be predictive of BN as compared to psychiatric controls. Hanna and Bond (2006) reported that, even after controlling for BMI, the frequency of negative messages is an important contributor to disordered eating symptomatology for both secondary school and university students. In a study by Wade, Bergin, Martin, Gillespie, Nathan, and Fairburn (2006) the number of lifetime eating disorder behaviors was associated with the degree of impaired functioning, which in turn was associated with conflict reported between parents and criticism from parents when growing up. In a survey of 210 undergraduate women at two universities, Botta and Dumlao (2002) tested the hypothesis that father-daughter communication and conflict resolution would be related to eating disordered behaviors. Results indicated that a lack of skilled conflict resolution and open communication between father and daughter could lead to disordered eating behaviors, and that the presence of such skills might offset the development of EDs.

In a two-part study Laliberte, Boland, and Leichner (1999) investigated variables thought to be more directly related to disturbed eating and bulimia as contributing to a "family climate for eating disorders." In the first study a nonclinical sample of 324 women who had recently left home for college and a sample of 121 mothers evaluated their families. Principal-components analyses revealed with three factors loading together for both students and mothers: Family Body Satisfaction, Family Social Appearance Orientation, and Family Achievement Emphasis. These factors represented the hypothesized "family climate for eating disorders" variable, while the rest of the variables loaded with more traditional family process variables (expressiveness, cohesion, and conflict), which represented more general family dysfunction. As hypothesized, the family climate for eating disorders factor score was a more powerful predictor of disturbed eating. The second study tested this finding in a clinical sample of bulimic patients (n = 40) and depressed patients (n = 17) and healthy controls (n = 27). Again, the bulimic group scored significantly higher on family climate variables than healthy controls as well as the depressed group after controlling for depression. One of the major findings in a large twin study (Kendler, MacLean, Neale, Kessler, Heath and Eaves, 1991) was that low paternal care was a risk factor for the later development of BN. Similarly, in a comparison study between 40 women with BN and their non-eating disordered sisters, insecure paternal attachment significantly predicted the risk for BN (Lehoux and Howe, 2007).

Annus, Smith, Fischer, Hendricks, and Williams (2007) reported that a history of food-related teasing from friends and family, negative maternal modeling, and friends' criticism of eating all related to both adult disordered behavior and adult eating and thinness expectancies.

Precipitating Biological Underpinnings

Dieting

Abundant evidence supports the contention that dieting is an important precursor of EDs, including BN. The onset of BN has been observed to occur either during a period of purposeful dieting (Mitchell, Hatsukami, Pyle and Eckert, 1986; Pyle, Mitchell and Eckert, 1981) or following weight loss (Garfinkel, Modolfsky, and Garner, 1980; Russell, 1979) for the vast majority of cases (73%-91%). While the studies by Mitchell, Hatsukami, Pyle and Eckert (1986) and Pyle, Mitchell and Eckert (1981) are rather nondescript about the chronological sequence of dieting and bingeing, more recent studies have validated the temporal precedence of dieting before bingeing in most BN subjects (Brewerton, Dansky, Kilpatrick and O'Neil, 2000; Haiman and Devlin, 1999; Mussell, Mitchell, Fenna, Crosby, Miller and Hoberman, 1997).

Experimental and laboratory-based studies on restrained eating and diet-induced binge eating yield further evidence for the relevance of this factor. One of the earliest, albeit uncontrolled studies demonstrating the effects of prolonged dieting in a non-clinical population was reported by Keys, Brozek, Hentschel, Mickelsen and Taylor (1950). Besides a variety of physical, emotional, and social changes following a prolonged period of semi-starvation and average weight decrease of 25%, binge eating was one of the behavioral changes reported, a phenomenon that had not been previously observed in the subjects before the study. Taken together, the cross-sectional research provides strong evidence of the temporal sequence of first dieting, then binge eating. In a study of risk factors for BN in a large group of twins, Kendler, MacLean, Neale, Kessler, Heath and Eaves (1991) found that risk factors for bulimia included a history of wide weight fluctuation, dieting, or frequent exercise.

A number of longitudinal studies have confirmed that dieting behavior, along with its associated weight concerns, such as negative body image and fear of weight gain, predicts the development of bulimic behaviors (Attie and Brooks-Gunn, 1989; Ghaderi and Scott, 2001; Graber, Brooks-Gunn, Paikoff, and Warren, 1994; Killen, Taylor, Hayward, et al., 1994; 1996; Leon, Fulkerson, Perry and Early-Zald, 1995; Leon, Fulkerson, Perry, Keel and Klump, 1999; Patton, Johnson-Sabine, Wood, Mann and Wakeling, 1990; Patton, Selzer, Coffey, Carlin and Wolfe, 1999; Vollrath, Koch and Angst, 1992). Patton, Johnson-Sabine, Wood, Mann and Wakeling (1990) reported that subjects classified as "dieters" at the outset were found to have nearly an 8 times higher risk of becoming "cases" than those originally classified as non-dieters.

Puberty

Based on evidence published by Graber, Lewinsohn, Seeley and Brooks-Gunn (1997) and Hayward, Killen, Wilson, et al. (1997), early sexual maturation or pubertal timing can be regarded as a non-specific risk factor for BN. Although this association between EDs and early sexual maturation has been hypothesized to be a function of increasing BMI (see obesity/BMI section), some studies don't support that relationship and some other aspect of puberty may play a role. Killen, Hayward, Litt, Hammer, Wilson, et al., (1992) examined the association between stage of sexual maturation and bulimic symptoms in a community-based sample of 971 adolescent girls enrolled in the sixth- and seventh-grades. Girls manifesting bulimic symptoms, while not older than their peers without such symptoms, were more developmentally advanced as determined using Tanner self-staging. The odds ratio for the association between sexual maturity and symptoms was 1.8 (95% confidence interval, 1.2 to 2.8), while the odds ratio for the association between BMI (adjusted for sexual maturity) and symptoms was 1.02 (95% confidence interval, 1.0 to 1.05). In addition, there was no independent statistical effect of age or of the interaction between age and sexual maturity index. In another study, Field et al. (1999) reported that girls who were further along in their maturational development were more likely than their less developed peers to begin purging at least once a month in order to control their weight. Taken together these results suggest that early puberty may be an important risk factor for the development of BN or bulimic symptoms independent of age and BMI.

Precipitating Psychological Underpinnings

Life Stressors

In a population-based study Welch, Doll and Fairburn (1997) reported that BN patients had more life events in the year preceding the onset of their disorder than age-matched normal controls (18% vs. 5% for $\geq$ 3 events). Adverse life events also differentiated eating disordered patients (mixed anorexic and bulimic) from both healthy and psychiatric controls (Horesh, Apter, Ishai, et al., 1996).

Schmidt, Slone, Tilley and Treasure (1993) reported that BN patients were significantly more likely to experience a "major difficulty" as well as "pudicity" problems. Taken together, there is some evidence that bulimic patients experience more severe life events than healthy controls.

Trauma/neglect/PTSD

Just as traumatic experiences may predispose to the subsequent development of BN, so can they also precipitate them acutely. The time period between traumatic experiences and the subsequent development of bulimic symptoms is extremely variable, with onset occurring anywhere from almost immediately in which vomiting may be in part a disgust reaction to years later. What determines this timing is likely to be a function of the interaction of other major risk factors for both BN and PTSD.

Precipitating Social Underpinnings

Peer Pressures

Both clinical experience and research reports indicate that some cases of BN begin with teasing about weight or appearance. In a study reported by Lehoux and Howe (2007) the role of perceived non-shared environmental influences in the risk of developing BN was compared in 40 women with BN and their non-eating disordered sisters. Perceptions of teasing distinguished bulimic women from their sisters. In a one year follow-up study of 6982 girls aged 9 to 14 years who denied vomiting, Field, Camargo, Taylor, Berkey, and Colditz (1999) found that the importance of thinness to peers (OR = 2.3; 95% CI, 1.8-3.0) was predictive of beginning to purge at least monthly. This finding was independent of age and Tanner stage of pubic hair development and suggests that peers can clearly exert a negative influence on girls' weight control beliefs and behaviors.

Media Messages

In their follow-up study of 6982 girls, Field, Camargo, Taylor, Berkey, and Colditz (1999) also demonstrated that trying to look like females on television, in movies, or in magazines (OR = 1.9; 95% CI, 1.6-2.3) was strongly predictive of beginning to purge at least monthly. This finding was also independent of age and Tanner stage of pubic hair development. In a related study, Field, Cheung, Wolf, Herzog, Gortmaker, Colditz, (1999) reported that the majority of preadolescent and adolescent girls studied in this school-based study of 548 5th through 12th graders were unhappy with their body weight and shape and that this discontentment was strongly related to the frequency of reading fashion magazines. The authors observed that the frequency of reading fashion magazines was positively related with the prevalence of dieting to lose weight, exercising to lose weight or improve body shape, dieting because of a magazine article, and deciding to exercise because of a magazine article.

Family Dynamics

In a study by Okon, Green, and Smith (2003), 20 adolescent girls diagnosed with BN completed questionnaires about bulimic symptoms and family "hassles" for one week, eight times daily, whenever contacted by pager. Statistical regression analyses found that "potent family hassles" were positive predictors of bulimic symptoms later that day, but this was only true for girls who perceived their family as having high levels of conflict or low levels of emotional expressiveness. Therefore, within the context of an apparent dysfunctional family environment, potent family hassles can predict intraindividual and interindividual bulimic symptoms that arise acutely for adolescent girls.

Perpetuating Biological Underpinnings

Starvation/Semi-Starvation
It is likely that disturbances in a number of neurotransmitters, neurohomones, peptides and neuromodulators act as important biological perpetuating factors

CNS Neurotransmitter Changes
There is considerable evidence for an impaired serotonergic responsiveness during the active phase of BN (Brewerton, 1995; Brewerton, Mueller, Lesem, et al., 1992; Goldbloom, Garfinkel, Katz and Brown, 1990; Kaye, Gendall, Fernstrom, Fernstrom, McConaha and

Weltzin, 2000; Kaye, Greeno, Moss, et al., 1998; Jimerson, Wolfe, Metzger, et al., 1997; Levitan, Kaplan, Joffe, Levitt and Brown, 1997; Monteleone, Brambilla, Bortolotti, Ferraro and Maj, 1998; Oldman, Walsh, Salkovskis, Fairburn and Cowen, 1995; Smith, Fairburn and Cowen, 1999; Weltzin, Fernstrom, Fernstrom, Neuberger and Kaye, 1995; Weltzin, Fernstrom, McConaha and Kaye, 1994). Studies have shown an inverse relationship between symptom severity and measures of serotonergic responsiveness (Jimerson, Lesem, Kaye and Brewerton, 1992; Monteleone, Brambilla, Bortolotti and Maj, 2000). In addition, there is evidence for an association between self-destructiveness, a history of sexual abuse, impulsivity and reduced serotonin function (Steiger, Gauvin, Israel, et al., 2001; Steiger, Koerner, Engelberg, et al., 2001; Steiger, Young, Ng Ying Kin, et al., 2001).

In addition to affecting eating behavior directly, alterations in CNS serotonin function may contribute to other psychological symptoms associated with BN. The diminished CNS serotonin could play a role in the high prevalence of depressive disorders in patients with BN. An impulsive-aggressive behavioral style, which is frequently seen in bulimic patients, may also be associated with diminished CNS serotonin function (Brewerton and Steiger, 2004).

Reduced CSF levels of the dopamine metabolite homovanillic acid (HVA) have been reported in BN patients with frequent binge-purge episodes (Kaye, Ballenger, Lydiard, et al., 1990; Jimerson, Lesem, Kaye and Brewerton, 1992) but not in those less severely ill. Furthermore, binge frequency has been reported to be inversely correlated with CSF HVA levels (Jimerson, Lesem, Kaye and Brewerton, 1992). Upon long-term recovery, normal concentrations of CSF HVA have been reported to normalize in BN (Kaye, Gendall and Strober, 1998). However, during the active phase of the illness these purported neurotransmitter abnormalities may drive the expression and continuation of symptoms.

Neuropeptide and Hormonal Alterations

Other neurochemical systems have been reported to be significantly different from controls in BN patients and may also contribute to the maintenance of symptoms. For example, CSF levels of cholecystokinin (CCK) have been reported to be significantly lower in BN patients, and levels were correlated with measures of anxiety (Lydiard, Brewerton, Beinfeld, Laraia, Stuart and Ballenger, 1993). In another study, BN patients showed significantly lower levels of beta-endorphin (B-END), which were correlated with measures of depression (Brewerton, Lydiard, Laraia, 1992).

It has also been shown that bulimic patients have significantly lower serum leptin concentrations in comparison to matched controls (Baranowska, Wolinska-Witort, Wasilewska-Dziubinska, Roguski, and Chmielowska, 2001; Brewerton, Lesem, and Garvey, 2000; Jimerson, Mantzoros, Wolfe, and Metzger, 2000; Monteleone, Bortolotti, Fabrazzo, La Rocca, Fuschino, Maj, 2000). Leptin levels appear to remain decreased even after sustained recovery in comparison to controls with matched percent BMI. This finding suggests that serum leptin levels may remain decreased and could be linked to decreased metabolic rate and a tendency to gain weight that is characteristic of BN

Plasma ghrelin concentrations have been reported to be significantly higher in bulimic patients as compared to healthy controls even though there was no difference between the BMIs between the groups (Tanaka, Naruo, Muranaga, Yasuhara, Shiiya, et al., 2002). These results suggest that not only BMI, but also disordered eating behavior characterized by bingeing and purging can influence circulating ghrelin levels.

Actively bulimic individuals have significantly higher plasma cortisol levels in comparison to controls (Brewerton et al, 1992; Brewerton, 1995). In addition, plasma cortisol levels have also been shown to be inversely correlated to serotonin receptor sensitivity. Therefore, the stresses of semi-starvation, bingeing and purging may lead

Perpetuating Psychological Underpinnings

Cognitive Distortions

One of the foremost clinical features of patients with EDs, including those with BN, is the presence of prominent cognitive distortions, in particular distorted self-statements or negative, self-deprecatory beliefs about oneself, e.g., "I am fat," "I am ugly," "I am unworthy," "I am inferior," etc. The success of cognitive behavioral therapy (CBT) for the treatment of BN, as well as many of its associated comorbid conditions, e.g., major depression, anxiety disorders, and substance use disorders, attests to the importance of addressing cognitive distortions. Failure to make an impact on this often resistant feature can result in the perpetuation of symptoms and/or behaviors that are "driven" by these illogical thoughts.

Interpersonal Problems

A related issue often associated with the maintenance of bulimic symptoms or nonresponsiveness to treatment is the failure to fully process or resolve challenging interpersonal issues. Such dynamics may often overlap or intersect with the cognitive distortions and negative affects noted elsewhere. Patients with BN are reported to have histories of more problematic social experiences, including histories of family dysfunction and interpersonal stressors that often lead to feelings of low self-esteem, social isolation, lack of perceived support, and poor coping and problem solving skills (Fairburn, Welch, Doll, Davies and O'Connor, 1997; Ghaderi and Scott, 1999; Grissett and Norvell, 1992; Gual, Perez-Gaspar, Martinez-Gonzalez, Lahortiga, Irala-Estevez and Cervera-Enguix, 2002; Herzog, Keller, Lavori and Ott, 1987; O'Mahony and Hollwey, 1995; Rorty, Yager, Buckwalter and Rossotto, 1999; Tiller, Sloane, Schmidt, Troop, Power and Treasure, 1997; Troop, Holbrey, Trowler and Treasure, 1994; Tuschen-Caffier and Vogele, 1999). Interpersonal Psychotherapy (IPT) seeks to enhance self-esteem, interpersonal functioning, and negative affect as they relate to each other and to bulimic symptoms.

Trauma, Neglect and PTSD

Trauma-related disorders, such as BN, major depression, and PTSD, may share common underlying factors that account for such interrelationships, including dysregulation in neuropsychobiological mechanisms that are triggered by gene expression and resultant underlying affective dysregulation, as well as common cognitive schemas involving issues of self-esteem, control, guilt and shame (Brewerton, 2004; 2007). This perspective is supported by several studies of mediating variables between previous abuse and later development of BN, which demonstrate that impulsivity and fundamental beliefs involving self-esteem, shame, and perceived control are important considerations in more completely understanding etiological mechanisms as well as treatment approaches (Andrews,1997; Brady, Killeen, Brewerton and Lucerini, 2000; Murray and Waller, 2002; Waller, 1998; Waller, Meyer, Ohanian, Elliott, Dickson and Sellings, 2001; Wonderlich, Crosby, Mitchell, Thompson, Redlin, Demuth and Smyth, 2001; Wonderlich, Crosby, Mitchell, et al., 2001). Rodriguez, Perez and Garcia (2005) reported that the highest likelihood of poor outcome was found in patients with sexual abuse and histories of other violent acts. In addition, this group of patients was at greatest risk for dropout and relapse following treatment.

Likewise, Anderson, LaPorte, Brandt and Crawford (1997) reported that sexually abused inpatients with BN exhibited higher levels of depression, anxiety, and eating disordered attitudes at each assessment point relative to nonabused subjects and that abused subjects were more likely to be re-hospitalized in the three month post-discharge period.

In another follow-up study of hospitalized bulimic patients, Fallon, Sadik, Saoud and Garfinkel (1994) reported that childhood PA and a family environment characterized by low cohesion and high control were significantly associated with poor outcome. The family environment characteristics seemed to have greater influence on clinical outcome than abuse per se. Gleaves and Eberenz (1994) also reported an association between sexual abuse history and poor prognosis in 464 bulimic women in residential treatment.

Schmidt, Slone, Tiller and Treasure (1993) compared the defensive styles of anorexic and bulimic patients and healthy female controls in an attempt to establish a link between early childhood adversity and later adult defensive style. BN patients were found to have a significantly less mature defense style than the other groups. In addition, excessive parental control during childhood was a negative predictor of mature defenses and physical abuse a positive predictor of immature defense style. The authors concluded that childhood adversity may constitute a vulnerability factor for the later development of BN, mediated by personality development.

Depression

There is some evidence that the presence of major depression or significant depressive symptoms interfere with either the engagement in treatment or with response to treatment. Maddocks and Kaplan (1991) studied 86 women with BN treated in a group program and found that depression and core symptoms of eating disorder best discriminated "positive" from "poor" treatment responders. In a one-year follow-up study of 100 bulimic patients who completed a clinical trial of CBT, the presence of major depression predicted poor outcome (Bulik, Sullivan, Joyce, Carter and McIntosh, 1998).

Personality Factors

A number of investigators have reported that bulimic patients with borderline personality disorder or so-called borderline features have a relatively poorer response to treatment (Herzog, Hartmann, Sandholz and Stammer, 1991).

Perpetuating Social Underpinnings

Cultural Effects

Western culture is a toxic environment for the individual recovering from BN. Pressures to be thin, young and physically attractive are ubiquitous in our culture, while at the same time exposure to highly palatable and readily available foods in large quantifies makes attaining abstinence from bingeing and purging and subsequent recovery difficult.

Social Reinforcement

Observations from clinical practice indicate that positive reinforcement for weight loss from others plays a powerful role in maintaining symptoms. Patients often irrationally fear weight gain following cessation of bingeing and purging.

Family Dysfunction

Blouin, Carter, Blouin, et al. (1994) studied potential prognostic indicators of short-term outcome in 69 women with BN who participated in a weekly 10-session structured CBT outpatient group program. The only significant predictor of improvement in binge frequency and bulimic cognitions was family environment. Controlling conflicted and over-organized family environments appeared to hinder improvements in not only binge frequency but bulimic cognitions as well. In an important study by Dancyger, Fornari, Scionti, Wisotsky, Sunday (2005), the mothers of ED patients were found to rate family functioning as significantly healthier and less chaotic than their daughters. Although there were fewer significant differences between maternal and paternal views of family functioning, there were no significant differences between fathers' and daughters' family perceptions. In addition, increased levels of depressive symptoms as reported by the daughters were linked to the perception of high family dysfunction. Differences in viewpoints between parents and daughters regarding family environment may negatively impact on the course of treatment and contribute to the continuation of dysfunctional family patterns.

FACTORS	BIOLOGICAL	PSYCHOLOGICAL	SOCIAL
PREDISPOSING	Genetics	Perfectionism/OCP traits	Pressures for Thinness
	Gender	Low self-esteem	Acculturation
	Trait-related diffs	Ineffectiveness	High achievement
	Age	Anxiety/mood D/O's	Athletic competition
	Ethnicity/race	Trauma/neglect/PTSD	Family dysfunction
	Prenatal/perinatal probs	Novelty/sensation seeking	
	Season of birth	Impulsivity	
	BMI/Obesity	Alexithymia	
	Pica/digestive problems		
	Family history of psychopathology		
PRECIPITATING	Puberty	Life stressors	Peer pressures
	Illness	Interpersonal dynamics	Media messages
	Dieting/weight loss	Trauma/neglect/PTSD	Family dynamics
PERPETUATING	Starvation effects	Cognitive distortions	Cultural effects
	CNS changes	Interpersonal problems	Social Reinforcement
	Peptide changes	Trauma/neglect/PTSD	Family dysfunction
	Hormone changes	Depression/Personality	

Figure 1. THE 3 "P's" across the bio-psycho-social spectrum.

Conclusion

In summary, there is no one cause of BN. Etiology is best seen using a biopsychosocial model along a neurodevelopmental continuum. The three P's are useful in thinking about etiology in any given individual. Latent vulnerability theory suggests strong genetic predisposing factors linked to anxiety, obsessive-compulsiveness which are exposed or triggered by behaviors leading to weight loss. Traumatic experiences often play important roles in predisposing, precipitating and perpetuating bulimic disorders, especially with comorbidity. Future research will uncover interactions among genetic and environmental factors (Caspi and Moffitt, 2006) in the tradition of newer integrative studies that assess gene-environment interactions such as those performed by Caspi and colleagues for major depression (Caspi, Sugden, Moffitt, Taylor, Craig, et al., 2003), antisocial behavior (Caspi, McClay, Moffitt, Mill, Martin, et al., 2002) and substance abuse (Caspi, Moffitt, Cannon, McClay, Murray, et al., 2005).

References

American Psychiatric Association (1994). *Diagnostic and Statistical Manual of Mental Disorders* (4th ed.). Washington, DC: APA.

American Psychiatric Association (1980). *Diagnostic and Statistical Manual of Mental Disorders* (3rd ed.). Washington, DC: APA.

American Psychiatric Association (1987). *Diagnostic and Statistical Manual of Mental Disorders* (3rd ed., revised). Washington, DC: APA.

Anderson-Fye, E.P., Becker, A.E. (2004). Sociocultural aspects of eating disorders. In Thompson, J.K. (Ed.). *Handbook of Eating Disorders and Obesity*. Hoboken, N.J., John Wiley and Sons, Inc. pp. 565-589.

Anderson, K.P., LaPorte, D.J., Brandt, H., Crawford, S. (1997). Sexual abuse and bulimia: response to inpatient treatment and preliminary outcome. *Journal of Psychiatric Research, 31*, 621-633.

Andrews, B. (1997). Bodily shame in relation to abuse in childhood and bulimia: a preliminary investigation. *British Journal of Clinical Psychology, 36*, 41-49.

Annus, A.M., Smith, G.T., Fischer, S., Hendricks, M., Williams, S.F. (2007). Associations among family-of-origin food-related experiences, expectancies, and disordered eating. *International Journal of Eating Disorders. 40*, 179-186.

Attie, I., and Brooks-Gunn, J. (1989). Development of eating problems in adolescent girls: A longitudinal study. *Developmental Psychology, 25*, 70-79.

Bailer, U.F., Price, J.C., Meltzer, C.C., Mathis, C.A., Frank, G.K., Weissfeld, L., McConaha, C.W., Henry, S.E., Brooks-Achenbach, S., Barbarich, N.C., Kaye, W.H. (2004). Altered 5-HT(2A) receptor binding after recovery from bulimia-type anorexia nervosa: relationships to harm avoidance and drive for thinness. *Neuropsychopharmacology, 29*, 1143-1155.

Baranowska B, Wolinska-Witort E, Wasilewska-Dziubinska E, Roguski K, Chmielowska M. (2001). Plasma leptin, neuropeptide Y (NPY) and galanin concentrations in bulimia nervosa and in anorexia nervosa. *Neuroendocrinology Letters, 22*, 356–358.

Becker, A.E., Burwell, R., Gilman, S.E., Herzog, D., Hamburg, P. (2002). Eating behaviors and attitudes following prolonged exposure to television among ethnic Fijian adolescent girls. *British Journal of Psychiatry*, 180, 509-514.

Berg, M.L., Crosby, R.D., Wonderlich, S.A., Hawley, D. (2000). Relationship of temperament and perceptions of nonshared environment in bulimia nervosa. *International Journal of Eating Disorders, 28*, 148-154.

Bloks, H., Hoek, H.W., Callewaert, I., van Furth, E. (2004). Stability of personality traits in patients who received intensive treatment for a severe eating disorder. *Journal of Nervous and Mental Disease, 192*, 129-138.

Blouin, J.H., Carter, J., Blouin, A.G., Tener, L., Schnare-Hayes, K., Zuro, C., Barlow, J., Perez, E. (1994). Prognostic indicators in bulimia nervosa treated with cognitive-behavioral group therapy. *International Journal of Eating Disorders, 15*, 113-123.

Boskind-Lodahl, M. (1976). Cinderella's stepsisters: a feminist perspective on anorexia nervosa. *Signs, 2*, 342-356.

Boskind-Lodahl, M., White, W.C. (1978). The definition and treatment of bulimiarexia in college women-a pilot study. *Journal of the American College Health Association, 27*, 84-97.

Botta, R.A., Dumlao, R. (2002). How do conflict and communication patterns between fathers and daughters contribute to or offset eating disorders? *Health Communication, 14,* 199-219.

Brady, K.T., Killeen, T.K., Brewerton, T., Lucerini, S. (2000). Comorbidity of psychiatric disorders and posttraumatic stress disorder. *Journal of Clinical Psychiatry, 61*, 22-32.

Brewerton, T.D. (1995). Toward a unified theory of serotonin dysregulation in eating and related disorders. *Psychoneuroendocrinology, 20*, 561-590.

Brewerton, T.D. (2002). Bulimia in children and adolescents. *Child and Adolescent Psychiatry Clinics of North America, 11*, 237-256.

Brewerton, T.D. (2004). Eating disorders, victimization and PTSD: principles of treatment. In Brewerton, T.D. (Ed.), *Clinical Handbook of Eating Disorders: An Integrated Approach.* New York: Marcel Dekker, Inc., pp. 509-545.

Brewerton, T.D. (2005). Psychological trauma and eating disorders. *Review of Eating Disorders, Part 1, 1*, 137-154.

Brewerton, T.D. (2007). Comorbid anxiety and depression and the role of trauma in children and adolescents with eating disorders. In Jaffa T. and McDermott B. (Eds.) *Eating Disorders in Children and Adolescents*. pp. 158-168.

Brewerton, T. D., Dansky, B. S., Kilpatrick, D. G., O'Neil, P. M. (2000). Which comes first in the pathogenensis of bulimia nervosa, dieting or bingeing? *International Journal of Eating Disorders, 28*, 259-264.

Brewerton, T. D., Dansky, B. S., O'Neil, P. M., Kilpatrick, D. G. (2007). Seasonal patterns of birth for bingers and purgers: results from the National Women's Study. *Syllabus 2007. Annual Meeting of the Academy of Eating Disorders.* Baltimore, MD, May 2007.

Brewerton, T.D., Hand, J.D., Bishop, E.M. (1993). The Tridimensional Personality Questionnaire in patients with eating disorders. *International Journal of Eating Disorders, 14,* 213-218.

Brewerton, T.D., Lesem, M.D., Kennedy, A., Garvey, W.T. (2000). Reduced plasma leptin concentration in bulimia nervosa. *Psychoneuroendocrinology, 25*, 649–658.

Brewerton, T.D., Lydiard, R.B. (1994). CSF cholecystokinin octapeptide in bulimia. *American Journal of Psychiatry, 151*, 1098.

Brewerton, T.D., Lydiard, R.B., Ballenger, J.C., Herzog, D.B. (1993). Eating disorders and social phobia. *Archives of General Psychiatry, 50*, 70.

Brewerton, T.D., Lydiard, R.B., Herzog, D.B., Brotman, A., O'Neil, P., Ballenger, J.C. (1995). Comorbidity of axis I psychiatric disorders in bulimia nervosa. *Journal of Clinical Psychiatry, 56*, 77-80.

Brewerton, T.D., Lydiard, R.B., Laraia, M.T., Shook, J., Ballenger, J.C. (1992). CSF beta-endorphin and dynorphin in bulimia nervosa. *American Journal of Psychiatry, 149*, 1086-1090.

Brewerton, T.D., Mueller, E.A., Lesem, M.D., Brandt, H.A., Quearry, B., George, D.T., Murphy, D.L., Jimerson, D.C. (1992). Neuroendocrine responses to m-chlorophenylpiperazine and l-tryptophan in bulimia. *Archives of General Psychiatry, 49*, 852-861.

Brewerton, T.D., Paolone, T.J., Soefje, S. (2001). The relationship between impulsivity, sensation seeking and obsessive-compulsive features in a clinical sample of eating disorder patients. *Annual Meeting of the Eating Disorders Research Society,* Bermalillo, New Mexico. November 28-December 1.

Brewerton, T.D., Steiger, H. (2004). Neurotransmitter dysregulation in anorexia nervosa, bulimia nervosa and binge eating disorder. In Brewerton, T.D. (Ed.), *Clinical Handbook of Eating Disorders: An Integrated Approach.* New York: Marcel Dekker, Inc., pp. 257-281.

Brooks-Achenbach, S., Barbarich, N.C., Kaye, W.H. (2004). Altered 5-HT(2A) receptor binding after recovery from bulimia-type anorexia nervosa: relationships to harm avoidance and drive for thinness. *Neuropsychopharmacology, 29*, 1143-155.

Bruch, H. (1973). *Eating disorders: Obesity, anorexia nervosa, and the person within.* New York: Basic Books.

Bulik, C.M., Devlin, B., Bacanu, S.A., Thornton, L., Klump, K.L., Fichter, M.M., Halmi, K.A., Kaplan, A.S., Strober, M., Woodside, D.B., Bergen, A.W., Ganjei, J.K., Crow, S., Mitchell, J., Rotondo, A., Mauri, M., Cassano, G., Kellp, P., Berrettini, W.H., Kaye, W.H. (2003). Significant linkage on chromosome 10p in families with bulimia nervosa. *American Journal of Human Genetics, 72*, 200–207.

Bulik, C. M., Sullivan, P. F., Fear, J. L., and Joyce, P. R. (1997). Eating disorders and antecedent anxiety disorders: a controlled study. *Acta Psychiatrica Scandinavica, 96*, 101-107.

Bulik, C.M., Sullivan, P.F., Carter, F.A., Joyce, P.R. (1997). Initial manifestations of disordered eating behavior: dieting versus binging. *International Journal of Eating Disorders, 22*, 195-201.

Bulik, C.M., Sullivan, P.F., Carter, F.A., Joyce, P.R. (1997). Lifetime comorbidity of alcohol dependence in women with bulimia nervosa. *Addictive Behaviors, 22*, 437-446.

Bulik, C.M., Sullivan, P.F., Carter, F.A., Joyce, P.R. (1997). Initial manifestations of disordered eating behavior: dieting versus binging. *International Journal of Eating Disorders, 22*, 195-201.

Bulik, C.M., Sullivan, P.F., Joyce, P.R., Carter, F.A., McIntosh, V.V. (1998). Predictors of 1-year follow-up in bulimia nervosa. *Comprehensive Psychiatry, 39*, 206-214.

Bulik, C.M., Sullivan, P.F., Kendler, K.S. (1998). Heritability of binge-eating and broadly defined bulimia nervosa. *Biological Psychiatry, 44*, 1210-1218.

Bulik, C.M., Sullivan, P.F., McKee, M., Weltzin, T.E., Kaye, W.H. (1994). Characteristics of bulimic women with and without alcohol abuse. *American Journal of Drug and Alcohol Abuse, 20*, 273-283.

Bulik, C. M., Sullivan, P. F., Wade, T. D., and Kendler, K. S. (2000). Twin studies of eating disorders: a review. *International Journal of Eating Disorders, 27*, 1-20.

Bulik, C.M., Sullivan, P.F., Weltzin, T.E., Kaye, W.H. (1995). Temperament in eating disorders. *International Journal of Eating Disorders, 17*, 251-261.

Button, E. J., Sonuga-Barke, E. J. S., Davies, J., and Thompson, M. (1996). A prospective study of self-esteem in the prediction of eating problems in adolescent schoolgirls: Questionnaire findings. *British Journal of Clinical Psychology, 35*, 193-203.

Calam, R., and Waller, G. (1998). Are eating and psychosocial characteristics in early teenage years useful predictors of eating characteristics in early adulthood? A 7-year longitudinal study. *International Journal of Eating Disorders, 24*, 351-362.

Caspi, A., McClay, J., Moffitt, T.E., Mill, J., Martin, J., Craig, I.W., Taylor, A., Poulton, R. (2002). Role of genotype in the cycle of violence in maltreated children. *Science, 297*, 851-854.

Caspi, A., Moffitt, T.E. (2006). Gene-environment interactions in psychiatry: joining forces with neuroscience. *Nature Reviews Neuroscience, 7*, 583-590.

Caspi, A., Moffitt, T.E., Cannon, M., McClay, J., Murray, R., Harrington, H., Taylor, A., Arseneault, L., Williams, B., Braithwaite, A., Poulton, R., Craig, I.W. (2005). Moderation of the effect of adolescent-onset cannabis use on adult psychosis by a functional polymorphism in the catechol-O-methyltransferase gene: longitudinal evidence of a gene X environment interaction. *Biological Psychiatry, 57*, 1117-1127.

Caspi, A., Sugden, K., Moffitt, T.E., Taylor, A., Craig, I.W., Harrington, H., McClay, J., Mill, J., Martin, J., Braithwaite, A., Poulton, R. (2003). Influence of life stress on depression: moderation by a polymorphism in the 5-HTT gene.[see comment]. *Science, 301*, 386-389.

Cassin, S.E., von Ranson, K.M. (2005). Personality and eating disorders: a decade in review. *Clinical Psychology Review, 25*, 895-916.

Chen, C. N., Wong, J., Lee, N., Chan-Ho, M. W., Lau, J. T., and Fung, M. (1993). The Shatin Community mental health survey in Hong Kong. II. Major findings. *Archives of General Psychiatry, 50*, 125-133.

Childress, A.C., Brewerton, T.D., Hodges, E.L., Jarrell, M.P. (1993). The Kids' Eating Disorders Survey (KEDS): results from a survey of middle school students. *Journal of the American Academy of Child and Adolescent Psychiatry, 32*, 843-850.

Cochrane, C.E., Brewerton, T.D., Hodges, E.L., Wilson, D. (1993). Alexithymia in the eating disorders. *International Journal of Eating Disorders, 14*, 219-222.

Cochrane, C.E., Malcolm, R., Brewerton, T.D. (1998). Eating disorders in cocaine abusers. *Addictive Disorders, 23*, 1-7.

Crago, M., Shisslak, C. M., and Estes, L. S. (1996). Eating disturbances among American minority groups: A review. *International Journal of Eating Disorders, 19*, 239-248.

Dancyger, I., Fornari, V., Scionti, L., Wisotsky, W., Sunday, S. (2005). Do daughters with eating disorders agree with their parents' perception of family functioning? *Comprehensive Psychiatry, 46,* 135-139.

Dansky, B.S., Brewerton, T.D., O'Neil, P.M., Kilpatrick, D.G. (1997). The National Women's Study: Relationship of crime victimization and PTSD to bulimia nervosa. *International Journal of Eating Disorders, 21,* 213-228.

Dansky, B.S., Brewerton, T.D., Kilpatrick, D.G. (2000). Comorbidity of bulimia nervosa and alcohol use disorders: results from the National Women's Study. *International Journal of Eating Disorders, 27,* 180-190.

Davis, C., and Katzman, M. A. (1999). Perfection as acculturation: Psychological correlates of eating problems in Chinese male and female students living in the United States. *International Journal of Eating Disorders, 25,* 65-70.

Emmons, L. (1992). Dieting and purging in Black and White high school students. *Journal of the American Dietetic Association, 92,* 306-312.

Espina, A. (2003). Alexithymia in parents of daughters with eating disorders: its relationships with psychopathological and personality variables. *Journal of Psychosomatic Research, 55,* 553-560.

Fairburn, C. G., Welch, S. L., Doll, H. A., Davies, B. A., and O'Connor, M. E. (1997). Risk factors for bulimia nervosa. A community-based case-control study. *Archives of General Psychiatry, 54,* 509-517.

Fallon, B.A., Sadik, C., Saoud, J.B., Garfinkel, R.S. (1994). Childhood abuse, family environment, and outcome in bulimia nervosa. *Journal of Clinical Psychiatry, 55,* 424-428.

Fassino, S., Abbate-Daga, G., Amianto, F., Leombruni, P., Boggio, S., Rovera, G.G. (2002). Temperament and character profile of eating disorders: a controlled study with the Temperament and Character Inventory. *International Journal of Eating Disorders, 32,* 412-425.

Fassino, S., Amianto, F., Gramaglia, C., Facchini, F., Abbate-Daga, G. (2004). Temperament and character in eating disorders: ten years of studies. *Eating and Weight Disorders: EWD, 9,* 81-90.

Favaro, A., Tenconi, E., Santonastaso, P. (2006). Perinatal Factors and the risk of developing anorexia nervosa and bulimia nervosa. *Archives of General Psychiatry, 63,* 82-88.

Fernandez-Aranda, F., Jimenez-Murcia, S., Alvarez-Moya, E.M., Granero, R., Vallejo, J., Bulik, C.M. (2006). Impulse control disorders in eating disorders: clinical and therapeutic implications. *Comprehensive Psychiatry, 47,* 482-488.

Field, A.E., Camargo, C.A., Taylor, C.B., Berkey, C.S., Colditz, G.A. (1999). Relation of peer and media influences to the development of purging behaviors among preadolescent and adolescent girls. *Archives of Pediatric and Adolescent Medicine, 153,* 1184-1189.

Field, A.E., Cheung, L., Wolf, A.M., Herzog, D.B., Gortmaker, S.L., Colditz, G.A. (1999). Exposure to the mass media and weight concerns among girls. *Pediatrics, 103,* E36.

Field, A.E., Colditz, G.A., Peterson, K.E., (1997). Racial/ethnic and gender differences in concern with weight and in bulimic behaviors among adolescents. *Obesity Research, 5,* 447-454.

Foley, D. L., Thacker, L. R., Aggen, S. H., Neale, M. C., and Kendler, K. S. (2001). Pregnancy and perinatal complications associated with risks for common psychiatric disorders in a population-based sample of female twins. *American Journal of Medical Genetics, 105*, 426-431.

Fornari, V., Kaplan, M., Sandberg, D., Matthews, M., Katz, J. (1992). The relationship between depression and anxiety disorders in anorexia nervosa and bulimia nervosa. *The International Journal of Eating Disorders, 12*, 21-29.

Garfinkel, Modolfsky, and Garner, (1980). The heterogeneity of anorexia nervosa: Bulimia as a distinct subgroup. *Archives of General Psychiatry, 37*, 1036-1040.

Ghaderi, A., Scott, B. (1999). Prevalence and psychological correlates of eating disorders among females aged 18–30 years in the general population. *Acta Psychiatrica Scandinavica, 99*, 261–266.

Ghaderi, A., and Scott, B. (2001). Prevalence, incidence and prospective risk factors for eating disorders. *Acta Psychiatrica Scandinavica, 104*, 122-130.

Gleaves, D.H., Eberenz, K.P. (1994). Sexual abuse histories among treatment-resistant bulimia nervosa patients. *International Journal of Eating Disorders, 15*, 227-231.

Goldbloom, D.S., Garfinkel, P.E., Katz, R., and Brown, G. (1990). The hormonal response to intravenous 5-hydroxytryptophan in bulimia nervosa. *Psychosomatic Medicine, 52*, 225-226.

Gowen, L. K., Hayward, C., Killen, J. D., Robinson, T. N. and Taylor, C. B. (1999). Acculturation and eating disorder symptoms in adolescent girls. *Journal of Research on Adolescence, 9*, 67-83.

Graber, J. A., Brooks-Gunn, J., Paikoff, R. L., and Warren, M. P. (1994). Prediction of eating problems: An 8-year study of adolescent girls. *Developmental Psychology, 30*, 823-834.

Graber, J. A., Lewinsohn, P. M., Seeley, J. R., and Brooks-Gunn, J. (1997). Is psychopathology associated with the timing of pubertal development? *Journal of the American Academy of Child and Adolescent Psychiatry, 36*, 1768-1776.

Grissett, N.L., Norvell, N.K. (1992). Perceived social support, social skills, and quality of relationships in bulimic women. *Journal of Consulting and Clinical Psychology, 60*, 293–299.

Gual ,P., Perez-Gaspar, M., Martinez-Gonzalez, M.A., Lahortiga, F., Irala-Estevez, J., Cervera-Enguix (2002). Self-esteem, personality, and eating disorders: baseline assessment of a prospective population-based cohort. *International Journal of Eating Disorders, 31*, 261–273.

Haiman, C., and Devlin, M. J. (1999). Binge eating before the onset of dieting: A distinct subgroup of bulimia nervosa? *International Journal of Eating Disorders, 25*, 151-157.

Halmi, K.A., Tozzi, F., Thornton, L.M., Crow, S., Fichter, M.M., Kaplan, A.S., Keel, P., Klump, K.L., Lilenfeld, L.R., Mitchell, J.E., Plotnicov, K.H., Pollice, C., Rotondo, A., Strober, M., Woodside, D.B., Berrettini, W.H., Kaye, W.H., Bulik, C.M. (2005). The relation among perfectionism, obsessive-compulsive personality disorder and obsessive-compulsive disorder in individuals with eating disorders. *International Journal of Eating Disorders, 38*, 371-374.

Hanna, A.C., Bond, M.J. (2006). Relationships between family conflict, perceived maternal verbal messages, and daughters' disturbed eating symptomatology. *Appetite, 47*, 205-211.

Hayward, C., Killen, J. D., Wilson, D. M., Hammer, L. D., Litt, I. F., Kraemer, H. C., Haydel, F., Varady, A., and Taylor, C. B. (1997). Psychiatric risk associated with early puberty in adolescent girls. *Journal of the American Academy of Child and Adolescent Psychiatry, 36*, 255-262.

Haiman, C., and Devlin, M. J. (1999). Binge eating before the onset of dieting: A distinct subgroup of bulimia nervosa? *International Journal of Eating Disorders, 25*, 151-157.

Herzog, T., Hartmann, A., Sandholz, A., Stammer, H. (1991). Prognostic factors in outpatient psychotherapy of bulimia. *Psychotherapy and Psychosomatics, 56*, 48-55. Herzog, D.B., Keller, M.B., Lavori, P.W., Ott, I.L. (1987). Social impairment in bulimia. *International Journal of Eating Disorders, 6*, 741–747.

Hodges ,E.L., Cochrane, C.E., Brewerton, T.D. (1998). Family characteristics of binge eating disorder patients. *International Journal of Eating Disorders, 23*, 145-151.

Hodges, E.L., Stellefson, E.J., Jarrell, M.P., Cochrane, C.E., Brewerton, T.D: (1999). Eating disorder pathology in a culinary arts school. *Eating Disorders: The Journal of Treatment and Prevention, 7*, 43-50.

Holland, A. J., Hall, A., Murray, R., Russell, G. F. M., and Crisp, A. H. (1984). Anorexia nervosa: a study of 34 twin pairs and one set of triplets. *British Journal of Psychiatry, 145*, 414-419.

Holland, A. J., Sicotte, N., and Treasure, J. (1988). Anorexia nervosa: evidence for a genetic basis. *Journal of Psychosomatic Research, 32*, 561-571.

Hooper, M. S. H., and Garner, D. M. (1986). Application of the eating disorders inventory to a sample of Black, White and Mixed race schoolgirls in Zimbabwe. *International Journal of Eating Disorders, 5*, 161-168.

Horesh, N., Apter, A., Ishai, J., Danziger, Y., Miculincer, M., Stein, D., Lepkifker, E., and Minouni, M. (1996). Abnormal psychosocial situations and eating disorders in adolescence. *Journal of the American Academy of Child and Adolescent Psychiatry, 35*, 921-927.

Hsu, L. K. G. (1996). Epidemiology of the eating disorders. *Psychiatric Clinics of North America, 19*, 681-700.

Hudson, J.I., Hiripi, E., Pope, H.G. Jr., Kessler, R.C. (2007). The prevalence and correlates of eating disorders in the National Comorbidity Survey Replication. *Biological Psychiatry, 61*, 348-358.

Jacobi, C., Hayward, C., de Zwaan, M., Kraemer, H. and Agras, W.S. (2004). Coming to terms with risk factors for eating disorders: application of risk terminology and suggestions for a general taxonomy. *Psychological Bulletin, 130*, 19-65.

Jacobi, C., Paul, Th., de Zwaan, M. Nutzinger, D.O. and Dahme, B. (2000). The specificity of self-concept disturbances in eating disorders. *International Journal of Eating Disorders, 5*, 204-210.

Jimerson, D.C., Lesem, D.T., Kaye, W.H., Brewerton, T.D. (1992). Low serotonin and dopamine metabolite concentrations in CSF from bulimic patients with frequent binge episodes. *Archives of General Psychiatry 49*, 132-138.

Jimerson, D.C., Mantzoros, C., Wolfe, B.E., Metzger, E.D. (2000). Decreased serum leptin in bulimia nervosa. *Journal of Clinical Endocrinology and Metabolism, 85*, 4511–4514.

Jimerson, D.C., Wolfe, B.E., Franko, D.L., Covino, N.A., Sifneos, P.E. (1994). Alexithymia ratings in bulimia nervosa: clinical correlates. *Psychosomatic Medicine, 56*, 90-93.

Jimerson, D. C., Wolfe, B. E., Metzger, E. D., Finkelstein, D. M., Cooper, T. B., and Levine, J.M. (1997). Decreased serotonin function in bulimia nervosa. *Archives of General Psychiatry, 54*, 529-534.

Johnson, J. G., Cohen, P., Kasen, S., and Brook, J. S. (2002). Childhood adversities associated with risk for eating disorders or weight problems during adolescence or early adulthood. *American Journal of Psychiatry, 159*, 394-400.

Johnson, C., Flach, A. (1985). Family characteristics of 105 patients with bulimia. *American Journal of Psychiatry, 142*, 1321-1324.

Johnson, C., Powers, P. S. and Dick, R. (1999). Athletes and eating disorders: The national collegiate athletic association study. *International Journal of Eating Disorders, 26*, 179-188.

Kaye, W.H., Ballenger, J.C., Lydiard, R.B., Stuart, G.W., Laraia, M.T., O'Neil, P., Fossey, M.D., Stevens, V., Lesser, S., Hsu, G. (1990). CSF monoamine levels in normal-weight bulimia: evidence for abnormal noradrenergic activity. *American Journal of Psychiatry, 147*, 225-229.

Kaye, W. H., Frank, G. K. W., Meltzer, C. C., Price, J. C., McConaha, C. W., Crossan, P. J., Klump, K. L., and Rhodes, L. (2001). Altered serotonin 2A receptor activity in women who have recovered from bulimia nervosa. *American Journal of Psychiatry, 158*, 1151-1154.

Kaye, W.H., Gendall, K.A., Strober, M. (1998). Serotonin neuronal function and selective reuptake inhibitor treatment in anorexia nervosa and bulimia nervosa. *Biological Psychiatry, 44*, 825-838.

Kaye, W. H., Greeno, C. G., Moss, H., Fernstrom, J., Fernstrom, M., Lilenfeld, L. R., Weltzin, T. E., and Mann, J. J. (1998). Alterations in serotonin activity and psychiatric symptoms after recovery from bulimia nervosa. *Archives of General Psychiatry, 55*, 927-935.

Kaye, W. H., Gendall, K. A., Fernstrom, M. H., Fernstrom, J. D., McConaha, C. W., and Weltzin, T. E. (2000). Effects of acute tryptophan depletion on mood in bulimia nervosa. *Biological Psychiatry, 47*, 151-157.

Kendler, K.S., Gardner, C.O., Prescott, C.A. (1998). A population-based twin study of self-esteem and gender. *Psychological Medicine, 28*, 1403-1409.

Kendler, K.S., MacLean, C., Neale, M., Kessler, R., Heath, A., Eaves, L. (1991). The genetic epidemiology of bulimia nervosa. *American Journal of Psychiatry, 148*, 1627-1637.

Kessler, R.C., Davis, C.G., Kendler, K.S. (1997). Childhood adversity and adult psychiatric disorder in the US National Comorbidity Survey. *Psychological Medicine, 27*, 1101-19.

Kessler, R.C., Sonnega, A., Bromet, E., Hughes, M., Nelson, C.B. (1995). Posttraumatic stress disorder in the National Comorbidity Survey. *Archives of General Psychiatry, 52*, 1048-60.

Keys, A., Brozek, J., Hentschel, A., Mickelsen, O., and Taylor, H. L. (1950). *The biology of human starvation*. Minneapolis: The University of Minnesota Press.

Killen, J.D. Hayward, C., Litt, I., Hammer, L.D., Wilson, D.M.,. Miner, B., Taylor, C.B., Varady, A., Shisslak, C. (1992). Is puberty a risk factor for eating disorders? *American Journal of Diseases of Children, 146,* 323-5, 1992

Killen, J.D., Taylor, C.B., Hayward, C., Haydel, K.F., Wilson, D.M., Hammer, L.D., Kraemer, H.C., Blair-Greiner, A., and Strachowski, D. (1996). Weight concerns influence the development of eating disorders: A 4-year prospective study. *Journal of Consulting and Clinical Psychology, 64*, 936-940.

Killen, J. D., Taylor, C. B., Hayward, C., Wilson, D. M., Haydel, K. F., Hammer, L. D., Simmonds, B., Robinson, T. N. Litt, I. Varady, A., and Kraemer, H. (1994). Pursuit of thinness and onset of eating disorder symptoms in a community sample of adolescent girls: A three year prospective analysis. *International Journal of Eating Disorders, 16*, 227-238.

Kleifield, E.I., Sunday, S., Hurt, S., Halmi, K.A. (1994). The Tridimensional Personality Questionnaire: an exploration of personality traits in eating disorders. *Journal of Psychiatric Research, 28*, 413-423.

Klump, K.L., Kaye, W.H., Strober, M. (2001). The evolving genetic foundations of eating disorders. *Psychiatric Clinics of North America, 24*, 215-225.

Klump, K.L., Strober, M., Bulik, C.M., Thornton, L., Johnson, C., Devlin, B., Fichter, M.M., Halmi, K.A., Kaplan, A.S., Woodside, D.B., Crow, S., Mitchell, J., Rotondo, A., Keel, P.K., Berrettini, W.H., Plotnicov, K., Pollice, C., Lilenfeld, L.R., Kaye, W.H. (2004). Personality characteristics of women before and after recovery from an eating disorder. *Psychological Medicine, 34,* 1407-1418.

Klump, K.L., Wonderlich, S., Lehoux, P., Lilenfeld, L.R., Bulik, C.M. (2002). Does environment matter? A review of nonshared environment and eating disorders. *International Journal of Eating Disorders, 31,* 118-135.

Lacey, J., Evans, C. (1986). The impulsivist: a multi-impulsive personality disorder. *British Journal of Addiction, 81,* 641-649.

Laliberte, M., Boland, F.J., Leichner, P. (1999). Family climates: family factors specific to disturbed eating and bulimia nervosa. *Journal of Clinical Psychology, 55*, 1021-1040.

Lilenfeld, L.R. (2004). Psychiatric comorbidity associated with anorexia nervosa, bulimia nervosa, and binge eating disorder. In Brewerton, T.D. (Ed.). *Clinical Handbook of Eating Disorders: An Integrated Approach.* New York: Marcel Dekker, Inc., pp. 183-207.

Lilenfeld, L.R., Kaye, W.H. (2004). Personality characteristics of women before and after recovery from an eating disorder. *Psychological Medicine, 34,* 1407-1418.

Kotler, L.A., Cohen, P., Davies, M., Pine, D.S., and Walsh, B.T. (2001). Longitudinal relationships between childhood, adolescent, and adult eating disorders. *Journal of the American Academy of Child and Adolescent Psychiatry, 40*, 1424-1440.

Le Grange, D., Telch, C.F., Tibbs, J. (1998). Eating attitudes and behaviors in 1435 South African Caucasian and non-Caucasian college students. *American Journal of Psychiatry, 155*, 250-254.

Leon, G. R., Fulkerson, J. A., Perry, C. L., and Early-Zald, M. B. (1995). Prospective analysis of personality and behavioral influences in the later development of disordered eating. *Journal of Abnormal Psychology, 104*, 140-149.

Leon, G. R., Fulkerson, J. A., Perry, C. L., Keel, P. K., and Klump, K. L. (1999). Three to four year prospective evaluation of personality and behavioral risk factors for later disordered eating in adolescent girls and boys. *Journal of Youth and Adolescence, 28*, 181-196.

Levine, M.P., Smolak, L. (2006). *The Prevention of Eating Problems and Eating Disorders: Theory, Research, and Practice*. Lawrence Erlbaum Associates, Inc.: Marwah, N.J.

Levitan, R.D., Kaplan A.S., Joffe R.T., Levitt, A.J., and Brown, G.M. (1997). Hormonal and subjective responses to intravenous meta-Chlorphenylpiperazine in bulimia nervosa. *Archives of General Psychiatry, 54*, 521-527.

Lewinsohn, P. M., Hops, H., Roberts, R. E., Seeley, J. R., and Andrews, J. A., (1993). Adolescent psychopathology: I. Prevalence and incidence of depression and other DSM-III-R disorders in high school students. *Journal of Abnormal Psychology, 102*, 133-144.

Lydiard, R.B., Brewerton, T.D., Beinfeld, M., Laraia, M.T., Stuart, G., Ballenger, J.C. (1993). CSF Cholecystokinin octapeptide in bulimia nervosa. *American Journal of Psychiatry, 150*, 1099-1101.

Maddocks, S.E., Kaplan, A.S. (1991). The prediction of treatment response in bulimia nervosa. A study of patient variables. *British Journal of Psychiatry, 159*, 846-849.archi, M., and Cohen, P. (1990). Early childhood eating behaviors and adolescent eating disorders. *Journal of the American Academy of Child and Adolescent Psychiatry, 29*, 112-117.

Mitchell, J. E., Hatsukami, D., Pyle, R. L., and Eckert, E. D. (1986). The bulimia syndrome: Course of the illness and associated problems. *Comprehensive Psychiatry, 27*, 165-170.

Mizushima, H., Ono, Y., Asai, M. (1998). TCI temperamental scores in bulimia nervosa patients and normal women with and without diet experiences. *Acta Psychiatrica Scandinavica, 98*, 228-230.

Molinari, E. (2001). Eating disorders and sexual abuse. Eating *and Weight Disorders: EWD, 6*, 68-80.

Monteleone, P., Brambilla, F., Bortolotti, F., Ferraro, C., and Maj, M. (1998a). Plasma prolactin response to D-fenfluramine is blunted in bulimic patients with frequent binge episodes. *Psychological Medicine, 28*, 975-983.

Monteleone, P., Brambilla, F., Bortolotti, F., and Maj, M. (2000). Serotonergic dysfunction across the eating disorders: relationship to eating behaviour, nutritional status and general psychopathology. *Psychological Medicine, 30*, 1099-1110.

Monteleone, P., Bortolotti, F., Fabrazzo, M., La Rocca, A., Fuschino, A., Maj, M. (2000). Plasma leptin response to acute fasting and refeeding in untreated women with bulimia nervosa. *Journal of Clinical Endocrinology and Metabolism, 85*, 2499–2503.

Mulder, R.T., Joyce, P.R., Sullivan, P.F., Bulik, C.M., Carter, F.A. (1999). The relationship among three models of personality psychopathology: DSM-III-R personality disorder, TCI scores and DSQ defenses. *Psychological Medicine, 29*, 943-951.

Murray, C., Waller, G. (2002). Reported sexual abuse and bulimic psychopathology among nonclinical women: the mediating role of shame. *International Journal of Eating Disorders, 32*, 186-191.

Mussell, M. P., Mitchell, J. E., Fenna, C. J., Crosby, R. D., Miller, J. P., and Hoberman, H. M. (1997). A comparison of onset of binge eating versus dieting in the development of bulimia nervosa. *International Journal of Eating Disorders, 21*, 353-360.

Nielsen, S. (1990). The epidemiology of anorexia nervosa in Denmark from 1973 to 1987: A nationwide register study of psychiatric admission. *Acta Psychiatrica Scandinavia, 81*, 507-514.

Ohzeki, T., Hanaki, K., Motozumi, H., Ishitani, N., Matsuda-Ohtahara, H., Sunaguchi, M., and Shiraki, K. (1990). Prevalence of obesity, leanness and anorexia nervosa in Japanese boys and girls aged 12-14 years. *Annals of Nutrition and Metabolism, 34*, 208-212.

Okon, D.M., Greene, A.L., Smith, J.E. (2003). Family interactions predict intraindividual symptom variation for adolescents with bulimia. *International Journal of Eating Disorders, 34,* 450-457.

Oldman, A., Walsh, A., Salkovskis, P., Fairburn, C. G., and Cowen, P. J. (1995). Biochemical and behavioural effects of acute tryptophan depletion in abstinent bulimic subjects: a pilot study. *Psychological Medicine, 25*, 995-1001.

O'Mahony, J.F., Hollwey, S. (1995). The correlates of binge eating in two nonpatient samples. *Addictive Behaviors, 20*, 471–480.

Patton, G. C., Johnson-Sabine, E., Wood, K., Mann, A. H., and Wakeling, A. (1990). *Psychological Medicine, 20*, 383-394.

Patton, G. C., Selzer, R., Coffey, C., Carlin, J. B., and Wolfe, R. (1999). Onset of adolescent eating disorders: population based cohort study over 3 years. *British Medical Journal, 318*, 765-768.

Polivy, J., and Herman, P. C. (1985). Dieting and bingeing. A causal analysis. *American Psychologist, 40*, 193-201.

Pumariega, A.J., Gustavson, C.R., Gustavson, J.C., Motes, P.S., Ayers, S. (1994). Eating attitudes in African-American women: The Essence Eating Disorders Survey. *Eating Disorders*, 2, 5-16.

Pyle, R.L., Mitchell, M.D., and Eckert, E.D. (1981). Bulimia: A report of 34 cases. *Journal of Clinical Psychiatry, 42*, 60-64.

Raffi, A. R., Rondini, M., Grandi, S., and Fava, G. A. (2000). Life events and prodromal symptoms in bulimia nervosa. *Psychological Medicine, 30*, 727-731.

Rodriguez, M., Perez, V., Garcia, Y. (2005). Impact of traumatic experiences and violent acts upon response to treatment of a sample of Colombian women with eating disorders. *International Journal of Eating Disorders, 37*, 299-306.

Rorty, M., Yager, J., Buckwalter, J.G., Rossotto, E. (1999). Social support, social adjustment, and recovery status in bulimia nervosa. *International Journal of Eating Disorders, 26*, 1–12.

Ruderman A. J. (1986). Dietary restraint: A theoretical and empirical review. *Psychological Bulletin, 99*, 247-262.

Russell, G. F. (1979). Bulimia nervosa: An ominous variant of anorexia nervosa. *Psychological Medicine, 9*, 429-448.

Schmeck, K., Poustka, F. (2001). Temperament and disruptive behavior disorders. *Psychopathology, 34*, 159-163.

Schmidt, U., Slone, G., Tiller, J., Treasure, J. (1993). Childhood adversity and adult defense style in eating disorder patients--a controlled study. *British Journal of Medical Psychology, 66*, 353-362.

Schmidt, U., Tiller, J., Blanchard, M., Andrews, B., and Treasure, J. (1997). Is there a specific trauma precipitating anorexia nervosa? *Psychological Medicine, 27*, 523-530.

Schotte, D. E., and Stunkard, A.J., (1987). Bulimia vs. bulimic behaviors on a college campus. *Journal of the American Medical Association, 258*, 1213-1215.

Smith, K. A., Fairburn, C. G., and Cowen, P. J. (1999). Symptomatic relapse in bulimia nervosa following acute tryptophan depletion. *Archives of General Psychiatry, 56*, 171-176.

Smith, J.E., Krejci, J. (1991). Minorities join the majority: eating disturbances among Hispanic and Native American youth. *International Journal of Eating Disorders, 10*, 179-186.

Smolak, L., Murnen, S.K. (2002). A meta-analytic examination of the relationship between child sexual abuse and eating disorders. *International Journal of Eating Disorders, 31*, 136-150.

Smolak, L., Murnen, S.K. (2004). A feminist approach to eating disorders. In Thompson, J.K., (Ed.). *Handbook of Eating Disorders and Obesity*. Hoboken, N.J., John Wiley and Sons, Inc., pp. 590-605.

Steiger, H., Bruce, K.R. (2007). Phenotypes, endophenotypes, and genotypes in bulimia spectrum eating disorders. *Canadian Journal of Psychiatry - Revue Canadienne de Psychiatrie, 52*, 220-227.

Steiger, H., Gauvin, L., Israel, M., Koerner, N., Ng Ying Kin, N. M. K., Paris, J., and Young, S.N. (2001a). Association of serotonin and cortisol indices with childhood abuse in bulimia nervosa. *Archives of General Psychiatry, 58*, 837-843.

Steiger, H., Gauvin, L., Joober, R., Israel, M., Ng Ying Kin, N.M., Bruce, K.R., Richardson, J., Young, S.N., Hakim, J. (2006). Intrafamilial correspondences on platelet [3H-]paroxetine-binding indices in bulimic probands and their unaffected first-degree relatives. *Neuropsychopharmacology, 31*, 1785-1792.

Steiger, H., Koerner, N., Engelberg, M. J., Israel, M., Ng Ying Kin, N. M. K., and Young, S. N. (2001b). Self-destructiveness and serotonin function in bulimia nervosa. *Psychiatry Research, 103*, 15-26.

Steiger, H., Young, S. N., Ng Ying Kin, N. M. K., Koerner, N., Israel, M., Lageix, P., and Paris, J. (2001c). Implications of impulsive and affective symptoms for serotonin function in bulimia nervosa. *Psychological Medicine, 31*, 85-95.

Steiger, H., Richardson, J., Israel, M., Ng Ying Kin, N.M., Bruce, K., Mansour, S., Marie Parent, A. (2005). Reduced density of platelet-binding sites for [3H]paroxetine in remitted bulimic women. *Neuropsychopharmacology, 30*, 1028-1032.

Stice, E., Maxfield, J., and Wells, T. (2003). Adverse effects of social pressure to be thin on young women: an experimental investigation of the effects of "fat talk". *International Journal of Eating Disorders, 34,* 108-117

Striegel-Moore, R., Smolak, L. (1996). The role of race in the development of eating disorders. In L. Smolak, M. P. Levine, and R. Striegel-Moore (Eds.), *The Developmental*

Psychopathology of Eating Disorders. 259-284. Mahwah, NJ: Lawrence Erlbaum Associates.

Strober, M., Freeman, R., Lampert, C., Diamond, J., Kaye, W. (2000). Controlled family study of anorexia nervosa and bulimia nervosa: evidence of shared liability and transmission of partial syndromes. *American Journal of Psychiatry, 157*, 393-401.

Sundgot-Borgen, J. (1994). Risk and trigger factors for the development of eating disorders in female elite athletes. *Medicine and Science in Sports and Exercise, 26*, 414-419.

Tanaka, M., Naruo, T., Muranaga, T., Yasuhara, D., Shiiya, T., Nakazato, M., Matsukura, S., Nozoe, S. (2002). Increased fasting plasma ghrelin levels in patients with bulimia nervosa. *European Journal of Endocrinology, 146*, R1–R3.

Tiller, J.M., Sloane, G., Schmidt, U., Troop, N., Power, M., Treasure, J.L. (1997). Social support in patients with anorexia nervosa and bulimia nervosa. *International Journal of Eating Disorders, 21*, 31–38.

Tomotake, M., Ohmori, T. (2002). Personality profiles in patients with eating disorders. *Journal of Medical Investigation, 49*, 87-96.

Treasure, J., Holland, A. (1989). Genetic vulnerabiltiy to eating disorders: evidence from twin and family studies. In Remschmidt, H., and Schmidt, M.H. (Eds.), *Child and Youth Psychiatry: European Perspectives*. New York: Hogrefe and Huber, pp. 59-68.

Troop, N.A., Holbrey, A., Trowler, R., Treasure, J.L. (1994). Ways of coping in women with eating disorders. *Journal of Nervous and Mental Disorders, 182*, 535–540.

Troop, N. A., Treasure, J. L. (1997). Psychosocial factors in the onset of eating disorders: Responses to life events and difficulties. *British Journal of Medical Psychology, 70*, 373-385.

Tuschen-Caffier, B., Vogele, C. (1999). Psychological and physiological reactivity to stress: an experimental study on bulimic patients, restrained eaters and controls. *Psychotherapy and Psychosomatics, 68*, 333–340.

Tuschl, R. J. (1990). From dietary restraint to binge eating: Some theoretical considerations. *Appetite, 14*, 105-109.

Vervaet, M., van Heeringen, C., Audenaert, K. (2004), Personality-related characteristics in restricting versus binging and purging eating disordered patients. *Comprehensive Psychiatry, 45*, 37-43,

Vollrath, M., Koch, R., Angst, J. (1992). Binge eating and weight concerns among young adults. Results from the Zurich Cohort Study. *British Journal of Psychiatry, 160*, 498-503.

Wade, T.D., Bergin, J.L., Martin, N.G., Gillespie, N.A., Fairburn, C.G. (2006). A transdiagnostic approach to understanding eating disorders. *Journal of Nervous and Mental Disease, 194*, 510-517.

Wade, T.D., Bulik, C.M., Prescott, C.A., Kendler, K.S. (2004). Sex influences on shared risk factors for bulimia nervosa and other psychiatric disorders. *Archives of General Psychiatry, 61*, 251-256.

Waller, G. (1998). Perceived control in eating disorders: relationship with reported sexual abuse. *International Journal of Eating Disorders, 23*, 213-216.

Waller, G., Meyer, C., Ohanian, V., Elliott, P., Dickson, C., Sellings, J. (2001). The psychopathology of bulimic women who report childhood sexual abuse: the mediating role of core beliefs. *Journal of Nervous and Mental Disorders, 189*, 700-708.

Walters, E. E., and Kendler, K. S. (1995). Anorexia nervosa and anorexic-like syndromes in a population-based female twin sample. *American Journal of Psychiatry, 152*, 64-71.

Webster, J. J., and Palmer, R. L. (2000). The childhood and family background of women with clinical eating disorders: a comparison with women with major depression and women without psychiatric disorder. *Psychological Medicine, 30*, 53-60.

Welch, S. L., Doll, H. A., and Fairburn, C. G. (1997). Life events and the onset of bulimia nervosa: A controlled study. *Psychological Medicine, 27*, 515-522.

Weltzin, T. E., Fernstrom, M. H., Fernstrom, J. D., Neuberger, S. K., and Kaye, W. H. (1995). Acute tryptophan depletion and increased food intake and irritability in bulimia nervosa. *American Journal of Psychiatry, 152*, 1668-1671.

Weltzin, T. E., Fernstrom, J. D., McConaha, C., and Kaye, W. H. (1994). Acute tryptophan depletion in bulimia: effects on large neutral amino acids. *Biological Psychiatry, 35*, 388-397.

Whitaker, A.H., Johnson, J., Shaffer, D., Rapoport, J. L., Kalikow, K., Walsh, B. T, Davies, M., Braiman, S., Dolinsky, A. (1990). Uncommon troubles in young people: Prevalence estimates of selected psychiatric disorders in a nonreferred adolescent population. *Archives of General Psychiatry, 47*, 487-496.

Wonderlich, S.A., Brewerton, T.D., Jocic, Z., Dansky, B.S., Abbott, D.W. (1997). The relationship of childhood sexual abuse and eating disorders: a review. *Journal of the American Academy of Child and Adolescent Psychiatry, 36*, 1107-1115.

Wonderlich, S., Crosby, R., Mitchell, J., Thompson, K., Redlin, J., Demuth, G., Smyth, J. (2001). Pathways mediating sexual abuse and eating disturbance in children. *International Journal of Eating Disorders, 29*, 270-279.

Wonderlich, S.A., Crosby, R.D., Mitchell, J.E., Thompson, K.M., Redlin, J., Demuth, G., Smyth, J., Haseltine, B. (2001). Eating disturbance and sexual trauma in childhood and adulthood. *International Journal of Eating Disorders, 30*, 401-412

Woodside, D. B. and Garfinkel, P. (1992). Age of onset in eating disorders. *International Journal of Eating Disorders, 12*, 31-36.

In: Evidence-Based Treatments for Eating Disorders   ISBN 978-1-60692-310-8
Author: Ida F. Dancyger and Victor M. Fornari   © 2009 Nova Science Publishers, Inc.

Chapter III

Overview of Evidence on the Underpinnings of Binge Eating Disorder and Obesity

Massimo Cuzzolaro[1] and Giuseppe Vetrone[2]
[1] University of Rome Sapienza, Roma, Italy
[2] University of Rome Tor Vergata, Roma, Italy

Abstract

Binge eating disorder (BED) is the most distinct subgroup in the diagnostic category of eating disorders not otherwise specified (EDNOS) and it is already accepted as an eating disorder (ED) in actual practice. However, it is not yet an approved DSM (Diagnostic and Statistical Manual of Mental Disorders) or ICD (International Classification of Diseases) diagnosis. Patients with both obesity and BED face many tasks: controlling their eating patterns and acquiring beneficial lifestyle changes, promoting and maintaining weight loss, improving their physical and psychological health and their quality of life. BED may benefit from specialized interventions, either psychosocial or pharmacological, in addition to standard behavioral weight control treatment. BED treatment programs have attempted to address these goals sequentially or in combination; they usually reduce binge eating, at least in the short term, but weight loss is insufficient or absent in most cases. After a brief account of current knowledge on epidemiology of BED, we will discuss in detail the nosological status of this possible new diagnostic category and its diagnostic criteria.

Introduction

The concept of binge eating disorder (BED) was introduced in the early 1990s (Spitzer, 1991). This symptom cluster presentation was formally recognized as a possible new diagnostic category only in 1994, in the fourth edition of the Diagnostic and Statistical Manual of Mental Disorders (DSM-IV) (American Psychiatric Association, 1994).

We enumerate three milestones that led to the proposal that BED should be added to the current list of mental disorders:

I. The first description of recurrent compulsive overeating as a clinical phenomenon probably dates back to 1932 (Stunkard, 1990; Wulff, 1932; Wulff, 2001) but the expression "binge eating" was coined half a century ago by Hyman Cohen (Stunkard, 1959). In the late 1950s the American psychiatrist Albert Stunkard (Stunkard, 2002; Stunkard, 1959) proposed the name of "binge-eating syndrome" for a possible new diagnostic category.

II. In 1979 the British psychiatrist Gerald Russell proposed naming "bulimia nervosa" (BN) a syndrome which he considered an "ominous variant" of anorexia nervosa (AN) (Russell, 1979). People with BN suffer from frequent binge eating attacks , regular compensatory behaviors, and morbid fear of fatness. Most of them maintain their weight within the normal range.

III. In the last two decades, clinicians increasingly reported on women and men who, engaged in recurrent binge eating but without the regular compensatory behaviors that characterize bulimia nervosa; most of these patients were overweight or obese. On the basis of these observations Spitzer and colleagues advanced the proposal of BED as a new diagnostic category (Spitzer, 1991; Spitzer, Devlin, Walsh, et al., 1992; Spitzer, Yanovski, Wadden, et al., 1993) and DSM-IV agreed with the suggestion.

We are now aware that binge eating as a symptom crosses the entire field of eating disorders (ED) and the whole spectrum of body weights (Fairburn and Wilson, 1993; Russell, 1997). However, BED is the name of a syndrome that in the DSM-IV and in the DSM-IV-TR (Text Revision) is defined as follows: "recurrent episodes of binge eating in the absence of the regular use of inappropriate compensatory behaviors characteristic of bulimia nervosa" (American Psychiatric Association, 1994; American Psychiatric Association, 2000). In the DSM-IV-TR, BED is proposed as an example of an eating disorder not otherwise specified (EDNOS) category. In addition, it is included in Appendix B (possible new diagnostic categories requiring further study). The Eating Disorders Work Group of the DSM-IV task force in conjunction with Spitzer and colleagues (1992) developed the provisional diagnostic criteria for BED on the basis of those for BN (American Psychiatric Association, 2000). No comparable diagnostic category related to BED exists in the tenth edition of the WHO International Classification of Diseases (ICD-10) (World Health Organization, 1992). The ICD-10 diagnosis for individuals who present with the clinical picture of BED may be Atypical Bulimia Nervosa (code number F50.3) or Eating Disorder, unspecified (code number F50.9) (World Health Organization, 1993). The DSM is one of the possible methods of classification of mental disorders but, since the publication of its third edition (1980), the taxonomy proposed by the American Psychiatric Association (APA) has become dominant. This event has probably contributed to the acceptance of the diagnostic category of BED.

BED has connected the psychiatric field of EDs with the medical area of obesity. The bridge drew more attention to the psychological and psychiatric aspects of obesity and contributed to the development of a multidimensional team approach to the assessment and treatment of eating and weight disorders. According to many handbooks and practice guidelines this approach appears now as the best therapeutic model for ED and obesity (American Psychiatric Association, 2006; Basdevant and Guy-Grand, 2004; Bosello, 2008; Fairburn and Brownell, 2002; Goldstein, 2005; Grilo, 2006; Lau, Douketis, Morrison, *et al*, 2007; Mitchell, Devlin, de Zwaan, et al., 2008; National Heart Lung and Blood Institute, (NHLBI), North American Association for the Study of Obesity, *et al*, 2000; National Institute for Clinical Excellence, 2004 January; Palmer and Norring, 2005; Wadden and Stunkard, 2002; Yager and Powers, 2007).

Although the conceptual issues and the diagnostic criteria of BED have not yet met sufficient agreement: in actual practice, BED is already accepted as an ED, and an increasing number of scientific articles have been devoted to it since 1991. Figure 1 illustrates the findings.

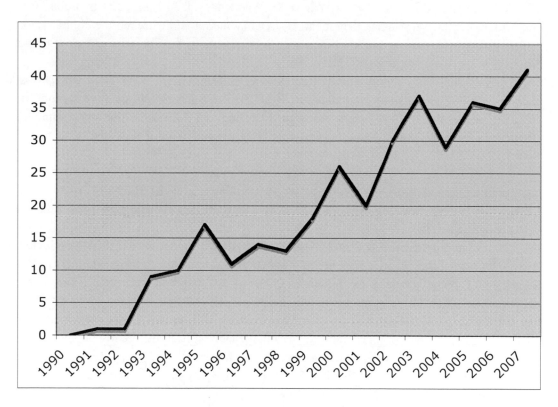

Figure 1. Number of PubMed references (1990-2007) that contain in the title the expression binge eating disorder (BED).

Epidemiological Research

Epidemiological research on BED has at least three major limitations: diagnostic status is recent, provisional and uncertain; many studies have assessed the disorder by self-report questionnaires rather than semi-structured clinical interviews; community-based investigations have examined samples of convenience rather than representative samples. For example, there is significant discrepancy in prevalence rates of BED as defined by self-report and interview assessment methods, with the interview method yielding lower estimates of prevalence (Varnado, Williamson, Bentz, et al., 1997).

Prevalence – International

BED seems to be significantly more prevalent than AN or BN, and is also almost as prevalent in males as in females. This is certainly in contrast to the sex ratio of females to males of 10:1 in AN. Studies based on community samples have indicated prevalence rates between 0.7 and 4 % (Striegel-Moore and Franko, 2003). According to Spitzer (Spitzer, Devlin, Walsh, et al., 1992; Spitzer, Yanovski, Wadden, et al., 1993), BED is probably 1.5 times more common in women than men. All EDs, including BED, are more common among white women than among black women with low treatment rates in both groups (Striegel-Moore, Dohm, Kraemer, et al, 2003).

The National Comorbidity Survey Replication (Hudson, Hiripi, Pope, et al., 2007) was a face-to-face household study, conducted in 2001-2003 in a large representative sample (n = 9282). The results of this recent research indicated the following lifetime community prevalence rates of DSM-IV-BED in USA: 3.5% in women and 2.0% in men; F to M ratio was 1.75 to 1.0.

An Italian three-phase community-based study evaluated 2,355 subjects representative of the population aged >14 years living in Sesto Fiorentino (Faravelli, Ravaldi, Truglia, et al., 2006). The authors found an overall lifetime prevalence of BED considerably lower than the American rate: 0.32%.

Lamerz and colleagues (Lamerz, Kuepper-Nybelen, Bruning, et al., 2005) conducted a cross-sectional survey in a German urban population of 6-year-old children and their parents. Episodes of binge eating were found in 2.0% of the children surveyed. There was a significant relationship between binge eating and obesity, but not between night eating and the child's weight. Furthermore, children's binge eating was strongly associated with eating disturbances on the part of their mothers. BED may manifest itself differently in children than adults. Shapiro and colleagues (Shapiro, Woolson, Hamer, et al., 2007) recently developed the Children's Binge Eating Disorder Scale (C-BEDS), a brief, structured, interviewer-administered scale to measure BED in children.

BED and Obesity: The Chicken or the Egg?

BED may especially be observed in overweight and obese individuals, and in Hudson et al.'s research (Hudson, Hiripi, Pope, et al., 2007), lifetime BED was significantly associated with current obesity class III (body mass index, BMI $\geq$ 40 kg/m^2). BED is much more frequent among treatment seeking obese subjects: up to 30% of participants in weight loss programs meet DSM-IV-TR criteria for BED. In France, for example, Basdevant et al. (Basdevant, Pouillon, Lahlou, et al., 1995) concluded that BED was very common (15%) in women seeking help for weight control, but extremely rare in a community sample of women (0.7%).

Subjects with obesity and BED, in an effort to feel better about themselves, often have become trapped in a cycle of attempting to diet, then losing control, binge eating, and gaining even more weight (Devlin, 2001; Polivy, 2001). However, it remains unclear which comes first: bingeing or dieting?

Some authors consider dieting as a precondition for the development of binge eating (Herman and Polivy, 1980; Herman and Polivy, 1990). It was recently suggested that a distinction between intention to restrict food intake and actual restrictive behavior may be useful to predict changes in overeating and BMI (Larsen, van Strien, Eisinga, et al., 2007).

Reas and Grilo examined a sample of 284 treatment-seeking adults with BED and found that weight problems preceded dieting and binge eating behaviors for a majority of patients (Reas and Grilo, 2007). In addition, proportionally more women than men reported that dieting preceded overweight or binge eating.

BED and Diabetes

There is a significant relationship between BED and type 2 diabetes.

A German multi-center study (Herpertz, Albus, Wagener, et al., 1998) explored the prevalence of ED (full and partial syndromes) in an inpatient and outpatient population of men and women with type 1 and type 2 diabetes. The overall prevalence range of current ED was 5.9-8.0% (lifetime prevalence 10.3-14.0%) without significant difference between the two types. However, the distribution of the EDs was different, with a predominance of BED in the type 2 diabetes sample. Patients with type 1 (5.9%) and type 2 (2.2%) diabetes, reported deliberate omission of insulin or oral agents in order to lose weight. In this research, BED seems to precede type 2 diabetes in most patients, and could be one of the causes of their obesity.

According to Herpertz and colleagues, BED is likely a risk factor for an accelerated weight gain, which often involves an increase of insulin resistance (Herpertz, Petrak, Kruse, et al., 2006).

BED and Psychiatric Comorbidity

BED is usually accompanied by co-morbid psychiatric disorders, especially depression, anxiety disorders, and substance abuse disorders (Guerdjikova, McElroy, Kotwal, et al., 2007; Stunkard, 2002; Stunkard and Allison, 2003; Wilfley, Friedman, Dounchis, et a.l, 2000). Hudson et al.'s study recently confirmed that lifetime BED is significantly associated with other psychopathology and role impairment (Hudson, Hiripi, Pope, et al., 2007).

Nosological Status of BED

May BED be Conceptualized as a Separate Syndrome?

BED is the most distinct EDNOS subgroup, however, it is currently not a diagnosis approved in either DSM or ICD. According to the current DSM-IV-TR definition, BED is characterized by repeated episodes of uncontrolled eating with excessive food intake and subjective distress but without subsequent compensatory weight loss mechanisms. The question remains, does BED represent a really separate diagnostic entity? In other words, is the concept of BED a reliable and valid diagnosis? We will report on some relevant studies that address this question.

In 1999 Williamson and Martin reviewed the first five years of research on BED and concluded that questions about the definition of BED remained (Williamson and Martin, 1999). The authors reported that binge eating is a common symptom associated with obesity. They also posited that BED may be conceptualized as a separate psychiatric syndrome, or it may be viewed as a behavioral symptom associated with obesity in a large number of cases.

Other researches supported the distinction between BED and BN. In 2000, Fairburn et al., published a paper on the relative course and outcome of BN and BED (Fairburn, Cooper, Doll, et al., 2000). They prospectively studied over a five-year period, two community-based cohorts of women, one with BN and the other with BED. BN and BED showed different courses of illness, with little movement of participants across the two diagnostic categories. The outcome of the BED cohort was better. Crow et al. examined a large sample of 385 women with full or partial AN, BN, or BED (Crow, Stewart Agras, Halmi, et al., 2002). Discriminant analysis demonstrated clear differences between full AN, BN, and BED, and this supported the distinction between BED and the other EDs.

However, Fichter et al. (Fichter, Quadflieg and Hedlund, 2008) recently found that course, outcome and mortality were similar for BED and BN-P with a diagnostic shift between them over time, "pointing to their nosological proximity".

In 2003, Devlin et al. (Devlin, Goldfein and Dobrow, 2003) evaluated four models relating to the nosological status of BED: a distinct disorder in itself; a variant of BN; a behavioral subtype of obesity; and a behavior that reflects psychopathology among the individuals with obesity (a psychopathological marker). According to the evidence, the authors wrote that BED "differs importantly from purging BN" but not from non-purging BN, and that BED "is not a strikingly useful behavioral subtype of obesity" because obese individuals with BED do not differ greatly from similar obese patients without BED in their response to obesity treatment. They concluded that it was not possible to determine the validity of BED as a distinct ED.

Stunkard, who originally described binge eating (Stunkard, 1959), defended with Allison a similar point of view in a thought-provoking article (Stunkard and Allison, 2003): the great variability of BED limits the implications that can be drawn from its diagnosis and, in particular, the presence or absence of BED is not a useful distinction in selecting treatment for obese individuals. BED may be more useful as "a marker of psychopathology" than as a new distinct diagnostic entity.

Walsh and Satir reviewing the literature published during the period 2002-2003 concluded that "a consensus does not yet appear to have formed in the field regarding the wisdom of formally designating BED as an eating disorder" (Walsh and Satir, 2005). Dingemans et al. (Dingemans, van Hanswijck de Jonge and van Furth, 2005) discussed the empirical status of BED after a decade of research in the light of Pincus et al.'s (Pincus, Frances, Davis, et al., 1992) general arguments for and against the inclusion of new diagnostic categories in the DSM. Unlike Walsh and Satir they concluded that "... there is evidence to suggest that BED represents a distinct eating disorder category" (p. 76).

More recently, Wilfley and colleagues, (Wilfley, Bishop, Wilson, *et al*, 2007) and Striegel-Moore and Franko (Striegel-Moore and Franko, 2008) supported the same point of view: BED should be made an official diagnosis in DSM-V.

It is probable that DSM-V will move some boundary lines in the section of ED. In particular, BN non-purging subtype (BN-NP) and BED give the impression of clinical pictures very close together. In 1998, Hay and Fairburn published the results of an interesting study designed to assess the validity of the DSM-IV classification of recurrent binge eating (Hay and Fairburn, 1998). They recruited a general population sample of 250 young women with recurrent binge eating and studied their eating habits and associated psychopathology by personal interviews. Subjects were reassessed one year later. The authors found that, on present state features, it was not possible to distinguish BED from the non-purging subtype of bulimia nervosa. However, these groups differed in their outcome at one year. Hay and Fairburn concluded that "the data on outcome support retaining a distinction between non-purging bulimia nervosa and binge eating disorder". In their opinion, bulimic eating disorders exist on a continuum of clinical severity, from BN purging type (most severe), through BN non-purging type (intermediate severity), to BED (least severe).

Other authors (Mond, Hay, Rodgers, et al., 2006), however, called into question the validity of subtyping of BN into purging and non-purging forms. In the opinion of Ramacciotti et al. (Ramacciotti, Coli, Paoli, et al., 2005) differences between BED and BN-NP seem to be more of degree than type and there seems little value in the separation between BED and BN-NP based on weight-shape concerns that substantially impair self-esteem. This construct seems core to both disorders and plays a substantial role in triggering and maintaining the binge-eating cycle.

Wilfley et al. (Wilfley, Bishop, Wilson, et al., 2007), in evaluating the current ED nosology on the basis of the available scientific evidence, concluded that in DSM-V it would be better to remove the subtypes both for AN and for BN. They also suggested that ED classification should be modified in DSM-V by retaining categories but adding a dimensional component.

Concerning this subject, let us mention that EDs have been conceptualized as discrete syndromes (or categories) and as dimensions that differ in degree among individuals. Schlundt and Johnson proposed in 1990 a three-dimensional model for ED: binge eating, fear of fatness, and body size (Schlundt and Johnson, 1990). Four years later, Beumont et al. suggested a unitary approach to ED diagnosis and proposed a slightly different three-dimensional model: binge eating, purging, and body size (Beumont, Garner and Touyz, 1994). However, which of these two models, categorical versus dimensional, is most valid?

Do the current classifications of EDs capture the natural clustering of eating-related pathology?

Some recent studies have directly and empirically addressed these questions.

Bulik et al. examined 2163 Caucasian female twins from a population-based registry (Virginia Twin Registry) and assessed bulimic and anorectic symptoms through personal interviews (Bulik, Sullivan and Kendler, 2000). The authors applied latent class analysis to nine symptoms of EDs; then they used demographic, personality, co-morbidity, and co-twin diagnosis data to validate the resultant classes and found three classes which largely correspond to the current diagnostic categories of AN, BN and BED. In particular, individuals in the three ED classes displayed differences in co-twin risk for AN, BN, and obesity.

Also Williamson et al. investigated "the question of whether the EDs vary along dimensions, with normalcy defining one end of the continuum, or whether the EDs are discrete categories" (Williamson, Womble, Smeets, et al., 2002). They explored the latent structure of ED symptoms, as defined by DSM-IV, in a group of 341 women with and without an ED diagnosis. The presence and severity of DSM-IV ED symptoms was assessed with a semi-structured interview and the data were subjected to a factor analysis. The results suggested that EDs may be conceptualized as having three primary features: binge eating, fear of fatness/compensatory behaviors, and drive for thinness. In addition, women with an ED diagnosis differed (at least partly) from women without an ED diagnosis "in kind rather than simply in degree". The three factors identified were then examined using taxometric analyses (statistical procedures used to discover whether the three factors varied along a continuum or detected the presence of latent classes). Taxometric tests found empirical support for conceptualizing BN and BED as discrete syndromes.

Williamson et al. recently reviewed a series of taxometric studies related to the validity of dimensional versus categorical models of ED and concluded that a conceptual representation of ED may involve at least a latent taxon (a taxon is any distinct group constituting a category within a system of classification), related to binge eating (and possibly purging), and one or more dimensions (Williamson, Gleaves and Stewart, 2005).

In summary, at this time, we suggest that more studies are required with large samples to empirically sort out which differences among the various EDs are qualitative and which differences are only quantitative (dimensional).

Does BED Represent a Stable Syndrome?

A number of studies and, in particular, those on the fate of untreated subjects and those on placebo responsiveness have raised concern about the diagnostic stability of BED and the question is still controversial (Stunkard, 2002).

Fairburn et al., studied prospectively a community based cohort over a five-year period and found that only 10% of subjects with BED at the beginning of the survey met criteria for this diagnosis five years later. The authors wrote that BED "is an unstable state with a strong tendency toward spontaneous remission" (Fairburn, Cooper, Doll, et al., 2000).

In contrast, Pope et al., in their retrospective research, found that BED is at least as chronic as AN and BN (Pope, Lalonde, Pindyck, et al., 2006). They interviewed 888 first-degree relatives of 300 overweight or obese probands (150 with BED and 150 with no lifetime ED) and discovered that the mean lifetime duration of illness among relatives with lifetime diagnoses of BED (N=131) was 14.4 years (SD=13.9). In the opinion of the authors, these results suggest that BED likely represents a stable syndrome.

Jacobs-Pilipski et al. studied sibutramine hydrochloride in a randomized controlled trial that included 451 participants (ages 19-63) with BED (Jacobs-Pilipski, Wilfley, Crow, et al., 2007). The investigators found that placebo responders (32.6%) exhibited significantly less symptom severity but, at follow-up, many of them reported continued symptoms. Therefore, placebo response in BED may be transitory or incomplete and the results seem to imply unpredictable stability in the BED diagnosis.

Diagnostic Criteria for BED

Should We Maintain DSM-IV Research Criteria for BED?

Diagnostic criteria are in a permanent state of revision and in the area of mental disorders they probably should be regarded as useful concepts and guidelines rather than as separate entities. In the last fifteen years, several authors have raised doubts about the DSM-IV research criteria for BED.

Criterion A (recurrent episodes of binge eating), in the opinion of Dingemans et al., "as currently defined should be maintained" (Dingemans, van Hanswijck de Jonge and van Furth, 2005). However, difficulties with diagnosis may arise from the precise identification of binge eating episodes in obese people. Three remarks may illustrate this point. The phenomenon of binge eating is described in DSM-IV-TR in the same way for BED and BN. Nevertheless, there are some differences (Wilfley, Schwartz, Spurrell, et al., 2000): for example, in BN, binge eating episodes usually happen in the context of overall dietary restraint and are easily identifiable, whereas, in most cases of BED, they occur in the background of habitual overeating and chaotic eating patterns. Raymond et al. recently compared energy intake in obese women with and without BED when they were allowed to have a binge eating episode in a laboratory setting (Raymond, Bartholome, Lee, et al, 2007). The BED obese group consumed significantly more total food in kilocalories (but not significantly more total grams of food) than the non-BED obese participants. Furthermore, the BED group consumed more dairy products and, in general, more kilocalories of fat. Bartholome et al. (Bartholome, Raymond, Lee, et al., 2006) evaluated multiple methods of assessing food intake in obese women with BED: laboratory binge eating episodes, 24-hour dietary recalls, and the Eating Disorder Examination (EDE) interview. The findings suggested only moderate agreement among these different methods.

With regard to criterion B (features associated with the binge-eating episodes) we agree with Dingemans et al.(Dingemans, van Hanswijck de Jonge and van Furth, 2005) who wrote that it is superfluous because it overlaps A and C criteria.

According to the same authors, criterion C (marked distress) should be revised to distinguish distress as an emotional state from distress as impairment in social or occupational functioning (Dingemans, van Hanswijck de Jonge and van Furth, 2005).

In the present form, criterion D (binge eating occurs at least two days a week for six months) may complicate the distinction between binge eating (acute and circumscribed attack with manifest loss of control) and compulsive overeating (urge to eat that may last an entire day). Therefore Dingemans et al. suggested "counting the number of binge-eating episodes rather than counting the number of days" (Dingemans, van Hanswijck de Jonge and van Furth, 2005).

Moreover, according to some researchers, it would be better to change the severity criterion and to move the boundary line between full-syndrome BED and sub-threshold BED (STBED). Striegel-Moore et al. (2000) compared 44 women with STBED and 44 women with BED and 44 healthy controls. The two ED groups did not differ significantly on measures of weight and shape concern, restraint, psychiatric distress, and history of seeking treatment for an eating or weight problem. The authors concluded that, given the importance of diagnostic status for access to treatment, the severity criterion specified for BED should be revised (Striegel-Moore, Dohm, Solomon, *et al*, 2000).

Also Crow and colleagues, in a study of 385 women with full or partial (sub-threshold) ED found that full and partial BED appear quite similar (Crow, Stewart Agras, Halmi, *et al*, 2002).

More recently, Friederich et al. compared eating-related and general psychopathology at baseline and in response to a multimodal treatment program in obese people with full syndrome BED, and STBED. They did not find differences between STBED and BED participants with regard to eating-related and general psychopathology at baseline and with regard to treatment outcome and concluded that a differentiation currently seems not to be of clinical significance (Friederich, Schild, Wild, et al., 2007).

We thus agree with Wilfley et al. who included among their specific recommendations for DSM-V, "unifying the frequency and duration cut-points for BN and BED to once per week for three months" (Wilfley, Bishop, Wilson, et al., 2007).

Criterion E (no regular use of inappropriate compensatory behaviors) tolerates unsafe compensatory behaviors on condition that they are infrequent (not "regular"). The elimination of the term "regular" may ensure a clearer distinction between BN and BED (Dingemans, van Hanswijck de Jonge and van Furth, 2005) but, on the other hand, this choice may increase the cumbersome residual category of EDNOS that is the most common diagnosis in clinical practice (Palmer and Norring, 2005).

Should New Diagnostic Criteria be Added for BED in DSM-V?

Body Image

The twentieth century has seen in Western countries, possible constant links between ED and body image disturbances (Habermas, 1989; Janet, 1903; Wulff, 1932). Unlike AN and

BN, current diagnostic criteria for BED focus completely on eating behavior and feelings about binge eating and do not include body image distortion and/or distress.

At this time, many studies have shown that obese individuals with BED present greater uneasiness and dissatisfaction about their body appearance, weight and shape than obese people without BED.

Marano et al. (Marano, Cuzzolaro, Vetrone, et al, 2007) recently investigated the psychometric properties of the Body Uneasiness Test (BUT) (Cuzzolaro, Vetrone, Marano, et al., 2006) in 1,812 adult subjects (18-65 years) with obesity seeking treatment, and evaluated the influence of gender, age and BMI on body image distress. Concurrent validity with Binge Eating Scale (BES) (Gormally, Black, Daston, et al., 1982) was evaluated, and the positive correlation between BUT and BES scores appears noteworthy.

Wilfley et al. (Wilfley, Schwartz, Spurrell, et al., 2000) compared five groups of women: patients with ED (AN, BN and BED), normal-weight and overweight control subjects. They found that patients with BED had weight and shape concerns comparable to BN patients and higher than AN patients.

More recently, Hrabosky et al. studied the excessive influence of shape or weight on self-evaluation (shape/weight overvaluation) in 399 consecutive patients with BED (Hrabosky and Grilo, 2007). Results showed that shape/weight overvaluation was unrelated to BMI but was strongly associated with psychometric measures of eating-related psychopathology and psychological functioning (higher depression and lower self-esteem). The authors concluded that shape/weight overvaluation "warrants consideration as a diagnostic feature for BED".

Some authors have compared males and females and have found that there are predictable gender differences. Reas et al. (Reas, White and Grilo, 2006) found that obese women with BED reported significantly greater levels of body checking than obese men with BED. Among women, the frequency of checking was related to younger age, lower BMI, body dissatisfaction, over evaluation of body shape and weight, greater depression, and lower self-esteem.

These sex related differences support Guerdjikova et al.'s results (Guerdjikova, McElroy, Kotwal, et al., 2007). The authors compared 44 obese males with BED with 44 age- and race-matched obese females with BED seeking weight loss treatment. They found that obese men and women with BED who presented for weight management were very similar in current and lifetime prevalence of psychiatric disorders, and metabolic abnormalities, but males had fewer previous attempts at weight loss or fewer help-seeking behaviors, possibly related to their less pronounced body dissatisfaction.

Obesity

Another matter of primary importance is the relationship between BED and obesity. In DSM-IV-TR obesity is not a criterion for the diagnosis of BED. Should obesity be included as a criterion for BED in DSM-V in the same way as underweight is a criterion for the diagnosis of AN? This question is still outstanding (Dingemans, van Hanswijck de Jonge and van Furth, 2005).

With regard to the nosological status of obesity, it is important to remember that this condition has traditionally been defined as a body-mass index (BMI) (the weight in kilograms divided by the square of the height in meters) of 30 or more kg/m^2. Excessive weight increases morbidity (e.g., hypertension, hyperlipidemia, cardiovascular disease, type 2 diabetes mellitus, numerous types of cancer, gallstones, and osteoarthritis) and the risk of death. For these reasons obesity has traditionally been classified among medical diseases.

However, Wooley and Garner's provocative statements appear still truthful: "Although millions seek treatments for obesity ... the majority of the obese struggle in vain to lose weight and blame themselves for relapses ... Many therapists may be contributing to this psychological damage by giving their patients false hope for success and by failing to recognize that seeking treatment for obesity may be triggered by psychological problems that are not addressed in obesity treatment" (Wooley and Garner, 1991). Furthermore, guidelines for the assessment, treatment and prevention of obesity and public health recommendations urge a focus not only on the degree of overweight and the obesity related medical complications; but also on lifestyle, eating behavior, motivation, social stigma, and mental health (Brownell, Puhl, Schwartz, et al., 2005; Herpertz, Kielmann, Wolf, et al., 2003; Lau, Douketis, Morrison, et al., 2007; Mitchell and de Zwaan, 2005; Mitchell, Devlin, de Zwaan, et al., 2008; National Heart Lung and Blood Institute, (NHLBI), North American Association for the Study of Obesity, et al, 2000; National Institutes of Health, 1998; World Health Organization, 2000).

On the other hand, considering obesity, or some aspect of obesity, as a mental (or behavioral) disorder has some merits but also raises many problems. In 2007 Devlin wondered if there is a place for obesity in DSM-V (Devlin, 2007). He divided into three groups the possible models of nonhomeostastic overeating that result in obesity: eating disorder models that stress the *form* of overeating; substance use disorder models that focus on its *consequences*; and affect regulation or stress response models that consider especially its *function*. The author concluded that to devise diagnostic criteria based on the above models raises multiple difficulties because the phenomena central to each model are basically dimensional. A more detailed understanding of the neurobiological relationships among eating behavior, reward systems, and affect regulation systems is needed.

In summary we suggest that a negative body image and a BMI value > 25 should be added as diagnostic criteria for BED in a future classification of ED.

Conclusion

In spite of many uncertainties, the concept of BED has been of increasing interest in the last fifteen years to both researchers and clinicians. The close relationship of BED with obesity has made it a field of study which has deeply involved and connected psychiatry, clinical psychology and internal medicine.

Acknowledgement

In memory of Professor Giuseppe Vetrone.

References

American Psychiatric Association (1994). *Diagnostic and Statistical Manual of Mental Disorders, DSM-IV* (4th edn). Washington, DC: American Psychiatric Association.

American Psychiatric Association (2000). *Diagnostic and Statistical Manual of Mental Disorders, DSM-IV-TR* (4th, Text Revised edn). Washington, DC: American Psychiatric Association.

American Psychiatric Association (2006). Practice Guideline for the Treatment of Patients with Eating Disorders (Third Edition). *American Journal of Psychiatry*, 163 (July Supplement), 1-54.

Bartholome, L. T., Raymond, N. C., Lee, S. S., *et al* (2006). Detailed analysis of binges in obese women with binge eating disorder: Comparisons using multiple methods of data collection. *International Journal of Eating Disorders*, 39, 685-693.

Basdevant, A. and Guy-Grand, B. (eds) (2004). *Médecine de l'obésité*. Paris: Flammarion.

Basdevant, A., Pouillon, M., Lahlou, N., *et al* (1995). Prevalence of binge eating disorder in different populations of French women. *International Journal of Eating Disorders*, 18, 309-315.

Beumont, P. J., Garner, D. M. and Touyz, S. W. (1994). Diagnoses of eating or dieting disorders: what may we learn from past mistakes? *International Journal of Eating Disorders*, 16, 349-362.

Bosello, O. (ed) (2008). *Obesità. Un trattato multidimensionale. 2^ ed*. Milano: Kurtis.

Brownell, K., Puhl, R., Schwartz, M., *et al* (eds) (2005). *Weight bias. Nature, consequences and remedies*. New York: Guilford.

Bulik, C. M., Sullivan, P. F. and Kendler, K. S. (2000). An empirical study of the classification of eating disorders. *American Journal of Psychiatry*, 157, 886-895.

Crow, S. J., Stewart Agras, W., Halmi, K., *et al* (2002). Full syndromal versus subthreshold anorexia nervosa, bulimia nervosa, and binge eating disorder: a multicenter study. *International Journal of Eating Disorders*, 32, 309-318.

Cuzzolaro, M., Vetrone, G., Marano, G., *et al* (2006). The Body Uneasiness Test (BUT): development and validation of a new body image assessment scale. *Eating and Weight Disorders*, 11, 1-13.

Devlin, M. J. (2001). Binge-eating disorder and obesity. A combined treatment approach. *Psychiatric Clinics of North America*, 24, 325-335.

Devlin, M. J. (2007). Is there a place for obesity in DSM-V? *International Journal of Eating Disorders*, S83-S88.

Devlin, M. J., Goldfein, J. A. and Dobrow, I. (2003). What is this thing called BED? Current status of binge eating disorder nosology. *International Journal of Eating Disorders*, 34 Suppl, S2-18.

Dingemans, A., van Hanswijck de Jonge, P. and van Furth, E. (2005). The empirical status of binge eating disorder. In *EDNOS, eating disorders not otherwise specified: clinical perspectives on the other eating disorders* (eds C. Norring and B. Palmer), pp. 63-82. Hove: Routledge.

Fairburn, C. and Brownell, K. (eds) (2002). *Eating Disorders and Obesity. A Comprehensive Handbook* (Second Edition edn). New York: Guilford.

Fairburn, C. G., Cooper, Z., Doll, H. A., *et al* (2000). The natural course of bulimia nervosa and binge eating disorder in young women. *Archives of General Psychiatry*, 57, 659-665.

Fairburn, C. G. and Wilson, G. T. (1993). Binge Eating: Definition and classification. In *Binge Eating. Nature Assessment and Treatment* (eds C. G. Fairburn and G. T. Wilson), pp. 3-14. New York: The Guilford Press.

Faravelli, C., Ravaldi, C., Truglia, E., *et al* (2006). Clinical epidemiology of eating disorders: results from the Sesto Fiorentino study. *Psychotherapy and Psychosomatics*, 75, 376-383.

Fichter, M. M., Quadflieg, N. and Hedlund, S. (2008). Long-term course of binge eating disorder and bulimia nervosa: Relevance for nosology and diagnostic criteria. *International Journal of Eating Disorders*, in press (published online: 12 May 2008).

Friederich, H. C., Schild, S., Wild, B., *et al* (2007). Treatment outcome in people with subthreshold compared with full-syndrome binge eating disorder. *Obesity (Silver Spring)*, 15, 283-287.

Goldstein, D. (ed) (2005). *The Management of Eating Disorders and Obesity. 2nd edition.* Totowa, NJ: Humana Press.

Gormally, J., Black, S., Daston, S., *et al* (1982). The assessment of binge eating severity among obese persons. *Addictive Behaviors*, 7, 47-55.

Grilo, C. (ed) (2006) *Eating and weight disorders.*

Guerdjikova, A. I., McElroy, S. L., Kotwal, R., *et al* (2007). Comparison of obese men and women with binge eating disorder seeking weight management. *Eating and Weight Disorders*, 12, e19-23.

Habermas, T. (1989). The psychiatric history of anorexia nervosa and bulimia nervosa: weight concerns and bulimic symptoms in early case reports. *International Journal of Eating Disorders*, 8, 259-273.

Hay, P. and Fairburn, C. (1998). The validity of the DSM-IV scheme for classifying bulimic eating disorders. *International Journal of Eating Disorders*, 23, 7-15.

Herman, C. P. and Polivy, J. (1980). Restrained eating. In *Obesity* (ed A. J. Stunkard), pp. 208-225. Philadelphia: Saunders.

Herman, C. P. and Polivy, J. (1990). From dietary restraint to binge eating: attaching causes to effects. *Appetite*, 14, 123-125; discussion 142-123.

Herpertz, S., Albus, C., Wagener, R., *et al* (1998). Comorbidity of diabetes and eating disorders. Does diabetes control reflect disturbed eating behavior? *Diabetes Care*, 21, 1110-1116.

Herpertz, S., Kielmann, R., Wolf, A. M., *et al* (2003). Does obesity surgery improve psychosocial functioning? A systematic review. *International Journal of Obesity and Related Metabolic Disorders,* 27, 1300-1314.

Herpertz, S., Petrak, F., Kruse, J., *et al* (2006). Eating disorders and diabetes mellitus. *Therapeutische Umschau*, 63, 515-519.

Hrabosky, J. I. and Grilo, C. M. (2007). Body image and eating disordered behavior in a community sample of Black and Hispanic women. *Eating Behaviors*, 8, 106-114.

Hudson, J. I., Hiripi, E., Pope, H. G., Jr., *et al* (2007). The prevalence and correlates of eating disorders in the National Comorbidity Survey Replication. *Biological Psychiatry*, 61, 348-358.

Jacobs-Pilipski, M. J., Wilfley, D. E., Crow, S. J., *et al* (2007). Placebo response in binge eating disorder. *International Journal of Eating Disorders*, 40, 204-211.

Janet, P. (1903). *Les obsessions et la psychasthénie: Vol 1, Section 5. L'obsession de la honte du corps*. Paris: Germer-Baillière.

Lamerz, A., Kuepper-Nybelen, J., Bruning, N., *et al* (2005). Prevalence of obesity, binge eating, and night eating in a cross-sectional field survey of 6-year-old children and their parents in a German urban population. *Journal of Child Psychology and Psychiatry*, 46, 385-393.

Larsen, J. K., van Strien, T., Eisinga, R., *et al* (2007). Dietary restraint: intention versus behavior to restrict food intake. *Appetite*, 49, 100-108.

Lau, D. C., Douketis, J. D., Morrison, K. M., *et al* (2007). 2006 Canadian clinical practice guidelines on the management and prevention of obesity in adults and children [summary]. *CMAJ: Canadian Medical Association Journal*, 176, S1-13.

Marano, G., Cuzzolaro, M., Vetrone, G., *et al* (2007). Validating the Body Uneasiness Test (BUT) in obese patients. *Eating and Weight Disorders*, 12, 70-82.

Mitchell, J. and de Zwaan, M. (eds) (2005). *Bariatric surgery. A guide for mental health professionals*. New York: Routledge.

Mitchell, J., Devlin, M., de Zwaan, M., *et al* (2008). *Binge eating disorder. Clinical foundations and treatment*. New York: Guilford.

Mond, J. J., Hay, P. J., Rodgers, B., *et al* (2006). Correlates of the use of purging and non-purging methods of weight control in a community sample of women. *Australian and New Zealand Journal of Psychiatry*, 40, 136-142.

National Heart Lung and Blood Institute, (NHLBI), North American Association for the Study of Obesity*, et al* (2000). *Practical Guide to the identification, evaluation and treatment of overweight and obesity in adults*. Bethesda: National Institutes of Health.

National Institute for Clinical Excellence (2004 January). Eating disorders: Core interventions in the treatment and management of anorexia nervosa, bulimia nervosa and related eating disorders. *Clinical Guideline 9. http://www.nice.org.uk/CG009NICEguideline*.

National Institutes of Health (1998). Clinical guidelines on the identification, evaluation and treatment of overweight and obesity in adults. The evidence report. *Obesity Research*, 6 Suppl 2, 51S-209S.

Palmer, B. and Norring, C. (2005). EDNOS - The other eating disorders. In *EDNOS, eating disorders not otherwise specified: clinical perspectives on the other eating disorders* (eds C. Norring and B. Palmer), pp. 1-9. Hove: Routledge.

Pincus, H. A., Frances, A., Davis, W. W., *et al* (1992). DSM-IV and new diagnostic categories: holding the line on proliferation. *American Journal of Psychiatry*, 149, 112-117.

Polivy, J. (2001) The false hope syndrome: unrealistic expectations of self-change. *International Journal of Obesity and Related Metabolic Disorders*, 25 Suppl 1, S80-84.

Pope, H. G., Jr., Lalonde, J. K., Pindyck, L. J., *et al* (2006). Binge eating disorder: a stable syndrome. *American Journal of Psychiatry*, 163, 2181-2183.

Ramacciotti, C. E., Coli, E., Paoli, R., *et al* (2005). The relationship between binge eating disorder and non-purging bulimia nervosa. *Eating and Weight Disorders*, 10, 8-12.

Raymond, N. C., Bartholome, L. T., Lee, S. S., *et al* (2007). A comparison of energy intake and food selection during laboratory binge eating episodes in obese women with and without a binge eating disorder diagnosis. *International Journal of Eating Disorders*, 40, 67-71.

Reas, D. L. and Grilo, C. M. (2007). Timing and sequence of the onset of overweight, dieting, and binge eating in overweight patients with binge eating disorder. *International Journal of Eating Disorders*, 40, 165-170.

Reas, D. L., White, M. A. and Grilo, C. M. (2006). Body Checking Questionnaire: psychometric properties and clinical correlates in obese men and women with binge eating disorder. *International Journal of Eating Disorders*, 39, 326-331.

Russell, G. (1979). Bulimia nervosa: an ominous variant of anorexia nervosa. *Psychological Medicine*, 9, 429-448.

Russell, G. (1997) The history of bulimia nervosa. In *Handbook of Treatment for Eating Disorders* (eds D. M. Garner and P. E. Garfinkel), pp. 11-24. New York: Guilford.

Schlundt, D. and Johnson, W. (1990). *Eating disorders: assessment and treatment*. Boston: Allyn and Bacon.

Shapiro, J. R., Woolson, S. L., Hamer, R. M., *et al* (2007). Evaluating binge eating disorder in children: development of the children's binge eating disorder scale (C-BEDS). *International Journal of Eating Disorders*, 40, 82-89.

Spitzer, R. L. (1991). Nonpurging bulimia nervosa and binge eating disorder. *American Journal of Psychiatry*, 148, 1097-1098.

Spitzer, R. L., Devlin, M., Walsh, B. T., *et al* (1992). Binge eating disorder: A multisite field trial of the diagnostic criteria. *International Journal of Eating Disorders*, 11, 191-203.

Spitzer, R. L., Yanovski, S., Wadden, T., *et al* (1993). Binge eating disorder: its further validation in a multisite study. *International Journal of Eating Disorders*, 13, 137-153.

Striegel-Moore, R. H., Dohm, F. A., Kraemer, H. C., *et al* (2003). Eating disorders in white and black women. *American Journal of Psychiatry*, 160, 1326-1331.

Striegel-Moore, R. H., Dohm, F. A., Solomon, E. E., *et al* (2000). Subthreshold binge eating disorder. *International Journal of Eating Disorders*, 27, 270-278.

Striegel-Moore, R. H. and Franko, D. L. (2003). Epidemiology of binge eating disorder. *International Journal of Eating Disorders*, 34 Suppl, S19-29.

Striegel-Moore, R. H. and Franko, D. L. (2008). Should binge eating disorder be included in the DSM-V? A critical review of the state of the evidence. *Annual Review of Clinical Psychology*, 4, 305-324.

Stunkard, A. (1990). A description of eating disorders in 1932. *American Journal of Psychiatry*, 147, 263-268.

Stunkard, A. (2002). Binge eating disorder and the night-eating syndrome. In *Handbook of obesity treatment* (eds T. Wadden and A. Stunkard), pp. 107-121. New York: Guilford.

Stunkard, A. J. (1959). Eating patterns and obesity. *Psychiatry Quarterly*, 33, 284-295.

Stunkard, A. J. and Allison, K. C. (2003). Binge eating disorder: disorder or marker? *International Journal of Eating Disorders*, 34 Suppl, S107-116.

Varnado, P., Williamson, D., Bentz, B., *et al* (1997). Prevalence of binge eating disorder in obese adults seeking weight loss treatment. *Eating and Weight Disorders*, 2, 117-124.

Wadden, T. and Stunkard, A. (eds) (2002). *Handbook of obesity treatment*. New York: Guilford.

Walsh, B. and Satir, D. (2005). Classification of eating disorders 2002-2003. In *Eating Disorders Review. Part 1* (eds S. Wonderlich, J. Mitchell, M. de Zwaan, *et al*), pp. 155-163. Oxford: Radcliffe.

Wilfley, D. E., Bishop, M. E., Wilson, G. T., *et al* (2007). Classification of eating disorders: Toward DSM-V. *International Journal of Eating Disorders*, 40 Suppl, S123-129.

Wilfley, D. E., Friedman, M. A., Dounchis, J. Z., *et al* (2000). Comorbid psychopathology in binge eating disorder: relation to eating disorder severity at baseline and following treatment. *Journal of Consulting and Clinical Psychology*, 68, 641-649.

Wilfley, D. E., Schwartz, M. B., Spurrell, E. B., *et al* (2000). Using the eating disorder examination to identify the specific psychopathology of binge eating disorder. *International Journal of Eating Disorders*, 27, 259-269.

Williamson, D. A., Gleaves, D. H. and Stewart, T. M. (2005). Categorical versus dimensional models of eating disorders: an examination of the evidence. *International Journal of Eating Disorders*, 37, 1-10.

Williamson, D. A. and Martin, C. K. (1999). Binge eating disorder: a review of the literature after publication of DSM-IV. *Eating and Weight Disorders*, 4, 103-114.

Williamson, D. A., Womble, L. G., Smeets, M. A., *et al* (2002). Latent structure of eating disorder symptoms: a factor analytic and taxometric investigation. *American Journal of Psychiatry*, 159, 412-418.

Wooley, S. C. and Garner, D. M. (1991). Obesity treatment: the high cost of false hope. *Journal of the American Dietetic Association*, 91, 1248-1251.

World Health Organization (1992). *The ICD-10 Classification of Mental and Behavioural Disorders. Clinical descriptions and diagnostic guidelines*. Geneva: World Health Organization.

World Health Organization (1993). *The ICD-10 Classification of Mental and Behavioural Disorders. Diagnostic Criteria for Research (ICD-10: DCR-10)*. Geneva: World Health Organization.

World Health Organization (2000). *Obesity: preventing and managing the global epidemic: report of WHO consultation*. Geneva: World Health Organ Tech Rep Ser.

Wulff, M. (1932). Über einen interessanten oralen Symptomen-Komplex und seine Beziehung zur Sucht. *Internationale Zeitschrift für Psychoanalyse*, 18, 281-302.

Wulff, M. (2001). Su un interessante complesso sintomatico orale e sui suoi nessi con la tossicomania (versione italiana a cura di G. Binni e M. Cuzzolaro di: Über einen

interessanten oralen Symptomen-Komplex und seine Beziehung zur Sucht, Internationale
Zeitschrift für Psychoanalyse, 18, 281-302, 1932). *Psicobiettivo*, 21, 73-88.

Yager, J. and Powers, P. (eds) (2007). *Clinical manual of eating disorders*. Washington, DC:
American Psychiatric Publishing.

In: Evidence-Based Treatments for Eating Disorders
Author: Ida F. Dancyger and Victor M. Fornari

ISBN 978-1-60692-310-8
© 2009 Nova Science Publishers, Inc.

Chapter IV

Research and Clinical Practice: A Dynamic Tension in the Eating Disorder Field

Judith D. Banker[1] and Kelly L. Klump[2]
[1] Center for Eating Disorders
Ann Arbor, Michigan
[2] Michigan State University
East Lansing, Michigan

Abstract

Recent research suggests that there is a "research-practice gap" in the field of eating disorders, as evidenced by discrepancies between the rate at which research results are produced and the rate at which the results are utilized in practice. Reasons for the gap, however, remain unclear. Even more uncertain are strategies that can be used to bridge this gap. Consequently, the purpose of the present chapter was to: 1) explore factors underlying the persistent research-practice gap in the eating disorders field; and 2) develop a "road map" for closing the gap. Data from an informal survey of members of the Academy for Eating Disorders were used to answer both questions. In addition, the learning and communication models of Innovation Diffusion Theory, Knowledge Transfer Theory, and the Evidence-Based Medicine movement were used to develop novel research-practice integration strategies for the eating disorders field. Findings from these data sources revealed that the primary reasons for the gap include an institutional, relational, and economically-driven separation between the research and practice communities; a perceived lack of generalizability of current empirically supported treatment (EST) research to clinical practice settings; the reliance on a one-directional research dissemination model of information transfer; and a lack of research translation training and education. To bridge the divide, it is recommended that the eating disorder field implement a long-range strategy, or road map, that fosters reciprocal communication and interaction between researchers and practitioners, institutional and organizational support of research-practice partnerships, and integration of interactive, rather than top-down, learning opportunities. Increased cross-talk and a respect for the value of research data and clinical observations will enhance efforts to close the research-gap and ultimately advance the treatment, research, and prevention of eating disorders.

It were not best that we should all think alike; it is difference of opinion that makes horse races.

– Mark Twain

Clinicians who treat people with eating disorders express frustration over pressure from researchers to provide empirically supported treatments (ESTs). Researchers scratch their heads over the seeming resistance of clinicians to stay current on the latest findings in research. Clinicians feel their expertise is dismissed by researchers; researchers feel their expertise is met with indifference from clinicians. We are witnessing, in the field of eating disorders, the classic research-practice gap, a long-standing phenomenon spanning fields as varied as medicine, engineering, education, public health, and even geography and library science. Indeed, a quick Google search of "research-practice gap" yielded over 17,000 hits, highlighting the universality of the gap in fields with both an applied and basic science component.

The phrase "research-practice gap" is frequently used to describe a research dissemination gap, i.e., the discrepancy between the rate at which research results are produced and the rate at which the results are utilized (Fain, 2003; Demaerschalk, 2004). Within this framework, solutions for bridging the gap focus on ways to enhance dissemination from a top-down or one-way knowledge transfer perspective (Haddow and Klobas, 2003; Schecter and Brunner, 2005). However, other references to the research-practice gap describe a broader, multivariate tension between researchers and practitioners that arises from a complicated array of factors, such as communication barriers (i.e., lack of shared language), economic and political influences, professional culture differences and "blindspots", and ineffective educational strategies (Robinson, 1998; Herle and Martin, 2002; McConnell, 2002; Botvin, 2004). It is into this latter group that we squarely place the research-practice gap in the field of eating disorders--where all of the above factors converge to create a rather sizeable "Bermuda Triangle", where valuable research findings disappear into the abyss along with the vital observations, techniques, and insights of experienced clinicians.

The debate surrounding the use of empirically supported treatments (ESTs) is perhaps the most glaring example of the gap that exists between research and practice in our field. Despite empirical support for the use of cognitive behavior therapy (CBT) in the treatment of eating disorders, in particular bulimia nervosa, research consistently shows that few clinicians use CBT as their primary treatment approach (Wilson, 1998; Crow et al., 1999; Mussell et al., 2000; Haas and Clopton, 2003; Von Ranson and Robinson, 2006; Tobin, Banker, Weisberg, and Bowers, 2007). Previous attempts to increase dissemination of ESTs have focused on the publication of treatment manuals (Agras and Apple, 1997; Lock, le Grange, Agras, and Dare, 2001; Fairburn, Marcus, and Wilson, 1993), conference workshops on treatment methods, and treatment plenary lectures. Nonetheless, despite best efforts, these strategies have generally failed, as the majority of clinicians do not use ESTs (Mussel et al., 2000).

The failure of these attempts to increase the utilization of ESTs prompted discussion at a recent international eating disorders research meeting that focused on how to improve our methods of research dissemination. One suggestion was to deliver the message about the importance of ESTs in a clearer way during joint meetings with practitioners. Clarifying and honing the message may be constructive. However, before refining previously ineffective methods and perhaps exacerbating the tension in the field, it seems ideal to take a step back and evaluate the utility of this one-directional approach, and to explore other frameworks for addressing research dissemination and the broader research-practice connection. Clearly, our field, our patients, and their families, would be significantly better off if the clinicians and researchers who are most invested in identifying effective treatments developed ways to interface around these critical issues. In fact, it is possible that while we are busy debating the best ways to disseminate ESTs, the adapted practices in the field may be as or even more effective than ESTs alone. Or maybe not. In any case, bridging the gap between research and practice by promoting a synthesis of research and clinical evidence could translate into significant breakthroughs for our patients and our treatment, research, and prevention efforts. With so much at stake, it is imperative that we, as a field, take stock of the factors that feed the tension between researchers and practitioners and start identifying strategies for constructing a much-needed bridge between these critical groups.

In this chapter, we hope to accomplish both of these goals by examining "data" from both within and outside of our field. The data from within the field come from a decidedly unscientific survey we conducted of the membership of the Academy for Eating Disorders (AED) asking them to comment on reasons for the gap and ways to overcome it. We will describe these "data" and the ways in which they can help us move forward in this age-old debate. In addition, we will use "data" from the education field, and principles from knowledge transfer, diffusion innovation theory, and the evidence-based practice (EBP) movement to propose a road map for bridging the schism between researchers and practitioners in the eating disorders field. We will end by discussing activities of the AED Research-Practice Task Force, a work group formed specifically to address the gap in our field.

The AED Survey

We start by looking within our own field to identify where and why tensions exist. We do this by capitalizing on our affiliations with the AED. As an international, multidisciplinary professional organization comprised of research scientists, clinicians, and various hybrids thereof, the AED has seen the research-practice gap played out in its own membership. Clinicians at times reported that they felt marginalized and unsupported, and researchers expressed frustration over the underutilization of empirical data. Professionally, we are representatives or even prototypes of these estranged groups. Kelly Klump is the 2007-2008 AED President and is a tenured faculty member at a major research university. She does not treat patients. Judith Banker was the 2008-2009 AED President and is a clinician and the founding director of an outpatient treatment center. She has only recently ventured into the world of conducting formal research. We decided to build on the differences in our roles within the AED and investigate the causes for, and possible solutions to, the research-practice gap in our field. Instead of carrying out the usual review of the empirical literature, we chose to do our own analysis by conducting an informal survey of our AED colleagues. This survey was humbly unscientific; however, it provided us with information on why the gap persists in our field, despite a long-standing literature on the topic (Arnow, 1999; Fairburn, 2005; Wilson, 1998).

The "research" questions were straightforward:

1) There appears to be a researcher-clinician gap in our field. What do you think is the main cause of this gap?
2) What is one step we can take to close the gap?

We emailed these questions to 32 AED colleagues from North America, Europe, Australia, and the U.K., half of whom do both research and clinical work. Of the half remaining, one quarter was strictly clinical practitioners and one quarter was strictly researchers. The response to our survey was overwhelming. We received all of the responses within one week. More importantly, the responses were uniformly thoughtful and united in their concern about this issue and about the importance to our field of finding effective ways to bridge the gap.

We reviewed these responses for common themes, but also for important differences that likely underscore the persistent gap. These commonalities and specific points of departure are delineated below, but we feel that we must make a "process" comment before proceeding. With few exceptions, the tone of the responses differed between researchers and clinicians. Clinicians clearly felt "under attack", as their responses included references to "a faith-based assault against clinicians" and the view that they are perceived as "unscientific charlatans". By contrast, the tone of responses from researchers was not of feeling attacked, but instead reflected a feeling of resignation and a bit of hopelessness that the gap could be closed.

What should we make of these differences in tone? We think they reflect the *perceived* power differential between clinicians and researchers and the tendency for researchers to be more commonly at the podium espousing the need for clinicians to change (rather than the reverse). Clinicians understandably feel attacked by this, while researchers feel hopeless, as the researchers' data fail to translate into new clinical practices. All of this points to a need to change our dialogue – change how it takes place, where it takes place, and the nature of the interchange. We will return to ideas about this change later. However, suffice it to say that the feelings about the gap and the history between "camps" runs deep and affects how we think and talk about the differences in our field.

Question #1: What Accounts for the Gap?

Commonalities

At least one structural obstacle to achieving optimal clinician-researcher collaboration was cited with startling uniformity: a lack of time and resources. This was the most frequent response for researchers and a common response for clinicians. Researchers noted that providing clinical care is not valued or rewarded at their academic institutions where publishing and grant funding are the standards by which they are evaluated. Likewise, researchers and clinicians acknowledged that clinicians neither have the time nor the resources to stay abreast of research in their practice where demands from managed care and/or other clinical pressures take precedence. The lack of funding for studies that involve clinician-researcher collaborations, as well as limited funding for translating research findings into practice, were also noted. Finally, clinicians pointed out several resource-based obstacles, including the lack of funding for long-term supervision for training in ESTs and time and financial constraints that tend to lower motivation to apply research to practice.

In addition to a lack of resources, clinicians and researchers perceived the differential "evidence" for good practice as key to the persisting gap. Respondents noted that researchers value data from randomized controlled trials (RCTs), whereas clinicians value clinical data from professional experience and observation. These different views about what is considered "evidence" were perceived as contributing to each side devaluing and "talking down" to the other rather than leading to an appreciation of the reasons why each side values different data. The perception of practitioners that research lacks relevance to clinical practice is a commonly cited factor contributing to a tension between research and practice in our field.

A final common finding of the survey focused on training. Researchers and clinicians both felt that they had received inadequate training to engage in integrated clinical-research activities. Respondents felt that researchers were not trained in how to disseminate research findings effectively and translate them into practice. Likewise, respondents felt that clinicians were not adequately trained in how to interpret and apply empirical data to their work. Deficits in each of these areas were thought to contribute to a resistance to change and a rigid either/or mentality that inhibits the integration of clinical and empirical data.

Differences

Aside from these commonalities, there were also some striking differences in clinician and researcher responses. While researchers overwhelmingly viewed a lack of resources and the differences in "evidence" as the primary obstacles to clinical-research collaboration, clinicians cited many more issues that needed to be addressed. This difference in the number and type of factors viewed as causative underscores our earlier comments about the differential experience of the gap in these two groups.

A number of clinicians reported feeling that the gap was due to a perception that most research findings are irrelevant for the realities of clinical practice. Respondents reported that exhortations from researchers to practice evidence-based treatment in the face of limited effectiveness for all eating disorder patients (e.g., for those with anorexia nervosa and/or extensive co-morbidity) leads to significant frustration and a sense of disconnect from the usefulness of empirical data. Clinicians reported that it is often necessary to blend a variety of treatment modalities in order to adapt to the shifting symptom picture and multiple disorders they encounter in their patients; yet, clinicians felt that few empirical guidelines exist for adapting ESTs to "real life" treatment and for changing course when ESTs are ineffective. Importantly, one researcher agreed with these responses, saying that researchers must do a better job of demonstrating generalizability of research findings to standard clinic populations. Likewise, two additional researchers felt that most eating disorders research lacks clinical relevance, as, in their view, the research focuses on issues that have little-to-no bearing on day-to-day practice.

Question #2: What can we do to close the gap?

Fortunately, the responses to this question were almost wholly uniform! First and foremost, our respondents believed that promoting institutional and organizational support for clinician-researcher interaction and collaboration is key to bridging the research-practice gap. Many suggestions centered on creating forums for open and honest discussions between clinicians and researchers. The most commonly cited venue for such discussions was the AED annual international conference. Both researchers and clinicians alike called for a stronger fusion of clinical and research data at these conferences, where ideally, presenters of empirical data would discuss clinical applications. Perhaps more importantly, respondents reported a strong desire for a greater prominence of purely clinical presentations at professional meetings. Finally, there was a desire for smaller, informal group discussions where professionals could discuss the "evidence" they value, the reasons for their opinions, and the ways in which the different forms of evidence inform, rather than contradict, each other. This coming together of the "minds" (aptly described by one clinician as a "researcher-clinician rapprochement") on the same playing field would serve to mitigate any perceived power differential or implied value placed on one type of evidence over another.

In addition to broadening the appeal of conferences, respondents felt that it would be useful to have regular clinical commentaries on empirical data in scientific journals (e.g., the *International Journal of Eating Disorders*) and professional newsletters (e.g., the AED *Forum*). Respondents also called for a need to lobby for funding for clinician-researcher collaborations and for translating research into patient care. Many felt that changes at the level of academic institutions or managed care would only occur if there were funding opportunities available for exploring clinical-research collaborations.

Respondents also felt that improvements in training could close the gap. Suggestions in this area included: 1) encouraging the inclusion of evidence-based interventions in clinician training to impart an appreciation for, rather than suspicion of, research; 2) changing training expectations by creating and encouraging "clinician investigator" job profiles rather than "clinician" OR "investigator" profiles; 3) providing refresher research design and statistics courses at conferences; and 4) teaching scientists to think like clinicians and vice versa.

Finally, clinicians made several suggestions for ways to increase the clinical relevance of research including testing treatments in randomized controlled trials (RCTs) and in "real life" treatment settings. Clinicians also stressed the importance of studying what clinicians do in their treatments rather than simply expecting clinicians to do what researchers study.

Developing a Road Map

It is clear from the responses of our survey that the dynamic tension between researchers and clinicians in the field of eating disorders is a multilayered, complex interaction of structural, institutional, relational and systemic factors. These "data" appear to strongly corroborate empirical findings, both within and outside of our field. Within our field, investigators have found that clinicians who treat individuals with eating disorders prefer to make treatment decisions based on their clinical experience rather than on the empirical literature (Haas and Clopton, 2003; Mussell et al., 2000; Von Ranson , 2005). Reasons cited for this include; a lack of a research emphasis in graduate training, a lack of EST training opportunities, inconsistency between ESTs and the clinician's preferred clinical approach, and the view that ESTs are not flexible enough to meet the treatment demands of patients typically seen in clinical practice (i.e., those with extensive co-morbidity, complex social histories, etc.). Overall, these findings are remarkably similar to the impressions of our AED colleagues described above.

These same tensions have been observed in other fields. For example, in software engineering, the underutilization of research findings in applied practice is reportedly due to: 1) an overemphasis on technology that lacks generalizability to applied settings; 2) a research focus that is too specialized and not interdisciplinary or problem-focused; and 3) a lack of incorporation of state-of-practice engineering into empirical research (Abrial, 2005). A similar situation exists in education, where empirically supported programs are not routinely implemented in schools because of a lack of training and support for teachers, competing demands for staff, limited resources (e.g., time, financial resources), and a failure of the programs to apply to the student populations they serve (Donovan, Brandsford, and Pellegrino, 2007). Thus, the research-practice divide, and reasons underlying the divide, appear to be universal phenomena. This means that effective strategies for overcoming the gap are unlikely to be specific to the eating disorders field, but will instead need to be broad-based efforts aimed at addressing core features underlying applied-research divides in all fields.

Fortunately, there are fields that are ahead of us in addressing these issues from whom we can borrow to develop our own road map. Three in particular, the education, organizational development, and medicine fields, offer theoretical models that seem especially relevant: Innovation Diffusion Theory, Knowledge Transfer Theory, and Evidence-Based Medicine.

Innovation Diffusion Theory

A number of fields (including education) have incorporated principles from innovation diffusion theory into their research-practice integration strategies. For the purposes of our discussion, we will cull the literature on these approaches down to core tenets.

Innovation diffusion, outlined in Everett Rogers' classic work *The Diffusion of Innovations* (1995), is the "process by which an innovation (an idea or practice perceived to be new) is communicated through certain channels over a period of time among the members of a social system." The communication in this process is based on *mutual exchange and understanding* between all stakeholders within a given system or culture. Innovation diffusion theorists stress that didactic, lecture-based presentations and lectures do very little to facilitate this mutual understanding and learning (O'Brien et al., 2001). Indeed, practices used to facilitate these key aspects of innovation diffusion tend to be highly experiential and interactive, including simulation (i.e., role playing), paired work (i.e., small group or paired training/discussion), guided experience or communities of practice (e.g., individual or peer supervision, special interest groups), work shadowing (i.e., learner observation), and narrative transfer (e.g., stories). Interestingly, in our field, we rarely utilize these interactive strategies, but instead rely on didactic, lecture-based presentations. According to innovation diffusion theory, these practices will do little to engender the effective learning and use of new knowledge generated by ESTs.

The interactive learning strategies described above can increase the chances that users will adopt the new innovation. During the learning process, users are theorized to progress through five stages in deciding whether to use the innovation in their everyday work/practice (Rogers, 1995):

1) *Knowledge* (awareness and basic understanding of the innovation)
2) *Persuasion* (the process of forming an attitude toward, or developing interest in, the innovation)
3) *Decision* (activities leading to a choice to either adopt or reject the innovation)
4) *Implementation* (putting the innovation into practice)
5) *Confirmation* (cost/benefit evaluation of on-going full use of the innovation).

In our field, we tend to view the decision making process for using ESTs as a discrete event, characterized primarily by stages 1 and 2. We have not moved forward in any significant way to: 1) develop processes that promote the evaluation of empirical research recommendations or clinical observational data (Stage 3); 2) develop guidelines for the integration of empirical research into clinical practice; or 3) translate clinical observation into treatment research (Stage 4). Clearly, as we embark on our attempts to integrate research and practice in our field, it is critical that we appreciate that the dissemination of information as a staged process, requiring a blend of experiential, collaborative, and interactive approaches.

Knowledge Transfer Theory

Organizational management guru Peter Drucker coined the terms "knowledge society" and "knowledge workers" in 1994 (Drucker, 1994), marking the beginning of the "knowledge field". The knowledge movement soon led to the general conceptualization of "knowledge transfer", or the transfer of best practices within an organization or firm (Szulanski, 2003). For our purposes, we will define knowledge transfer as the process of transferring or conveying knowledge, skills, and competence from those who generate this knowledge to those who will utilize the knowledge. What is important for us to note is that within the framework of knowledge transfer, equal value is placed on the transfer of "explicit knowledge" (i.e., research findings, hard facts, material for guidelines and protocols) and the transfer of "tacit knowledge" (i.e., clinical "know-how", expertise, unwritten, practical, contextual knowledge) (Nonaka and Takeuchi, 1995). Currently, our field tends to view explicit knowledge (e.g., ESTs) as the only knowledge, with a decidedly one-directional pattern of knowledge transfer. However, theorists have highlighted several different models of knowledge transfer that are not limited to this uni-directional pattern. For example, Reardon, Lavis, and Gibson (2006) propose three models of knowledge transfer:

1) *Producer Push*: The producers of the knowledge explicitly plan and implement strategies to push that knowledge towards audiences they identify as needing to know.
2) *User Pull:* The users of the knowledge deliberately plan and implement strategies to pull knowledge from sources they identify as producing information useful to their own decision-making.
3) *Exchange*: Relationships are built and nurtured between those who produce the knowledge and those who might use the knowledge, to facilitate the exchange of information, ideas, and experience. Integral to the exchange are producers helping users to build the capacity to integrate the knowledge and users helping producers' work be more relevant.

To date, our field has primarily adhered to the "Producer Push" model of knowledge transfer, with researchers encouraging and, at times, demanding clinicians to adopt ESTs. It has been a stunningly ineffective model for research dissemination (see data on rates of EST use above). By contrast, the exchange model appears to be ideal for our field, as relationships foster the mutual dissemination of both *explicit* (research) and *tacit* (clinical) knowledge, which should result in stronger alignment of research and practice. Research from a wide range of fields supports this model in showing that knowledge is most effectively assimilated and integrated when there is buy-in from key stakeholders (O'Brien et al., 2001; Donovan et al., 2007; Reardon et al., 2006).

Evidence-Based Practice

The Evidence-Based Practice (EBP) movement, begun in the medical field in the U.K., has become ubiquitous in the field of medicine. EBP is defined as "the integration of best research evidence with clinical expertise and patient values" which leads to optimized clinical outcomes and quality of life (Sackett et al., 2000). The basic principles of EBP have common-sense appeal. We include it here because EBP has frequently become synonymous with the use of ESTs and, therefore, could be a tempting model for our field to turn to for guidance on research dissemination.

Within this model, it is the responsibility of the clinician to seek the current, best research evidence for their practice following five steps (Sackett et al., 2000):

1) Convert one's need for information into an answerable question.
2) Track down the best clinical evidence to answer that question.
3) Critically appraise that evidence in terms of its validity, clinical significance, and usefulness.
4) Integrate this critical appraisal of research evidence with one's clinical expertise and the patient's values and circumstances.
5) Evaluate one's effectiveness and efficiency in undertaking the four previous steps, and strive for self-improvement.

Literature in the field of medicine emphasizes ways to streamline this process, educating practitioners on how to access and streamline their literature research (Fain, 2003; Straus et al., 2005). Although clinical judgment, expertise, and experience are taken into account in EBP, this model places the brunt of the dissemination burden on the practitioner. Our current one-directional, "Producer-Push" model of research dissemination fits with the EBP model, i.e., researchers produce ESTs and provide descriptions and recommendations about them in the form of papers in research journals and conference presentations. It is then incumbent upon clinicians to seek out information about ESTs , avail themselves of expert training and supervision on the use of ESTs, and successfully integrate these practices into their treatment of patients. However, as we have seen, this approach has resulted in a research-practice stalemate in our field. Clinicians continue to rely more on their own clinical experience and judgment, and ESTs remain underutilized. Importantly, the American Psychological Association (Levant, 2006) has developed guidelines for Evidence-Based Practice in Psychology (EBPP) that offer an expanded definition of evidence and research designs that reinforces the contribution of clinical expertise within the EBP model.

The Road Map

In order to organize the theories and principles reviewed above into our own road map, we again look to the field of education to provide us with a unifying framework. This field has been addressing its own research-practice gap for over a decade and has been a forerunner in integrating knowledge transfer and innovation diffusion principles into its strategies for overcoming research-practice gaps (Warford, 2005; Love, 1985). In their seminal report, Donovan et al. (2007) present an extensive set of steps, strategies, and directives that aim to promote dissemination within, and integration of research findings with, applied practice. As we are at the beginning stages of this process, we must move in a thoughtful, deliberate way to create a similarly layered, thematic map tailored to the dynamics unique to our field. We selected three fundamental guidelines from the education report to organize our initial phase of research-practice integration:

1) Research findings and clinical knowledge need to be organized and communicated in a way that is easy to understand and integrate.
2) Implementation of a new model for research-practice integration must be viewed as a long-term, five to ten year process.

3) Research-practice collaboration will require a fundamental change in the relationship between the two groups.

All three steps include elements of innovation diffusion, knowledge transfer, and EBP discussed above. Thus, these recommendations provide an excellent framework within which to integrate what we have learned from our own field and others into a road map for moving forward. We outline recommended guidelines below, accompanied by specific action items and strategies. Notably, we describe these guidelines within the context of the AED, as we feel this organization is in the best position to charter the implementation of the suggested strategies.

The AED Research-Practice Integration Guidelines

Guideline #1. Research findings and clinical practice information need to be organized and communicated to practitioners and researchers, respectively, in a way that is easy to comprehend and to integrate into their thinking.

- Provide plain language summaries (similar to the practice of The Cochrane Library[1]) for empirical articles in AED publications, including the *International Journal of Eating Disorders*
- Form "clinical topics" committees to translate and describe clinical practices to researchers. These committees can serve as liaisons between clinical and research communities, promote the clinical practice of formulating and seeking answers to "answerable questions", and model writing up case studies, conducting single-case experiments, and pioneering other ways to convey clinical or "tacit" knowledge.
- Create interactive learning opportunities for disseminating research as well as clinical evidence These techniques should include those recommended by innovation diffusion theory (see above), including mentoring, guided experience and experimentation, simulation, work shadowing, paired work, communities of practice, and narrative transfer.
- Support and encourage the development of AED conference workshops that integrate participatory learning methods.
- Support and encourage translational research.

Guideline #2. Given that it will take five to ten years to build the bridge between research and practice, we must remain consistent and persevere in our methods of approach.

---

[1]The Cochrane Collaboration is a non-profit organization dedicated to improving healthcare decision-making globally, through systematic review of the effects of healthcare interventions published in The Cochrane Library (see www.cochrane.org)

- Sustain, augment, and ensure the quality of the "bridge" by maintaining a research-practice oversight group to monitor and evaluate the process, to review the literature, and to continue to strategize ways to further facilitate research-practice integration.
- Regularly review the AED Research-Practice Integration Guidelines on a member-wide basis (through the AED general listserv, website, and/or *Forum*) to ensure relevance and scope.
- Develop mechanisms that promote and strengthen full AED membership buy-in into the research-practice integration process over time.
- Build on existing organizational infrastructure (e.g., AED Special Interest Groups, committees, member listserv, publications, education and training programs) to support and integrate research-practice linkages throughout the AED membership.

Guideline #3. Research-practice collaboration will require a fundamental change in the relationship between the two groups.

- Expand definitions of current terminology to embrace the range of experience and values of both partner groups.
- Support the American Psychological Association's (see Levant, 2006) endorsement of a) an expanded understanding of "research evidence" that includes multiple types of evidence (e.g. efficacy, effectiveness, epidemiological, treatment utilization, etc.) drawn from a range of potential sources (e.g., laboratory and clinical settings, assessments, etc.); and b) the position that evidence-based practice is not confined to RCTs alone, but rather multiple research designs contribute to effective treatment
- Support the recognition that clinical observation, judgment and experience (tacit knowledge) contribute to the knowledge base in our field.
- Encourage research funding mechanisms that: 1) address what clinicians are doing in their treatment practices; 2) provide resources for clinicians to learn and be supervised in ESTs; 3) support researcher-clinician partnerships that field test ESTs as well as clinical interventions derived solely from clinical practice; and 4) support research conducted by practicing clinicians.
- Foster the development of a common language by discouraging the use of jargon.
- Develop AED conference sessions that foster researcher-practitioner dialogue and collaborations.
- Create researcher-practitioner columns and news pieces in the AED *Forum*.
- Continue the researcher-practitioner model for AED conference plenaries and keynote addresses.

Guideline Implementation

Given the scope, variety, and complexity of some of the strategies outlined above, it is critical that the implementation of the guidelines is monitored, as described in the first directive under Guideline #2. The formation of an oversight group would be the first step in the implementation process. Members of this group should represent the domains of research and practice, and should be professionals who share a long-term commitment to strengthening the research-practice interface. Exposure to, and on-going education in, the areas of knowledge transfer, diffusion theory, and interactive learning methods will be necessary so that members of the group understand how to establish effective implementation priorities, strategies, and methods for evaluating the process.

The AED, as a representative of the field, has taken this initial step by forming a Research-Practice Task Force[2]. Comprised of an international, cross-section of seasoned researchers, researcher-practitioners, and practitioners, the mandate of the task force is to develop strategies (including those outlined above) to foster research-practice integration within the AED and the field at large. Begun in 2007, the task force is implementing preliminary steps by promoting researcher-clinician dialogue in interactive formats into the AED International Conference on Eating Disorders. For example, the task force hosted the 2008 World Summit on Eating Disorders entitled "Let's Talk: Advancing the Research-Practice Partnership". This summit session included researchers and clinicians from around the globe who discussed their own perspectives for closing the gap. Several of the strategies outlined above were described and beginning action plans were developed. In the future, the task force will continue to oversee the implementation and on-going review of research-practice integration within the AED, expanding on the guidelines outlined above.

Conclusion

In ending, it is clear that the research-practice gap is a universal phenomenon that exists within virtually all professions that have an applied and basic science component. Given the universality of the causes of the tension and the barriers to integration, it is likely that the basis of the gap lies somewhere in human nature and somewhere in the character of organizational systems (both quite daunting variables with which to tamper). Nonetheless, the resounding enthusiasm of our colleagues for developing ways to address the research-practice gap is heartening and, given the guidance and experience of other fields, it is incumbent upon us to move forward in this direction. However, before we are able to enact the larger structural changes described above, we must first focus on the fundamental steps involved in establishing on-going opportunities for clinician-researcher *dialogue and collaboration.*

The AED Research-Practice Integration Guidelines set forth a range of actions we can implement to strengthen the research-practice partnership in the AED. These guidelines are by no means exhaustive or set in stone. Rather, they are intended to provide a work-in-progress that will stimulate an on-going conversation between researchers and practitioners about the sources and types of knowledge, tools, processes, and initiatives that will promote the most effective practices in our field.

Despite our quite different professional experiences, we, the authors, developed mutual trust and respect for each other through our AED opportunities to work closely and talk together about our perspectives. Dialogue, shared experience, and support bridged any gap that may have initially existed between us. The AED and professionals in our field can similarly help close the gap by using dialogue, collaboration, mutual support, and respect to bring researchers and clinicians together. In joining the richness of clinical observation with the world of formal scientific investigation, the quality of our research and treatments will improve. Our community of professionals and the quality of the lives of people with eating disorders will be all the better for it.

References

Abrial, J.R., Issarny, V., Ghezzi, C., and Parnas, D. (2005). Fundamental Research in Software Engineering, Long Term Session, Report V1.0, European Commission, Software Technologies, Brussels, Belgium.

Agras, W.S., and Apple, R. (1997). *Overcoming Eating Disorders: A Cognitive-Behavioral Treatment for Bulimia Nervosa and Binge-Eating Disorder: Therapist Guide.* U.S.Graywind Publications, Inc.

Arnow, B.A. (1999). Why Are Empirically Supported Treatments for Bulimia Nervosa Underutilized and What Can We Do About It?, *In Session: Psychotherapy in Practice*, 55, 769-779.

Bero, L., Grilli, R., Grimshaw, J., Harvey, E., Oxman, A., and Thomson, M. (1998). Closing the Gap Between Research and Practice: An Overview of Systematic Reviews of Interventions to Promote the Implementation of Research Findings, *BMJ*, 317, 465-468.

Botvin, G.J. (2004). Advancing Prevention Science and Practice: Challenges, Critical Issues, and Future Directions, *Prevention Science*, 5(1), 69-72.

Crow, S.J., Mussell, M.P., Peterson, C.B., Knopke, A. J, and Mitchell, J. E. (1999). Prior Treatment Received by Patients with Bulimia Nervosa, *International Journal of Eating Disorders*, 25, 39-44.

Demaerschalk, B.M. (2004). Evidence-Based Clinical Practice Education in Cerebrovascular Disease, Stroke: *Journal of the American Heart Association,* 35, 392-396.

Donovan, M.S., Bransford, J.D., and Pellegrino, J.W. (Eds.), (2007). *How People Learn: Bridging Research and Practice*, Committee on Learning Research and Educational Practice, Commission on Behavioral and Social Sciences and Education, National Research Council, National Academy Press, Washington DC.

Drucker, P.F. (1994). The Age of Social Transformation, *The Atlantic Monthly*, 274, 53-80.

Fain, J. (2003). *Reading, Understanding, and Applying Nursing Research: A Text and Workbook*, Philadelphia, Pennsylvania, F.A. Davis Co.

Fairburn, C.G. (2005). Let Data Guide Tx of Eating Disorders, Guest Editorial, *Clinical Psychiatry News*, 7.

Fairburn, C.G., Marcus, M.D., and Wilson, G.T. (1993). Cognitive–Behavioral Therapy for Binge Eating and Bulimia Nervosa: A Comprehensive Treatment Manual. In C.G.

---

[2] 2007-2008 AED Research-Practice Task Force members are Drew Anderson, Judith Banker, Kelly Klump, Dianne Neumark-Sztainer, Robert Palmer, Susan Paxton, Jill Pollack, Howard Steiger, Lucene Wisniewski. & Kathryn Zerbe.

Fairburn and G.T. Wilson (Eds.), *Binge Eating: Nature, Assessment, and Treatment* (pp. 361-405). New York. TheGuilford Press.

Haas, H.L., and Clopton, J.R. (2003). Comparing Clinical and Research Treatments for Eating Disorders, *International Journal of Eating Disorders*, 33, 412-420.

Haddow, G., and Klobas, J.E. (2004). Communication of Research and Practice in Library and Information Science: Closing the Gap, *Library and Information Science Research*, 26, 29-43.

Herle, M., and Martin, G.W. (2002). Knowledge Diffusion in Social Work: A New Approach to Bridging the Gap, *Social Work*, 47(1), 85-95.

Levant, R. F. (2006). APA Presidential Task Force Report on Evidence-Based Practice, Evidence-Based Practice in Psychology, *American Psychologist*, 61(4), 271-285.

Lock, J., le Grange, D., Agras, W.S., and Dare, C. (2001). *Treatment Manual for Anorexia Nervosa: A Family-Based Approach*. New York. Guilford Press.

Love, J.M. (1985). Knowledge Transfer and Utilization in Education, *Review of Research in Education*, 12, 337-386.

McConnell, S. (2002). Closing the Gap, From the Editor, *IEEE Software*, 19(1), 3-5.

Mussell, M.P., Crosby, R.D., Crow, S.J., Knopke, A.J., Peterson, C.B., Wonderlich, S.A., and Mitchell, J.E. (2000). Utilization of Empirically Supported Psychotherapy Treatments for Individuals with Eating Disorders: A Survey of Psychologists, *International Journal of Eating Disorders*, 27, 230-237.

Nonaka, I., and Takeuchi, H. (1995). *The Knowledge Creating Company*, New York. Oxford University Press.

O'Brien, M.A., Freemantle, N., Oxman, A.D., Wolf, F., Davis, D.A., and Herrin, J. (2001). Continuing Education Meetings and Workshops: Effects on Professional Practice and Health Care Outcomes, *Cochrane Database of Systematic Reviews*, (2).

Reardon, R., Lavis, J., and Gibson, J. (2006). *From Research to Practice: A Knowledge Transfer Planning Guide*, Toronto, Ontario, Canada, Institute for Work and Health.

Robinson, V.M.J. (1998). Methodology and the Research-Practice Gap, *Educational Researcher*, 27(1), 17-26.

Rogers, E.M. (1995). *Diffusion of Innovations*, Fourth Edition, New York. The Free Press.

Sackett, D.L., Straus, S.E., Richardson, W.S., Rosenberg, W., and Haynes, R.B. (2000). *Evidence-based Medicine: How to Practice and Teach EBM (*Second Edition). Edinburgh. Churchill Livingstone.

Schecter, C., Brunner, S.M. (2005). Bridging the Gap Between Public Health Research and Practice: Lessons from the Field, Position Paper, Washington DC, Academy for Educational Development, AED Center for Health Communication.

Straus, S.E., Richardson, W.S, Glasziou, P., and Haynes, R.B. (2005). *Evidence-Based Medicine: How to Practice and Teach EBM* (Third Edition). Edinburgh. Churchill Livingstone.

Szulanski, G. (2003). *Sticky Knowledge: Barriers to Knowing in the Firm*. London. Sage Publications.

Thompson-Brenner, H., and Westen, D. (2005). A Naturalistic Study of Psychotherapy for Bulimia Nervosa, Part 2: Comorbidity and Therapeutic Outcome, *Journal of Nervous and Mental Disorders*, 193, 573-594.

Tobin, D.L., Banker, J.D., Weisberg, L., and Bowers, W. (2007) I Know What You Did Last
     Summer (and It Was Not CBT): A Factor Analytic Model of International
     Psychotherapeutic Practice in the Eating Disorders, *International Journal of Eating
     Disorders*, 40, 754-757.
Von Ranson, K.M. and Robinson, K.E. (2006). Who is Providing What Type of
     Psychotherapy to Eating Disorder Clients?: A Survey, *International Journal of Eating
     Disorders*, 39, 27-34.
Wilson, G.T. (1998). The Clinical Utility of Randomized Controlled Trials, *International
     Journal of Eating Disorders*, 24, 13-29.
Warford, M.K. (2005). Testing a Diffusion of Innovations in Education Model (DIEM), *The
     Innovation Journal: The Public Sector Innovation Journal,* 10 (3), Article 32,
     warformk@buffalostate.edu.

In: Evidence-Based Treatments for Eating Disorders   ISBN 978-1-60692-310-8
Author: Ida F. Dancyger and Victor M. Fornari   © 2009 Nova Science Publishers, Inc.

Chapter V

Inpatient Psychiatric Treatment of Adolescents and Adults with Eating Disorders

Parinda Parikh, Dara Bellace and Katherine Halmi
Weill Cornell Medical College
White Plains, New York, USA

Abstract

Although eating disorders (EDs) have been described in the literature for over a millennium there are no standardized, universally accepted, evidence based criteria for the inpatient treatment of patients with EDs. This may be due to the ethical conundrum involved in enrolling medically compromised ED patients in randomized controlled trials where urgent medical stabilization often takes precedence over conducting a regimented research treatment protocol, as the latter may expose the patient to undue clinical risk. Most clinicians specializing in EDs rely on their clinical training and experience along with the treatment guidelines published by the American Psychiatric Association (2006) in managing and determining the level of care needed for their patients. In the United States, managed care companies and other health maintenance organizations use their own heterogeneous cost-efficiency driven criteria in determining the level and length of inpatient care, with mostly unknown but sometimes documented poor long-term outcomes.

This chapter discusses the inpatient management of anorexia nervosa (AN) and bulimia nervosa (BN) for adolescent and adult patients. Any reputable treatment program should emphasize a multidisciplinary approach integrating comprehensive diagnostic evaluation, medical management, pharmacotherapy, individual psychotherapy, group psychotherapy, family therapy, nutritional counseling and comprehensive discharge planning.

Introduction

Patients suffering from AN, BN, and ED Not Otherwise Specified (ED NOS) often experience significant medical and psychiatric complications, in addition to having other co-morbid psychiatric illnesses. This chapter will discuss the clinical manifestations and the medical complications of EDs along with pertinent medico-legal issues and evidence in the literature regarding treatment recommendations for the inpatient management of adolescents and adults diagnosed with EDs.

General Issues for AN Patient Hospitalization

There is little research data comparing the efficacy of different inpatient treatment protocols for AN. In determining a patient's appropriateness for an inpatient level of care, it is important to consider the patient's overall medical condition, psychiatric symptoms, psychological well-being, social support network, prior treatment response or failure, and the patient's commitment to treatment. Many of the symptoms of AN are ego-syntonic, which often leads to complete denial of the illness and failure in seeking the proper treatment. As a result, an emaciated, medically compromised AN patient will often continue to refuse treatment for weight restoration. The dropout rate from voluntary inpatient treatment programs is reported to be as high as 51%. (Woodside, Carter and Blackmore, 2004).

This the 12th inpatient hospitalization for Laura, a 16-year-old Caucasian female first diagnosed with her ED 3 years ago. She usually gets readmitted at a BMI of 13 in a severely emaciated state, with electrolyte imbalance from diuretic abuse and water loading. During her inpatient stay, she complies with the weight restoration program and reaches a BMI of 18.5 only to lose a significant amount of weight within 3 months after discharge. There are multiple psychosocial stressors contributing to her disorder but various treatment teams at different hospitals have been unsuccessful in resolving them. During the last admission, Child Protective Services were involved because of concerns of medical neglect and it was recommended that Laura enter a residential program away from home. That was the first time Laura was able to maintain her weight for over a year. She stated that she "always wanted to lose weight but could not do it" and "was waiting to get out of there." When she was given a Thanksgiving pass to come home for few hours, she convinced her parents that she did not need to return to the residential program. At that point, her case slipped through the cracks in the vast maze of Child Protective Services. Laura lost 40 pounds in 2 months and was re-hospitalized for her ED.

Clinical presentations similar to Laura's are no longer an exception. Increasingly, young adolescents presenting with an earlier onset of ED's have repeated hospitalizations before they reach adulthood. In addition to weight restoration and pharmacological management, we need to fully examine, identify and try to resolve any contributing perpetuating psychological and social stressors.

Jenny, a 35-year-old married female, had a prior history of an ED was taken to a nearby emergency room after a family member called 911 stating that she had "passed out" at home. Upon arrival at the hospital emergency department, the patient was noted to be severely emaciated. She weighed only 69 pounds and was 5 feet 3 inches tall (BMI 12.2 kg/m^2). Jenny was found to be orthostatic, bradycardic (with pulse of 42), hypothermic and cognitively compromised. After initiation of intravenous hydration and immediate stabilization, she was admitted to a medical floor of the hospital for management of electrolyte abnormalities and further cardiac monitoring. One week later, even though her condition improved, Jenny was still unable to eat any food or accept any liquid supplements. When the internist discussed the option of admission to an ED unit for weight restoration, Jenny attempted to get up from her bed and threatened to walk out of the hospital against medical advice. A psychiatric consultant was called in to assess Jenny's judgment and her capacity to understand the risks and benefits of undergoing treatment and the consequences of her treatment refusal. When talking with her husband, the treatment team realized that he had made several attempts to have her hospitalized for her ED with no success. An application for involuntary admission to an inpatient ED unit at a psychiatric hospital was made by the treating psychiatrist. This application was supported by assessments from three other independent psychiatrists, as required by state law.

In the United States, patients can voluntarily consent to be admitted to a psychiatric unit. When a patient is in imminent danger to herself or others, an involuntary commitment is available when clinically necessary. Few studies have compared the rates and outcomes of voluntary versus involuntary inpatient treatment of AN patients. Follow-up studies have shown that involuntarily hospitalized patients were eventually thankful to the people who intervened during the time of their initial treatment refusal (Russell, 2001).

Often a severely emaciated AN patient who presents to an emergency room with electrolyte abnormalities, autonomic instability, and electrocardiogram changes requires involuntary commitment.

Criteria for Inpatient Hospitalization for Patients with AN

For adults, the physiological parameters that are considered important for inpatient admission include the rate and amount of weight loss, the presence of autonomic instability, as well as the patient's metabolic and electrolyte status. Generally, adult patients who weigh significantly less than 85% of the weight recommended for their height and body frame (BMI < 17.5) have tremendous difficulty gaining weight outside of a highly specialized and intensely structured inpatient program. This is due to the poor insight and judgment, lack of motivation (Ametller, Castro, Serrano, et al, 2005), and lack of physical and emotional resources that tend to characterize this group of patients. At times, this type of inpatient setting may also be medically and psychiatrically necessary for patients above 85% of their targeted body weight, especially if they are having medical complications or are not responding to outpatient treatment.

The clinician's threshold for admitting an adolescent patient with AN is usually lower than that for adults, regardless of the patient's percent body weight and/or BMI, as research has shown that early intervention in adolescents improves outcomes (Lindblad, Lindberg and Hjern, 2006). For instance, an adolescent's unexplained, rapid weight loss over a short period of time (greater than 8-10 lbs every month), coupled with a refusal to eat, may necessitate a brief inpatient stay for immediate stabilization.

For all AN inpatients, it is necessary to obtain a complete blood analysis including complete blood count with differential; a metabolic panel including sodium, potassium, chloride, bicarbonate, glucose, magnesium, phosphorus and calcium; a liver function panel; thyroid function tests; iron studies; pregnancy test (for females); an electrocardiogram; and a consultation with an inte rnist for medical clearance to rule out any organic etiology contributing to symptoms of AN. Other co-morbid psychiatric conditions like worsening depression, psychotic symptoms or serious suicidality are also likely to warrant hospitalization. Patients with AN are candidates for inpatient admission if they show poor progress in the outpatient setting or if they do not have access to a partial program or a day treatment program. Other psychosocial factors supporting the decision for an inpatient admission may include a chaotic family environment; substance abuse by the patient or other family members; physical, sexual or emotional abuse; other family members with psychiatric or medical problems; medical neglect; and lack of resources.

Table 1 and Table 2 outline some common medical indicators for inpatient admission and common laboratory findings in AN, respectively.

Table 1. Common Medical Indicators for Inpatient Hospitalization for AN

Clinical Condition	Features
Autonomic Instability	Heart rate < 40bpm; BP < 90/60 mm Hg; blood glucose < 60 mg/dl; uncontrolled diabetes; electrolyte imbalance
Weight (% of healthy body weight)	In adults, < 85% and refusal to gain weight in outpatient setting; In children and adolescents, rapid weight loss and/or refusal to eat, regardless of % of healthy weight
Outpatient Compliance	Poor
Behaviors	Purging Starvation
Dangerousness	Refusal of treatment; Dangerousness to self and/or others

(Adapted from the American Psychiatric Association, (1))

Nutritional Rehabilitation and Medical Monitoring of AN Inpatients

When an adult patient with AN is admitted to an inpatient ED unit, an appropriate target weight range should be established. To do so, clinicians should take into consideration factors such as the patient's height, age-appropriate weight, current weight and menstrual history (for females).

Table 2. Common Laboratory Findings Related to Restricting Behaviors/Starvation

- Hyponatremia
- Low T3 and T4 levels
- Low estrogen, low luteinizing and follicle-stimulating hormone, low testosterone
- Hyperadrenocortisolemia
- Leukopenia, anemia, thrombocytopenia
- Hypophosphatemia
- Elevated liver function tests (AST, ALT, GGT, Alkaline phosphatase)
- Elevated serum cholesterol
- Increased ventricular-brain ratio on brain imaging
- Sinus bradycardia, arrhythmias, prolonged QTc
- Hypoalbuminemia

(Parikh and Halmi, 2006).

To establish a target weight range for adolescent patients with AN, one should consider the patient's menstrual history (for females with secondary amenorrhea), mid-parental heights (average of the heights of both parents), and skeletal frame. The Center for Disease Control (CDC) growth charts can also be helpful in establishing a target weight range (Kuczmarski, Ogden, Grummer-Strawn, et al, 2000). Patients must always be given a target weight range rather than a specific target weight, as multiple factors including dehydration, vomiting, laxative abuse, diuretic abuse and other causes of fluid shift may contribute to weight fluctuations. Most multidisciplinary treatment programs have a registered dietitian who can design each patient's meal plans according to their caloric needs, and individual preferences. Prior to discharge, the dietician can also prepare a structured meal plan that can ensure nutritional adequacy once the patient begins treatment in an outpatient setting.

Published guidelines recommend a weight gain of 1.1 to 2.2 kg per week for hospitalized AN patients (British-Psychological-Society, 2004). The weight restoration process typically starts at 30–40 kcal/kg/day (i.e., approximately 1,000–1,600 kcal/day), however this rate may need to be slowed in more severely ill patients who are below 70% of their ideal body weight. Intake can then be progressively increased to 70–100 kcal/kg/day, while monitoring their total daily intake, 24-hour urine output, vital signs, electrolytes (i.e., sodium, potassium, phosphorus, magnesium, calcium), and liver function tests. AN patients should also be monitored for any edema or electrocardiogram changes.

Studies have shown that it is more efficient, effective and easier for severely emaciated patients to take high-calorie liquid supplements divided into six small feedings throughout the day, rather than consuming the same amount of solid food calories, in order to maintain the same rate of weight gain (Okamoto, Yamashita, Nagoshi, et al, 2002). As the patient's weight continues to increase, they can be gradually introduced to solid foods. This process should start with 'partial trays' consisting of approximately 1,000 calories per day in solid foods, accompanied by six small liquid feedings. When patients start achieving healthier eating patterns, with better perceptions of hunger and satiety, and are improving medically, they can progress to higher-calorie trays (up to 2,400 kcal per day) with liquid supplements at snack time depending on their metabolic needs.

All inpatient feedings must be done in a supervised setting, monitored by trained nursing staff who record each patient's food and fluid intake. Bathrooms on the unit should be locked at all times, except for 6 to 8 designated "commode times" during the day. During these times, a nursing staff member should monitor each patient and record her urine output as well as any bowel movements. Constipation is a major complication of restrictive eating as well as laxative abuse, and often becomes problematic during the weight restoration process. Using a gentle stool softener along with a fiber supplement may therefore be helpful. Occasionally a patient may complain of impaction which requires immediate medical attention and possible use of stronger laxatives or manual disimpaction to avoid further complications like obstipation or more rarely colonic obstruction. Inpatients should be weighed daily in a hospital gown prior to morning showers and after they have voided. Staff members should be aware that many AN patients will frequently engage in behaviors to manipulate their weights, such as hiding coins or weights in their gowns, intentionally retaining urine, or water loading. Such possible behaviors must be monitored closely and addressed by the treatment team.

Each patient's internist or pediatrician (for adolescent patients) should be consulted by the inpatient treatment team and involved in the treatment process where appropriate. Occasionally a cardiologist will need to be consulted for any unresolved electrocardiogram changes. An orthopedist may need to be consulted when there are any concerns about fractures and bone loss. It is important for clinicians treating these complicated patients to realize that most abnormal laboratory findings will start improving gradually as nutritional rehabilitation progresses. However, some complications such as severe osteoporosis may be irreversible.

Inpatient nutritional rehabilitation programs should attempt to create a milieu that incorporates emotional nurturance. Such programs should also implement a combination of reinforcers that link each patient's activity level and other unit privileges to appropriate weight gain and desired improvement in negative behaviors, while avoiding power struggles with patients. Daily feedback during morning rounds concerning any changes in weight, privilege status and other observable parameters is also helpful for these patients.

Psychosocial Treatments for AN Inpatients

Individual, group and family therapy are all utilized within the inpatient setting. Cognitive and behavior therapy principles can be applied in both inpatient and outpatient settings. Individual behavior therapy has been reported to successfully restore weight in AN patients (Halmi, 1985). In controlled inpatient studies of AN, behavior therapy was found to be effective in inducing weight gain (Wulliemier, Rossel and Sinclair, 1975). Behavior therapy is important in the treatment of AN patients as it can mitigate some of the symptoms arising from the emaciated, malnourished state such as irritability, depression, preoccupation with food, cognitive impairments and sleep disturbances. Individual cognitive therapy focuses on severe cognitive distortions related to food and body image, although success with this technique can be achieved only after some weight gain in a severely underweight patient (Garner, 1986). More recent modifications of these therapies are well described in the literature (Kleifield, Wagner and Halmi, 1996). Two techniques often used in cognitive therapy are cognitive restructuring and problem solving. AN patients usually have a rigid style of thinking and perceiving their world, characterized by dichotomous, "all-or-nothing" thinking. These distorted thoughts are present primarily in relation to food and weight, but also around issues of self-esteem and self-concept, with pervasive feelings of ineffectiveness often accompanied with an extreme drive for perfectionism. These cognitive distortions are best addressed in individual cognitive therapy.

Family therapy and family groups are also utilized on most inpatient units. As a general rule, a family assessment should be done on all AN patients living with their families regardless of the age the patient. For adolescent AN patients, family therapy is an essential element of management (Eisler, Dare and Russell, 1997). Family support groups facilitated by clinicians are also helpful in educating other family members regarding the illness.

During inpatient stay, the patient should participate in group therapy sessions, including those geared toward body image and specific ED problems; self-esteem, self-confidence, and self-expression; gender specific issues; nutrition; and medication education. These groups, along with substance abuse counseling groups and controlled exercise groups, are all proven to be helpful in educating patients about the different aspects of recovery from AN. Separate body image groups and peer support groups for adolescent patients are especially useful in addressing their age-specific issues.

Psychopharmacology for AN Inpatients

Pharmacotherapy is not the first line of treatment for AN. However, medications may be helpful in treating the comorbid psychiatric conditions that many AN patients experience, such as anxiety disorders, mood disorders, and psychotic symptoms. For further discussion on this topic, please refer to the chapter by Mitchell and colleagues.

Discharge Planning for the Hospitalized AN Patient

To date, there are no studies to provide evidence-based discharge criteria for AN patients. The ideal discharge criteria, if permitted by managed care, are as follows: 1) achieving and maintaining normal weight range for at least one week in patients who are repeatedly hospitalized for treatment of AN or attaining 90% of normal weight in patients with first episode of inpatient hospitalization; 2) significant improvement in other ED behaviors such as purging, over-exercising, laxative abuse, and binge eating; 3) medical stability (e.g., stable vitas signs, normal electrocardiogram and lab work); and 4) no suicide risk or overt psychiatric symptoms warranting continued inpatient stay. Discharge planning should consider transition to a partial hospitalization program or a day treatment program especially if the patient has had repeated relapses or in the case of an adolescent patient with lack of structure at home. Comprehensive multifaceted treatment must be continued with experienced professionals including an internist or a pediatrician for medical care, individual cognitive psychotherapist, and a family therapist especially for patients under age 18.

Criteria for Inpatient Hospitalization for BN

The majority of BN patients can be treated effectively in an outpatient community setting. The main clinical indications for inpatient hospitalization are often medical or psychiatric instability. Medical hospitalization is usually a consequence of purging behaviors, such as frequent vomiting, laxative abuse, and/or abuse of diet pills or diuretics, which can create serious electrolyte imbalances and dehydration, as described in Table 3. These patients are usually referred to an inpatient ED unit by their families or an emergency room clinician. These patients may present with complaints of weakness and lethargy and are at risk for developing cardiac arrhythmias. A serum potassium below 2.5 mEq/L requires medical admission for electrolyte correction. Other situations that can present as medical emergencies are severe abdominal pain, gastric dilation, intractable vomiting, bloody vomitus, and cardiac problems from ipecac intoxication. The most serious consequence of gastric dilatation is gastric rupture (Matikainen, 1979). Esophageal tears and rupture due to severe vomiting are also life threatening complications (Mitchell, Pyle and Miner,1982).

Psychiatric symptoms requiring inpatient hospitalization for BN include a severe mood disorder, substance abuse or dependence, and concerns of suicidal or repeated parasuicidal behaviors. Over 30% of patients with BN have co-morbid depression, which is also accompanied by suicidal ideation (Braun, Sunday and Halmi, 1994). Bulimic patients who become dysfunctional in their work, social, or personal lives, and who spend most of their income on financing their binges, will benefit from hospitalization. A course of intensive, closely monitored inpatient treatment can help these patients to break the binge-purge cycle and establish healthier routines.

Table 3. Medical Findings Related To Purging Behaviors (Vomiting And Laxative Abuse)

- Dehydration (evident by elevated sodium)
- Hypokalemia (diagnosed by low potassium, can induce cardiac arrhythmias)
- Metabolic alkalosis (diagnosed by elevated serum bicarbonate, decreased chloride and decreased potassium)
- Hypomagnesaemia, hypophosphatemia, hypochloremia,
- Hyperamylasemia (salivary or pancreatic amylase hypersecretion)
- Esophageal tears, gastric ruptures
- Pneumomediastinum
- Skeletal or cardiac myopathies (syrup of ipecac-induced)
- Metabolic seizures (from electrolyte abnormalities)
- Mild neuropathies
- Cognitive impairment
- Chronic constipation, loss of normal bowel functioning (may need colon resection and colostomy in severe cases)

(Parikh and Halmi, 2006).

Although, the length of stay for a bulimic patient is now mainly dictated by the managed care companies and health maintenance organizations, treatment based on expert clinical consensus may be far more clinically advantageous for patients. Generally, an inpatient ED hospital stay of 7-10 days is approved by insurance companies for bulimic patients experiencing one or more of the above mentioned complications. Such approval is granted if the patient was treated and failed multiple levels of care in the community setting (i.e., outpatient, partial hospitalization and day treatment programs).

A comprehensive psychiatric evaluation along with a thorough family assessment is especially important for a bulimic adolescent or adult patient living at home. Vocational assessment and training are also useful for a dysfunctional bulimic patient who has been unable to cope with her home, work and social life.

Nutritional Rehabilitation and Medical Monitoring of BN Inpatients

The first goal of treatment is to stop the binge-purge behaviors. This can be done by providing maintenance calories in supervised meals, sometimes divided into six small meals for breakfast, lunch, dinner, and three small snacks over the course of the day. Patients must be observed during meals as well as for several hours after meals. This approach of preventing a vomiting response to eating is known as response prevention behavior therapy (Leitenberg, Rosen, Gross, et al, 1988). Because bulimic patients will tend to surreptitiously vomit in their room, bathroom, or in any non-monitored place, it is important to supervise their bathroom and room access. Frequent monitoring of serum amylase level, bicarbonate, chloride, and potassium can be helpful in assessing their vomiting behaviors as well. Under the guidance of a registered dietitian, patients are trained to identify their binge-inducing foods and challenge their binge practices, learning to eat these foods in smaller amounts while in a supervised setting. Once the BN patient is able to establish normal eating behaviors in a supervised setting, she is given increasing freedom to select her own meals.

Weekly electrolyte assessment and electrocardiograms are helpful in monitoring and correcting abnormal laboratory values. Positive urine toxicology upon admission must be followed with a repeat drug and urine test to ensure that the patient has not been abusing any illicit substances during their inpatient stay. Patients with a history of laxative abuse will report constipation and constantly seek laxatives to relieve the unpleasant "feeling of fullness". This should be monitored by the bathroom log, medical examination and x-rays of abdomen, if indicated. Using a stool softener and a fiber supplement may help these patients regulate their bowels, while training them to stop abusing stimulant and osmotic laxatives.

Psychosocial Treatments for BN Inpatients

Among the different psychotherapy approaches that have been rigorously studied, cognitive behavioral therapy has been shown to be the most effective for BN patients (Fairburn, Kirk, O'Connor, et al, 1986). This approach to treatment helps these patients to focus on personal psychological issues, interpersonal relationships, and development of social skills, as well as stabilizing their eating behaviors. Common psychological issues that tend to arise with this population are an inability to express anger and other feelings appropriately; depression stemming from feelings of guilt, abandonment, losses and trauma; and dependency and control issues.

Bulimic patients are often found to exhibit severe impulsivity, which includes engaging in a range of antisocial behaviors (e.g., lying and shoplifting) complicated by substance abuse and mood dysregulation. Even though a significant number of BN patients also meet criteria for avoidant personality disorder (Braun, Sunday and Halmi, 1994), borderline personality traits (e.g., splitting; projection) are more frequently observed in the inpatient setting. For these patients, food often becomes an escape medium from the discomfort and dissatisfaction they feel within their personal lives. In the inpatient unit, it is common to see these patients "acting out" in other ways when their relationship with food is being supervised, monitored and restructured. Frequently, patients will rebel and may at times leave the hospital prematurely prior to completion of the treatment, resulting in frequent relapses and poorer long-term prognosis. Concepts derived from skills training groups (Linehan, Heard and Armstrong, 1993) are therefore used to enhance competence in regulating affect, interpersonal relationships, problem solving, and distress tolerance – all of which can be helpful in teaching these patients effective coping skills.

It is common to see adolescents with BN secretly engaging in bulimic behaviors, frequently isolating themselves from the rest of their family. Family therapy and family groups must be included for all adolescent and adult patients living at home (Eisler, Simic, Russell, et al, 2007). This often helps to elucidate the precipitating and perpetuating factors of their binge/purge behaviors. In addition, a "family contract" can be used effectively in helping patients and families take responsibilities for their behaviors and adopt healthier coping mechanisms.

Medication Treatments for BN Inpatients

Compared to AN, the pharmacological interventions for BN have been more extensively studied and published in the literature. Various agents that have found to be useful are antidepressant medications such as the tricylic antidepressants (TCAs), the serotonin specific reuptake inhibitors (SSRIs) and other newer agents. For further discussion on this topic, please refer to the chapter by Mitchell and colleagues.

Discharge Planning for the Hospitalized BN Patient

In the absence of evidence-based studies evaluating discharge criteria, the ideal discharge criteria, if permitted by managed care, are as follows: 1) achieving and maintaining a binge-purge free period for at least a week, if this is the patient's first inpatient hospitalization, and longer for relapsing patients; 2) medical stability (e.g., stable vital signs, normal electro-cardiogram and serum electrolytes); 3) successful pharmacological treatment of psychiatric symptoms, and 4) no suicide risk or overt co-morbid psychiatric symptoms warranting a continued inpatient hospital stay. Discharge planning should consider transition to a partial hospitalization program or a day treatment program for adult BN patients who have had repeated relapses, or for adolescent BN patients who lack structure at home.

> Erika is a 21-year-old adult female who was transferred from a medical hospital for further treatment of her ED on a 'voluntary' legal status. One week prior to her transfer, she had walked into the emergency room with complaints of dizziness, light headedness and palpitations. Metabolic panel revealed sodium and potassium of 129 and 2.6mg/dl respectively. Erika admitted that she has been drinking 4-5 liters of water along with diet sodas and coffee to suppress her appetite. She proudly reported that she managed to lose 20 lbs in just one month using this strategy. She was at BMI of 17.5 on admission. Later she also admitted to purging behaviors (6-8 times daily) which started 4 weeks before admission, when she was having feelings of gastric fullness while consuming large amounts of fluids. She also endorsed symptoms of depression and anxiety, and admitted that she had been binge drinking alcohol with friends on the weekends. She is currently a second year law student who feels overwhelmed, juggling her studies and a part-time job at a corporate law firm.
>
> At the advice of her psychiatrist, Erica admitted herself voluntarily in an inpatient ED unit once she was medically stabilized. However, she reported tha she "felt better" within 3 days and wanted to leave the hospital. The treating psychiatrist discussed with her the possibility of staying for at least for 1 week to "interrupt the purging cycle" but Erika was focused on not missing work and school. As she was not deemed to be psychotic, suicidal or homicidal, she was discharged against medical advice with referral to an outpatient ED program. Within a 6-month span, she was rehospitalized 3 times to different inpatient ED units for similar symptoms of purging, physical complaints suggestive of electrolyte abnormalities, bloody vomitus and refusal to eat adequately.

Conclusion

EDs including AN, BN and their variants are psychiatric disorders with high morbidity and mortality from medical complications. The etiology of these disorders is mutifactorial, with a prominent biologic diathesis interacting with environmental factors facilitating its development and progression. As described earlier, certain patients do require an inpatient level of care due to the severity of their symptoms. Even though the length of an inpatient stay is primarily determined by the constraints of insurance limitations, clinicians should utilize guidelines based on current expert clinical consensus. Despite considerable research in the treatment of these disorders, a significant number of patients do not recover completely and the course of their illness is marked by life long relapses and frequent inpatient hospitalizations. Outcome is favorable in over 50 % of those treated. For an adolescent patient, it is even more important to restore weight to a near-optimum level so as to restore menses and ovulation in female patients and prevent long-term irreversible damage from osteoporosis. Hospitalization for these patients provides them with numerous advantages including: 1) rapid restoration of weight for an AN patient; 2) medical and psychiatric stabilization for both AN and BN patients; 3) interruption of self-harming behaviors; and 4) comprehensive evaluation and treatment of previously undiagnosed psychiatric co-morbidities. Current good clinical practice recommendations include a multidisciplinary approach integrating nutritional rehabilitation, medical stabilization, pharmacotherapy, psychotherapy, various group therapies, with appropriate aggressive care in order to improve outcome and prevent morbidity and mortality from the ED.

References

American Psychiatric Association. (2006). *Practice Guideline for the Treatment of Patients with Eating Disorders. 3rd Edition* ed. Washington DC: American Psychiatric Press.

Ametller L, Castro J, Serrano E, Martinez E, Toro J. (2005). Readiness to recover in adolescent anorexia nervosa: prediction of hospital admission. *Journal of Child Psychology and Psychiatry, and Allied Disciplines*, 46(4), 394-400.

Braun DL, Sunday SR, Halmi KA. (1994). Psychiatric comorbidity in patients with eating disorders. *Psychological Medicine*, 24(4), 859-67.

British-Psychological-Society. (2004). Eating disorders. Core interventions in the treatment and management of anorexia nervosa, bulimia nervosa and related eating disorders. *Leicester* (UK).

Eisler I, Dare C, Russell GF, Szmukler G, le Grange D, Dodge E. (1997). Family and individual therapy in anorexia nervosa. A 5-year follow-up. *Archives of General Psychiatry*, 54(11), 1025-30.

Eisler I, Simic M, Russell GF, Dare C. (2007). A randomised controlled treatment trial of two forms of family therapy in adolescent anorexia nervosa: a five-year follow-up. *Journal of Child Psychology and Psychiatry, and Allied Disciplines*, 48(6), 552-60.

Fairburn CG, Kirk J, O'Connor M, Cooper PJ. (1986). A comparison of two psychological treatments for bulimia nervosa. *Behaviour Research and Therapy*, 24(6), 629-43.

Garner DM. (1986). Cognitive therapy for bulimia nervosa. *Adolescent Psychiatry*, 13, 358-90.

Halmi, KA. (1985). Behavioral management of anorexia nervosa. In: Garner, DM, Garfinkel, PE, eds. *Handbook of Psychotherpay for Anorexia Nervosa and Bulimia*. New York: Guilford Press :147-59.

Kleifield EI, Wagner S, Halmi KA. (1996). Cognitive-behavioral treatment of anorexia nervosa. *The Psychiatric Clinics of North America*, 19(4), 715-37.

Kuczmarski RJ, Ogden CL, Grummer-Strawn LM, Flegal KM, Guo SS, Wei R, et al. (2000). CDC growth charts: United States. *Advance Data*, 314, 1-27.

Leitenberg H, Rosen JC, Gross J, Nudelman S, Vara LS. (1988). Exposure plus response-prevention treatment of bulimia nervosa. *Journal of Consulting and Clinical Psychology*, 56(4), 535-41.

Lindblad F, Lindberg L, Hjern A. (2006). Improved survival in adolescent patients with anorexia nervosa: a comparison of two Swedish national cohorts of female inpatients. *The American Journal of Psychiatry*, 163(8), 1433-5.

Linehan MM, Heard HL, Armstrong HE. (1993). Naturalistic follow-up of a behavioral treatment for chronically parasuicidal borderline patients. *Archives of General Psychiatry*, 50(12), 971-4.

Matikainen M. (1979). Spontaneous rupture of the stomach. *American Journal of Surgery*, 138(3), 451-2.

Mitchell JE, Pyle RL, Miner RA. (1982). Gastric dilatation as a complication of bulimia. *Psychosomatics*, 23(1), 96-7.

Okamoto A, Yamashita T, Nagoshi Y, Masui Y, Wada Y, Kashima A, et al. (2002). A behavior therapy program combined with liquid nutrition designed for anorexia nervosa. *Psychiatry and Clinical Neurosciences*, 56(5), 515-20.

Parikh P, Halmi KA. (2006). Anorexia Nervosa. *Current Psychosis and Therapeutics Reports*, 4, 121-7.

Russell GF. (2001). Involuntary treatment in anorexia nervosa. *The Psychiatric Clinics of North America*, 24(2), 337-49.

Woodside DB, Carter JC, Blackmore E. (2004). Predictors of premature termination of inpatient treatment for anorexia nervosa. *The American Journal of Psychiatry*, 161(12), 2277-81.

Wulliemier F, Rossel F, Sinclair K. (1975). A comparison of two different treatments of anorexia nervosa. *Journal of Psychosomatic Research*, 19(4), 267-72.

In: Evidence-Based Treatments for Eating Disorders
Author: Ida F. Dancyger and Victor M. Fornari

ISBN 978-1-60692-310-8
© 2009 Nova Science Publishers, Inc.

Chapter VI

Day Treatment for Anorexia Nervosa*

Ida F. Dancyger, Victor M. Fornari and Jack L. Katz
New York University School of Medicine
New York, New York, USA

Abstract

This chapter examines the emergence during the past 25 years of day treatment as an intensive therapeutic alternative to hospital inpatient care for patients with anorexia nervosa. The scientific literature regarding the inpatient treatment of eating disorder patients, whether on a general medical, general psychiatric, pediatric, or specialized eating disorders unit, is reviewed. A summary of the research describing the use of a day treatment model for anorexia nervosa is then provided. Criteria for admission or exclusion and the unique challenges and pitfalls with the different care options, including the authors' own experience with eating disorder populations in various clinical settings, are presented. Two cases of young women with anorexia nervosa are described to highlight the complex clinical and pragmatic considerations in selecting a treatment setting. It is noted that economic (that is., managed care) constraints have played an increasingly important role in the decisions regarding level of care. Future research efforts should help to provide an evidence-based framework to inform clinical decision-making regarding the optimal treatment setting for individuals with anorexia nervosa at different stages of their illness.

Introduction

When should a person with anorexia nervosa (AN) be treated in the hospital? How does one decide what the suitable level of care is? When does one decide to end a certain level of care and either transfer a patient to a less or more restrictive program or discharge her to services in the community? How do mental health providers balance the often conflicting

---

* Parts of this chapter were previously published and are reprinted here with permission from NOVA Publishers.

viewpoints of patients and their families (not to mention managed care companies)? These questions will be examined in this chapter as it addresses day treatment in the spectrum of care for the treatment of AN. The clinical evaluation and care of individuals with AN is sufficiently complex so as to present a major challenge for any practitioner treating these patients. Families, many health professionals, and much of the lay public do not sufficiently appreciate the serious nature of eating disorders (ED). Despite what is often viewed as simply a self-imposed dietary restriction, EDs are serious conditions that carry a high rate of medical complications and substantial risk of death.

Current Trends

Treating patients in a managed care environment has strongly influenced the site of treatment in the continuum from inpatient to day treatment to outpatient care. Overall, a wide range of treatment options is available on an outpatient level for those individuals who can manage safely outside of an inpatient or partial hospitalization /day program setting (per criteria to be discussed). Outpatient care for AN and/or bulimia nervosa can and often does include some combination of the following modalities: individual or group psychotherapy, family therapy, nutritional counseling, medical monitoring, and/or psychopharmacology. Recently, treatment for many adolescents/ adults with EDs has shifted from an inpatient setting to a more cost effective day hospital approach. But first we will examine the parameters of inpatient care for EDs.

Inpatient Treatment of Anorexia Nervosa on a General Psychiatric or a Specialized Eating Disorders Unit

Introduction and Clinical Issues

While outpatient treatment represents the most commonly employed approach for the management of AN (Robinson, 1993), there can occur circumstances that suggest or even mandate treatment in an inpatient setting. Whether this will be on a medical (or adolescent) unit, a general psychiatric unit, or a dedicated ED unit will reflect not only certain clinical considerations but also facility availability and insurance constraints.

The clinical considerations in outpatient vs. inpatient treatment relate to the severity of the symptoms of AN and their biological concomitants, co-morbidity concerns, the course of the illness, and the degree of compliance with and response to prior treatment. The behavioral aspects of the disorder, namely, the self-starvation, the eating rituals, the excessive exercise, and the possible purging activities will typically fall along a spectrum of severity, as will the consequent physiological aberrations. When the latter become potentially life threatening (see section on treatment in a general medical or adolescent unit), the priority obviously exists for biological intervention. When the behavioral issues are particularly prominent, admission to an inpatient unit, whether general or specialized, becomes more logical (Vandereycken, 2003).

Indications for Psychiatric Admission

Probably the most clear cut indication of a need for psychiatric admission is the presence of suicidality. As perhaps 50% of ED patients meet criteria for co-morbid major depression at some time during the course of illness (Cooper, 1995; Halmi et al., 1991), suicidal ideation can occur; the presence of intent, and certainly a plan, requires urgent psychiatric admission. But more common are the other indications. These include: significant weight loss, either gradually to below 75% of ideal body weight (IBW), or more acutely to 85% to 75% of IBW (APA Guidelines, 2006); poor motivation to participate in outpatient treatment with progressive overall downhill course; declining ability to function in activities of daily life because of the patient's preoccupation with her diet, weight, appearance, etc.; exercise that has become so frenetic that the patient frequently borders on a state of exhaustion or is unavailable for other obligations; purging with emetics, laxatives, or diuretics that has gotten so out of hand as to threaten the patient's physiological homeostasis; and, finally, family turmoil consequent to the patient's ED which in turn is further aggravating matters and from which the patient must be extricated to have any chance of being stabilized. The presence of co-morbid substance abuse, if severe enough in its own right, might also mandate inpatient admission.

General Psychiatric Unit vs. Specialized Eating Disorder Unit

Because of the clinical expertise and formalized treatment protocols that characterize most dedicated ED units, admission to such a setting might seem the obvious choice for inpatient treatment. Nevertheless, there are considerations that can lead instead to admission to a general psychiatry unit. The first of these is, quite simply, lack of availability. Not all regions have a specialized ED unit, whereas general psychiatry units are more widely distributed; moreover, admission waiting time may be shorter for a general unit because of the more rapid turnover rate characteristic of acute inpatient services. The second consideration is insurance coverage, as this might not be approved for an ED unit, which can require a specific minimum length of stay to facilitate treatment protocols and thus optimize outcome.

From a clinical standpoint, there is also a potential downside to an ED unit stay in that younger patients may learn "anorectic techniques" (e.g., purging mechanisms, how to hide one's purging, methods to artificially elevate one's weight, etc.) from their more seasoned fellow patients. Furthermore, as mentioned above, active suicidality in an anorectic patient is probably best treated on a general psychiatric unit because of the familiarity of such units with this problem. Finally, general psychiatry units are typically locked while ED units may or may not be. For the suicidal, uncooperative, or even psychotic AN patient, a locked unit clearly has advantages.

Pitfalls and Exclusionary Criteria for a Psychiatric Unit Admission

While psychiatric admission is indicated by the above considerations, it should not be assumed that it is without its own possible perils. Particularly noteworthy is the impact on self-esteem. Moreover, if the hospitalization proves unsuccessful in reversing the patient's downward spiral, it may contribute to a sense of total hopelessness in patient and family about possible recovery in the future.

Very young patients (e.g., those under 16 years of age) should probably not be admitted to a general adult unit but rather to an adolescent medicine unit. The presence of highly disturbed adults and the absence of age-appropriate peers would likely be deleterious to the youthful patient's course.

Finally, not all general psychiatric units are experienced in treating eating disordered patients. Staff may be readily deceived by the anorectic (or bulimic) patient's manipulations. Angry countertransferences may develop in response to a starving anorectic patient's adamant refusal to eat. There may even be some staff envy of the seeming impenetrable will power of the starving anorectic patient to continue dieting in the face of available food and external pressure to resume normal eating.

The Advantages of Treatment on an Eating Disorders Unit

A specialty unit is obviously organized to deal with the special pathology to which it is dedicated. An Eating Disorders Unit (EDU) staff is prepared to provide multi-modal treatment that can address the multiple facets of AN. This will include such approaches as: individual therapy, family therapy, group therapy, therapeutic activities, psychoeducation, nutritional counseling, and pharmacotherapy. Moreover, behavior therapy that provides both positive and negative reinforcers to promote weight gain, whether via access to or restrictions from exercise, visitors, or off-unit privileges, is comfortably employed by an EDU staff. An appropriate dietary schedule (often with small multiple feedings), use of liquid nutritional supplements, and prevention of bathroom access by purgers after meals are also standard operating procedures for an EDU. Similarly, the common weekly weight gain target (of 2.0 – 3.0 lbs) is well known to the staff and carefully monitored.

In addition, the availability of a full unit of eating-disordered patients facilitates group therapy, both cognitive-behavioral and insight oriented. And a nutritionist, in light of the serious nutritional needs of these patients, becomes a funded and visible member of the permanent staff, a circumstance that would not exist on a general psychiatric unit.

Finally, the staff members of an EDU are savvy. They are sophisticated in their knowledge of the tricks and maneuvers employed by anorectic patients to hide their weight loss, non-eating, and purging. Patients are carefully weighed, watched, and monitored.

Pitfalls and Disadvantages of Treatment on an Eating Disorders Unit

If an EDU presents all of the above advantages, why is it not the perfect place for treatment of AN (managed care considerations aside)? Ironically, it is precisely because the unit contains perhaps one to two dozen ED patients housed together that problems occur.

Frequently, because of the resistance of AN patients to gain weight, there can be an "Us vs. Them" atmosphere on the unit. If the staff is knowledgeable about deceptive techniques, the patients are equally shrewd, often leading to a competition as to who is in charge and more iron-willed.

Also, as stated above, patients learn anorectic techniques from each other. They can also become competitive about their thinness with each other. Not surprisingly, some patients prove treatment resistant and will eventually be discharged with negligible improvement in any sphere, which can have a demoralizing effect on the other patients. Even amongst those who have improved, there is no guarantee of sustained improvement. Indeed, Bruch argued that patients who gain weight principally as a consequence of behavioral reinforcers are particularly likely to relapse following discharge (Bruch, 1974).

Finally, because EDs are so pernicious and frustrating to treat, staff burnout can become a problem on an EDU. The staff itself needs periodic "feeding" to maintain morale and motivation in working with such resistant patients day after day.

Weight Gain Parameters

While severe weight loss need not be the only reason for inpatient admission, it is commonly the most glaring concern and thus merits particular attention. Techniques for promoting weight gain include: behavioral reinforcers, small but frequent feedings, use of liquid nutritional supplements, and a structured daily meal plan. (Purgers are also not permitted bathroom privileges for about two hours after meals.)

If the patient is fully uncooperative with the treatment regimen and her weight continues to fall, the staff must be prepared to take more aggressive steps to insure adequate re-nourishment. Two techniques are available: nasogastric feeding and total parenteral nutrition. Neither is without its dangers (e.g., severe fluid retention with its consequences) and both must be administered carefully, expertly, and only when urgently needed. (Nasogastric feedings will have a secondary benefit in that the N-G tube discomfort provides a negative reinforcer for ongoing avoidance of eating.) Also, additional electrolyte and mineral supplements, particularly potassium and phosphorous, may be required in those who have been extensive purgers (Halmi et al., 1991).

A goal weight restoration to at least 90% of ideal body weight (a percentage at which regular menstruation is likely to resume) is typically set (Golden at al., 1997). The rate of weight gain is usually targeted at no more than 2.0 – 3.0 lbs./week (Halmi et al., 1991). This is to minimize the possibility of re-feeding edema and also to allow the patient to feel that her weight restoration is not going to go out of control and that the treatment weight goal is not one which will result in her now perceiving herself as being "fat."

Research Findings

While there is a paucity of research on the efficacy of inpatient treatment for AN, a few studies have examined certain aspects of this modality. At least two studies (Wiseman et al., 2001; Baron et al., 1995) have described a greater rate of relapse among anorectic patients who were discharged at lower than target weights. Lower weights were associated with briefer hospital stays (often due to managed care pressures), rather than with more severe presenting symptomatology. There is a virtual absence of controlled studies that examine the effectiveness of treatment on an EDU vs. that on a general psychiatric inpatient unit.

A randomized controlled study of treatment efficacy for AN on ED inpatient units vs. in outpatient settings could not establish a significant outcome difference between the two after five years (Crisp et al., 1991). But such comparisons are difficult because of the possible range of treatment modalities in both settings (individual, family, group, dynamic, interpersonal, behavioral, cognitive-behavioral, pharmacologic, etc.), differing durations of treatment, differences in treatment adherence, differences in pre-treatment symptoms, and symptom severity and duration. Nevertheless, in life threatening situations, it would be difficult to justify withholding or even delaying inpatient admission for the patient with AN.

Other Types of Inpatient Care: General Medicine and Adolescent Medicine Units

Introduction

Individuals with EDs who require acute physiological stabilization, due to a variety of serious complications, are generally admitted to medical units of general hospitals. Interestingly, weight gain can vary dramatically between treatment sites (Goldberg et al., 1980). However, closer analysis suggests that differences are linked primarily to prognostic indicators in the patients admitted to each site. There is a lack of empirical data to support the possibility that the type of unit the ED patient enters makes a difference in outcome. Except for the Crisp and colleagues (1991) study referred to previously, there has not been any other randomized controlled trials of inpatient versus outpatient treatment of AN (Meads, Gold and Burns, 2001).

Clinical Considerations

The location of inpatient treatment in the spectrum of care for AN often depends more on chance than scientifically validated data (Vandereycken, 2003). There is currently no clear-cut clinical consensus regarding the major treatment questions, including that of when to admit to an inpatient setting. The lack of controlled research limits the availability of evidence-based practice in this regard. What is more evident is that economic restraints posed by managed care limit the length of inpatient care, which leads to early discharge at lower body weights and thus greater likelihood of relapse and chronicity. When comparing the clinical experience among the United Kingdom, the United States, and Australia, variations in clinical practice exist depending upon the health care system of the country. Therapists dealing with the seriously ill anorectic patients have to face difficult decisions, ethically as well as clinically.

Locus of Control: Whose Responsibility Is It Anyway?

The age of the patient may determine where the locus of responsibility lies. Refusal of life saving care can become a clinical concern. Parents of minors must provide the appropriate care for their dependent children and provide consent for treatment. Rarely, if ever, do families refuse to co-operate. Only one report in the literature that we could find addressed the role of parental medical neglect in two cases reported to the child protective agency in that locale (Fornari et al., 2001). The situation with adult patients can be more problematic but they usually have someone who is significantly involved with them. Parents, siblings, and, when married, spouses are the ones to request and/or petition for care when their ill family member refuses treatment and faces a life-threatening situation. On occasion, it may be necessary to petition for emergency care even over the objection of the family member when it appears that the family is not able to provide for the safe treatment for their loved one. It may be that family members become fatigued after a long illness in their child or sibling or spouse and relinquish hope. In certain situations, it may also be that the identified patient is the victim of abuse and the family will not acknowledge this, but would rather opt for allowing the patient to die. Thus, the clinical decision-making requires an understanding of the history of the illness, as well as familiarity with the family structure, history, and dynamics. Although some investigators question the role of the family in the evaluation and treatment of adults with AN, in our experience, it is important for the understanding and ultimate recovery of the patient (Dancyger et al., 2005).

Specialized Day Treatment for Eating Disorders

Emergence of Day Programs

There is support in the literature for the use of day treatment/partial hospitalization as an alternative to inpatient hospitalization for patients with serious mental illnesses (Orgrodniczuk and Piper, 2001). The first day hospital for general psychiatric illnesses was founded in 1937 (Dzhagarov, 1937) and, about 50 years later, the first specialized day/partial hospital program for EDs was developed in Toronto, Canada (Piran et al., 1989). Other programs soon followed in Australia, Germany, Israel, and the USA.

Fiscal Constraints and Third Party Payers

The costs of day treatment for EDs are substantially lower than those for inpatient care and are more likely to be covered by insurance companies and HMOs. As patients are living and sleeping at home, beds/laundry/housekeeping and overnight staff are not needed. Furthermore, in most programs, at least one meal/snack per day is usually eaten outside the facility, so food/cafeteria costs are also reduced. This makes this type of approach more affordable to a wider range and a larger number of individuals and their families (Zipfel et al.,2002). Also some programs will permit a three day per week attendance, thus allowing individuals to continue with aspects of work or school, which may be advantageous in the long-term to them and their families in terms of income or completion of studies.

Clinical Advantages

One clinical advantage of day treatment for some individuals with EDs is that they are not removed from their usual evening/weekend environment and can continue thereby to receive support of family and friends. They can also maintain the opportunity to function normally in at least certain areas of their lives, separate from their illness (e.g., part-time work or school). For these individuals, regression and dependence on the inpatient unit may be avoided, as the individual is required to self-regulate and self-monitor whenever not in the day program. Thus, during evening hours, weekends, and holidays, these patients can remain involved with their ongoing lives, roles, and relationships. This may contribute to more independence and also to more ready generalization of newly learned behaviors, attitudes, skills, and strategies from treatment setting to real life setting. At the same time, the patient has the support of the group treatments and the program staff to help process, understand, and manage the difficulties of everyday living in the community. Relationship problems, self-esteem issues, self-control concerns, social pressures, etc., all can be brought back to the program and worked through on an ongoing basis (Zipfel et al., 2002).

Pitfalls

For some individuals, the advantages turn into disadvantages if they are unable to keep themselves from the self-destructive behaviors when outside of the day treatment program. That is to say, some individuals may continue to engage in disordered eating, starving, bingeing, and purging on the outside and keep these behaviors hidden and secret from day program staff. In addition, the families of these patients may not be able to manage their out of control behaviors in the home environment (Zipfel et al., 2002).

For some adolescents who need transportation to the day program, the requirement of daily attendance may be a hardship or even an impossibility due to the distance from the facility or the transportation costs or the tensions that emerge in the time spent driving with a parent to and from the program.

Inclusion Criteria

Clinically, treaters often turn to day programs for those patients for whom outpatient care has not been intensive enough or with sufficient structure to provide for improvement or at least prevent deterioration.

The individual needs to be evaluated by a physician to assess overall medical stability and to rule out such medical concerns as dehydration, electrolyte disturbances, cardiac problems, and acute medical complications of malnutrition.

Weight requirements may vary from program to program but generally those who are less than 75% of ideal body weight for height would be better suited for inpatient care (APA Practice Guidelines, 2006) and should not be considered for Day Treatment until weight has been stabilized and restored to at least 75% of IBW and probably higher. In one of the few studies to examine this, Howard and colleagues (1999) found that, when patients were below 90% of IBW at time of transfer from Inpatient to Day Treatment, they were nine times more likely to be unsuccessfully treated than were those who were above 90% of IBW at time of transfer.

Exclusion Criteria

Acute medical conditions, as described above, including severe starvation/ severe emaciation, that is, weight less than 75%IBW or BMI below 16, can be considered contra-indications for treatment in a day program. In addition, serious cardiovascular complications, for example, dysrhythmia or cardiac failure, cannot be managed in a day treatment setting. Similarly, serious gastrointestinal complications may require fulltime attention. Acute psychiatric conditions/emergencies, such as acute psychosis, are an indication for inpatient care. Serious substance abuse, including serious drug/substance use complications, first requires specialty treatment, as these individuals are not able to make good use of a day program. Suicidal or parasuicidal crises, which require a safe and contained environment for the individual, cannot be managed in a day treatment facility in light of the lack of 24/7 monitoring of the patient.

Transition Considerations

Transition from one level of care to another requires consideration of a variety of factors. The "how, what, where, and when" of the practical decision making process concerning day program or partial hospital has not been well defined in the literature. For some, it may rest on the availability of these services in their community. For others, it may be determined by what the insurance carrier stipulates that the patient's benefits allow. The admission to a day program has been most successful in our own experience when it serves as a transition from inpatient care (Dancyger et al., 2003). Generally, we have observed that, following inpatient care, anorectic patients tend to be less resistant to the day program than those who were not hospitalized. Following discharge, individuals are often delighted to be out of the hospital and able to sleep at home and resume their "normal" lives. When the day program is integrated with the inpatient program, it can provide a natural progression and be seamless. When it involves a hospital discharge and transfer to another day treatment setting, it may require more careful transition planning in order to enhance continuity of care and thereby increase the likelihood of cooperation and eventual recovery.

In our own experience, it is often difficult to achieve the bulk of the weight restoration for severely malnourished individuals in a day treatment setting. Generally, achieving the last 10% of weight restoration is more attainable, although there have been individuals who were able to gain the majority of their weight in a day program setting. However, each person's motivational level and family environment needs to be appreciated. Careful monitoring of the course of treatment allows for the possibility of re-hospitalizing those individuals who fail to meet their treatment goals in a day program.

Day treatment can also be an intensification of an outpatient plan that failed to accomplish the goals of care, as outlined in the APA practice guideline. (APA, 2006, Table 8, pp. 37-39). If outpatient goals are not attained or safety concerns arise, the patient might then be referred to a day program, provided that there are no acute life-threatening indications for emergency inpatient admission. In practice, this shift from outpatient to a more intensive level of care is often met with resistance. Not uncommonly, the clinical situation deteriorates further, thereby necessitating an inpatient admission. If there is co-operation, outpatients whose clinical status begins to deteriorate might be able to be adequately served in a day program. Johnson and colleagues have described their comprehensive program, in which there is flexibility of care along the continuum of inpatient, day program, and outpatient settings, including an individual psychotherapist who continues with the patient throughout her course of treatment (Johnson and Sansone, 1993).

Research Findings

There is good support in the literature for patients with serious mental disorders, who in the past would have been in inpatient programs, being treated successfully in day treatment/partial hospitalization programs. This type of treatment seems to be most beneficial for the more psychologically minded patients (Orgrodniczuk and Piper, 2001). (See Table 1 for a summary of day treatment research for a wide range of subjects but mainly female adolescents and adults with EDs.) Differences across programs, including age groups, criteria for admission and discharge, clinical emphases, and international differences in health care environments, require that further research be conducted to clarify the nature and effectiveness of this relatively new treatment approach to EDs (Zipfel et al., 2002).

Table 1. Studies of day treatment of eating disorders

Authors	Subjects (Mean age in years)	Diagnosed	Findings	Follow-up
Danziger, et al. (1988)	32 adolescents	AN	84% reached IBW, 89% resumed menses, 59% overcame body image distortions, 88% stopped ritualistic exercise	
Woodside, et al. (1995)	91 pts	BN	BN displayed noticeable improvement in BP and weight gain after discharge of DTP	
Kaplan, Olmsted, Molleken, (1997)	527 pts. (25 yrs)	AN, ANBN, BN	AN- 88% MPMW >50% -no B and P	2 years later – 80% remain asymptomatic
Gerlinghoff, et al. (1998)	106 pts.(3 males) (23.3 yrs)	AN, BN, EDNOS	AN-64% weight gain, BN-significant decrease in binges	Mean of 17.2 months later– 64% were evaluated,7% still AN, 4% still BN
Olmsted and Kaplan, (1999)	Adult females	AN, BN	AN-49-58% weight restored.BN-44% abstained from binges and purges	
Howard, et al. (1999)	59 females, (24.8 yrs)	AN	24% were failures and required IP or left AMA	
Olmsted and Kaplan, (1999)	Adult females	AN, BN	AN-49-58% weight restored.BN-44% abstained from binges and purges	
Dare and Eisler, (2000)	14 adolescents	AN, BN	Some symptomatic improvement	

Table 1. (Continued)

Authors	Subjects (Mean age in years)	Diagnosed	Findings	Follow-up
Tasca, Flynn, Bissada, (2002)	61 females (28.9 yrs)	AN, BN, EDNOS	ED DTP proved more engaged and avoiding than gen. psychiatric DTP	
Dancyger, et al. (2003)	82 females. (17.9 yrs)	AN, BN, EDNOS	49% successful, 13% required IP	
Robinson (2003)	Female patients	AN	There is no conclusive evidence that inpatient care is more beneficial than outpatient care. However, high-quality outpatient care can make inpatient care unnecessary.	
Franzen, et al. (2004)	125 pts. (1male) (22.7 yrs)	AN, BN, EDNOS	106 completers, 19 non-completers (15.2%) had more severe bulimic sxs.	
Zeeck, et al. (2004)	18 females (27.1 yrs.)	BN	27.8% complete remission at discharge, 50% still BN	1.5 years later - 50% complete remission, 21.4% still BN
Gowers and Bryant-Waugh (2004)	Child and adolescent patients	AN, BN, EDNOS	Younger patients can have their ED managed on an outpatient basis with inpatient care reserved for AN patients with serious complications.	
Schmidt and Asen, (2005)	Adolescents and Adults	AN	Multi-family day treatment therapy is an effective alternative compared to IT for AN	

Authors	Subjects (Mean age in years)	Diagnosed	Findings	Follow-up
Kong (2005)	50 females (25.8 yrs.)	AN, BN, EDNOS	Day treatment showed greater improvements re: frequency of BandP, BMI, depression and self-esteem than the control group (OP).	

Clinical Vignettes

Ms. B

Ms. B was a 19 year-old college student with no history of being overweight, who had been referred for evaluation of a possible ED.

Ms. B had been notably thinner for three years but, while away at boarding school and her first year of college, her parents thought that she "looked fabulous, in fact, never better!" It was only during her summer vacation at home that her parents began to note that she hardly ate, and they arranged for an evaluation. At the consultation, Ms. B's dad proclaimed that, "we are just here for you to tell our daughter what she needs to eat!" Ms. B appeared sad and annoyed, as she did not think that there was a problem being five-foot eight-inches and weighing ninety-eight pounds.

Ms. B had little to report other than that she was "fine." The family had endured numerous losses and tragedies: a cousin had killed herself at age twenty, the family business was near bankruptcy, the housekeeper of twelve years had just died, and the family dog had been run over accidentally by a neighbor. It sounded overwhelming, and yet the parents were amazed that the therapist thought these circumstances constituted "a big deal."

Ms. B reluctantly opened up and described her ambivalent relationship with her powerful father whom she feared and revered and she recounted the sadness she felt for her mother who lived in a loveless marriage. Ms. B revealed that not only were there things that she was not prepared to discuss, but that she could not even trust her own memory. The patient then shared a series of vivid childhood traumatic memories. At the same time, she wondered whether they could be "a figment of my imagination." It was clear that this sensitive and vulnerable young woman had a complex story with traumatic elements. The therapist's impression was that Ms. B had had AN for several years, coupled with depression. He recommended that she be hospitalized to initiate nutritional rehabilitation in a structured adolescent medicine unit that specialized in EDs. The family was reluctant. As her vital signs were stable, and the weight loss was not acute, the therapist arranged to see Ms. B several days later.

The therapist encouraged her to consider a trial of outpatient nutritional rehabilitation coupled with individual psychotherapy. Although Ms. B stated that she was "confused," she reluctantly agreed to accept the proposed plan. Despite her cooperative stance, however, weight gain was not accomplished during the first four weeks of outpatient treatment, and she then agreed to inpatient care. Ms. B was hospitalized for six weeks on an inpatient adolescent medical unit. Weight gain was targeted at approximately 2.5 pounds per week. During the first month, however, only five pounds were gained, and she was transferred to an EDs unit.

The patient spent three months on the locked EDs unit at a tertiary care, university-based psychiatric hospital. Weight gain to the goal set was accomplished with a liquid diet. The patient was then transferred to the EDs day treatment program. This program operated five days per week from 8:30 am until 5:30 pm. It included three meals and two snacks daily, as well as therapeutic activities, and individual, group, and family psychotherapy. Ms. B struggled upon returning home, and her weight quickly plummeted. Day treatment appeared not to provide sufficient structure to prevent relapse. Following three weeks in the day program, the patient was re-admitted to the medical unit with dehydration and then transferred to the general psychiatric unit following disclosure of suicidal intent.

The family struggled with the treatment team and worried that "nothing was helping!" During the inpatient psychiatric admission, the patient disclosed that she was drinking alcohol heavily and was treated with an alcohol withdrawal protocol to prevent the emergence of withdrawal symptoms. The patient was then referred for aftercare to the drug treatment program. During this period, the patient formed a close working alliance with her drug treatment counselor, and managed to maintain her weight.

At follow-up, although the patient has struggled with her low weight for many years, she has managed to remain outside of a hospital for the past ten years. Treatment has focused on her sobriety and her need to maintain her weight. Despite having a Body Mass Index of only 16, the patient has maintained regular menses.

Ms. M

Ms. M was eleven years old when she first presented to the ED program at a tertiary care university medical center in suburban New York. Prepubertal, she had failed to make the expected weight gain necessary for growth. Her parents were reluctant to allow her to be hospitalized even though she had refused to cooperate with a weight restoration plan on an outpatient basis. It was a challenge to set limits for her on the adolescent medical unit, as she would call her parents who would then call the administration of the hospital, requesting a different approach and undermining the care. Family meetings attempted to engage the family and educate them about EDs, but were unsuccessful. The patient was discharged home and outpatient care was initiated, but was unsuccessful. Upon re-admission, the parents were more cooperative with the treatment team.

Despite this, they continued to undermine the therapeutic plan. The parents demanded a change of psychiatrists after their daughter complained. Not surprisingly, the patient continued to fail to make her weight goals and was not satisfied with her new psychiatrist. The patient was once again discharged home at the parents' insistence. Several weeks later, the patient was readmitted. Over the course of the first year of care, the patient was admitted five times.

It was later learned that the mother had a brother who had been hospitalized psychiatrically as a teenager and was now a chronic psychiatric patient living in a state psychiatric hospital. The patient had not known about her uncle. The parents believed that the uncle would have been "better off dead" than alive in a psychiatric hospital.

The patient was eventually transferred to a psychiatric unit where she reached her goal weight by age thirteen. Menarche followed, the patient was horrified, and she proceeded to lose weight until she was readmitted to an ED unit in a private freestanding psychiatric hospital. The patient was then admitted to a day program where she proceeded to lose the weight once again. Despite intensive individual psychotherapeutic efforts, family treatment, and pharmacological approaches, the patient was hospitalized over twenty times in five years. By the age of eighteen, she had osteopenia and chronic amenorrhea. The family was exhausted by her frequent crises. They began to make hopeless remarks such as, "If she doesn't wish to recover, what can we do?" They stated that not every person can be "saved." Despite our efforts to achieve weight restoration, it appeared that the patient, now a young adult, was headed for chronicity and eventual death. At the time of this writing, the patient is thirty years old and has severe osteoporosis. Wheel chair bound, the patient remains at a chronically low weight.

These two cases highlight the severity and complexity of the clinical course of individuals with AN. Ms. B had co-morbid depression and alcohol dependence, but after numerous treatment programs has managed to remain at a stable low weight with regular menses and working fulltime. Ms. M demonstrates chronic relapsing AN with poor outcome, despite intensive treatment over a long period of time, including all levels of medical and psychiatric care.

Conclusion

Although there are neither well established evidence based guidelines nor systematic controlled research studies, clinical decisions about patients and their families regarding the type and location and duration of treatment are made every day in this country and around the world. In this chapter, we have attempted to address the place of day treatment as a more recent therapeutic modality available to some individuals in some cities. The treatment of EDs is not unlike treatment of many other psychiatric illnesses in that "surveys conducted in academic centers have found that up to 40% of clinical decisions are unsupported by evidence from the research literature" (Geddes et al, 1996; Gray, 2004; Greenhalgh, 2001).

Although more research is needed to address the many still unanswered questions, we have directed our attention to some of the recent clinical and research issues concerning day treatment of eating disorders. While recognition of the limits of our knowledge is important, particularly in light of the paucity of scientifically based evidence to inform the decision-making process, growing clinical experience does suggest that day treatment is a valuable new modality in the spectrum of care for individuals with AN.

References

American Psychiatric Association. (2006). Practice guideline for the treatment of patients with eating disorders (revision). *American Journal of Psychiatry,* 157, (May Supplement), 11-65.

Anderson, A. E., Bowers, W., and Evans, K. (1997). Inpatient Treatment of Anorexia Nervosa. In D. M. Garner, and P. E. Garfinkel (Eds.), *Handbook of treatment for eating disorders* (2nd edition), 327-353). New York, NY: The Guilford Press.

Baron, S.A., Weltzin, J.E., and Kaye, W.H. (1995). Low discharge weight and outcome in anorexia nervosa. *American Journal of Psychiatry*, 152, 1070-1072.

Bruch, H. (1974). Perils of behavior modification in treatment of anorexia nervosa. *Journal of the American Medical Association*, 230, 1419-1422.

Cooper, P.J. (1995). Eating disorders and their relationship to mood and anxiety. In K.D. Brownell, and C.G Fairburn, (Eds.), *Eating disorders and obesity: A comprehensive handbook*. New York, NY: Guilford Press; 159-164.

Crisp, G.H., Norton, K., and Gowers S., (1991). A controlled study of the effect of therapies aimed at adolescent and family psychopathology in anorexia nervosa. *British Journal of Psychiatry,* 159, 325-333.

Dancyger, I., Fornari, V., Scionti, L., Wisotsky, W., and Sunday, S. (2005). Do daughters with eating disorders agree with their parents' perception of family functioning? *Comprehensive Psychiatry*, 46, 135-139.

Dancyger,I., Fornari, V., Schneider, M., Fisher, M., Frank, S., Goodman, B., Sison, C., and Wisotsky, W. (2003). Adolescents and eating disorders: An examination of a day treatment program. *Eating and Weight Disorders: Studies on Anorexia, Bulimia and Obesity,* 8, 242-248.

Danziger, Y., Carol, C.A., Varsono, I., Tyano, S., and Mimouni, M. (1988). Parental involvememt in treatment of patients with anorexia nervosa in a pediatric day-care unit. *Pediatrics*, 81,159-162.

Dare, C., and Ivan, E. (2000). A multi-family group day treatment programme for adolescent eating disorder. *European Eating Disorders Review*, 8, 4-18.

Fornari, V., Dancyger, I., Schneider, M., Fisher, M., Goodman, B., and McCall, A. (2001). Parental medical neglect in the treatment of adolescents with anorexia nervosa. *International Journal of Eating Disorders,* 29, 358-362.

Franzen, U., Backmund, H., and Gerlinghoff, M. (2004). Day treatment group programme for eating disorders: Reasons for dropout. *European Eating Disorders Review,* 31, 105-117.

Geddes, J.R., Game, D., Jenkins, N.E., et al. (1996). What proportion of primary psychiatric interventions are based on evidence from randomized controlled trials? *Quality in Health Care,* 5, 215-217.

Gerlinghoff, M., Backmund, H., and Franzen, U. (1998). Evaluation of a day treatment programme for eating disorders. *European Eating Disorders Review,* 6, 153-158.

Goldberg, S.C., Eckert, E.D., Casper, R.C., Halmi, K.A., Davis, J.D., and Roper, M.T., (1980). Factors influencing hospital differences in weight gain in anorexia nervosa. *Journal of Nervous and Mental Disease,* 168, 181-183.

Golden, N.H., Jacobsen, M.S., Schebendach, J., Solanto, M.V., Hertz, S.M., and Shenker, J.R. (1997). Resumption of menses in anorexia nervosa. *Archives of Pediatric and Adolescent Medicine*, 151, 16-21.

Gowers, S., and Bryant-Waugh, R. (2004). Management of child and adolescent eating disorders: the current evidence base and future directions. *Journal of Child Psychology and Psychiatry*, 45(1), 63-83.

Gray, G.E. (2004). *Concise guide to evidence-based psychiatry.* Washington DC: American Psychiatric Press.

Greenhalgh, T. (2001). *How to read a paper: The basics of evidence based medicine,* 2nd edition, London: BMJ Books.

Halmi, K. (2001). Inpatient treatment of eating disorders. In G. Gabbard (Ed.), *Treatment of psychiatric disorders* (3rd edition), 2119-2126. Washington DC: American Psychiatric Press.

Halmi, K.A., Eckert, E., Marchi, P., Sampugnaro, V., Apple, R., and Cohen, J. (1991). Comorbidity of psychiatric diagnoses in anorexia nervosa. *Archives of General Psychiatry*, 48, 712-718.

Herzog, D. B. (1988). Eating disorders. In A.J. Nicholi, (Ed.) *The new Harvard guide to psychiatry* (434-445). Cambridge, MA: The Belknap Press of the Harvard Press.

Herzog, W., and Beaumont, P. (2002). Day hospitalization programs for eating disorders: A systematic review of the literature. *International Journal of Eating Disorders*, 31, 1-5-117.

Howard, W., Evans, K., Quintero-Howard, C., Bowers, W., and Andersen, A. (1999). Predictors of success or failure of transition to day hospital treatment for inpatients with anorexia nervosa. *American Journal of Psychiatry*, 156,1697-1702.

Johnson, C.L. and Sansone, R.A. (1993). Integrating the twelve-step approach with traditional psychotherapy for he treatment of eating disorders. *International Journal of Eating Disorders*, 14(2), 121-134.

Kaplan, A. S., and Olmsted, M.P. (1997). Partial hospitalization. In D. M. Garner, and P. E. Garfinkel (Eds.), *Handbook of treatment for eating disorders* (2nd edition), 354-360. New York: The Guilford Press.

Kaplan, A. S., Olmsted, M.P., Carter, J.C., and Woodside, B. (2001). Matching patient variables to treatment intensity: The continuum of care. *Psychiatric Clinics of North America*, 24, 281-292.

Kong, S. (2005). Day treatment programme for patients with eating disorders: randomized controlled trial. *Journal of Advanced Nursing*, 51(1), 5-14.

Meads, C., Gold, L., and Burls, A. (2001). How effective is outpatient care compared to inpatient care for the treatment of anorexia nervosa? A systematic review. *European Eating Disorders Review*, 9, 229-241.

Olmsted, M., McFarlane, T., Molleken, L., and Kaplan, A.S. (2001). Day hospital treatment of eating disorders. In G. Gabbard (Eds.), *Treatment of psychiatric disorders* (3rd edition), 2119-2126. Washington DC: American Psychiatric Press.

Olmsted, M., and Kaplan, A.S. (1999). Relative effectiveness of a 4-day vs. 5-day hospital program. *Paper presented at the Eating Disorder Research Society Meeting*, San Diego, CA.

Piran, N., Langdon, L., Kaplan, A., and Garfinkel, P.E. (1989). Evaluation of a day hospital program for eating disorders. *International Journal of Eating Disorders,* 8, 523-532.

Robinson, P. (1993). Treatment of eating disorders in the United Kingdom. Part I. A Survey of Specialist Services. *Eating Disorders Review*, 1, 4-9.

Robinson, P. (2003). Day treatments. *Handbook of Eating Disorders*, 333-347.

Schmidt, U., and Asen, E. (2005). Editorial: does multi-family day treatment hit the spot that other treatments cannot reach? *Journal of Family Therapy,* 27, 101-103..

Tasca, G., Flynn, C., and Bissada, H. (2002). Comparison of group climate in an eating disorders partial hospital group and a psychiatric partial hospital group. *International Journal of Group Psychotherapy*, 52(3).

Thornton, T., Beumont, P., and Touyz, S. (2002). The Australian experience of day programs for patients with eating disorders. *International Journal of Eating Disorders, 32,* 1-10.

Vandereycken, W. (2003). The placement of inpatient care in the treatment of anorexia nervosa: Questions to be answered. *International Journal of Eating Disorders, 34*, 409-422.

Williamson, D.A., Thaw, J.M., and Varnado-Sullivan, P.J. Cost-effectiveness analysis of a hospital-based cognitive-behavioral treatment program for eating disorders. *Behavior Therapy,* 32, 459-477.

Wiseman, C.V., Sunday, S.R., Klapper, F., Harris, W.A., and Halmi, K.A. (2001). Changing patterns of hospitalization in eating disorder patients. *International Journal of Eating Disorders,* 30, 69-74.

Woodside, D., Wolfson, L., Garfinkel, P., Olmsted, M., Kaplan, A., and Maddocks, S (1995). Family interactions in bulimia nervosa I: study design, comparisons to established population norms, and changes over the course of an intensive day hospital treatment program. *International Journal of Eating Disorders,* 17(2), 105-115.

Zeeck, A., Herzog, T., and Hartmann, A. (2004). Day clinic or inpatient care for severe bulimia nervosa? *European Eating Disorders Review, 12,* 79-86.

Zipfel, S., Reas, D., Thornton, C., Olmsted, M., Williamson, D., Gerlinghoff, M., et al. (2002). Day hospitalization programs for eating disorders: a systematic review of the literature. *International Journal of Eating Disorders*, 31, 105-117.

In: Evidence-Based Treatments for Eating Disorders
Author: Ida F. Dancyger and Victor M. Fornari

ISBN 978-1-60692-310-8
© 2009 Nova Science Publishers, Inc.

Chapter VII

Medical and Nutritional Treatment of Children, Adolescents and Young Adults with Eating Disorders

Martin Fisher
New York University School of Medicine
New York, New York, USA

Abstract

During the past decade, several consensus statements have been published describing a team approach to the treatment of children, adolescents and young adults with EDs. This chapter utilizes these statements, along with the clinical experience of the author, to summarize four key areas in the state of knowledge of the medical and nutritional care of patients with EDs: (1) Issues of epidemiology and diagnosis are discussed, highlighting the difficulties in using strict DSM criteria in the younger age groups and the high frequency of EDNOS in adolescents. (2) A series of clinical issues are explored, including optimal goal weights, approaches to nutritional rehabilitation, criteria for hospital admission and discharge, the refeeding syndrome, and the role of behavior modification with younger patients. (3) Medical issues are reviewed, focusing on electrolyte disturbances and cardiovascular abnormalities; endocrine disorders and osteopenia / osteoporosis; other organ system (including gastroenterologic, neurologic, hematologic, immunologic and dermatologic) findings; and the medical work-up. And (4) The outcome literature for patients with EDs is summarized, demonstrating the improved outcome found in adolescents compared to adults.

While much of the treatment of patients with eating disorders (EDs) is performed by mental health professionals, the medical and nutritional aspects of care are often provided by physicians specializing in Pediatrics, Family Practice or Internal Medicine. These physicians are frequently joined by colleagues in nutrition or nursing to offer a comprehensive team approach. Many of the practitioners of this team approach are specialists in Adolescent

Medicine, who run several of the largest programs for the treatment of (EDs) in the United States and world-wide. These specialists treat children, adolescents and often young adults, in coordination with psychiatrists, psychologists, and social workers who provide the mental health care.

In 1995, the Society for Adolescent Medicine published a Position Statement and Background Paper describing this team approach and summarizing the state of knowledge on the treatment of EDs in children, adolescents and young adults to that point (Society for Adolescent Medicine, 1995; Fisher, et al., 1995). The Statement was updated in 2003, (Society for Adolescent Medicine, 2003) and the team approach it described was also included in statements by the American Psychiatric Association in 1993 and 2000 and the American Academy of Pediatrics in 2003 (American Psychiatric Association, 1993; American Psychiatric Association, 2000; American Academy of Pediatrics, 2003). The treatment approaches endorsed by these statements are based on expert opinion; there are very few studies that have been performed to provide specific evidence-based approaches in the medical and nutritional management of EDs in children and adolescents. This chapter will provide an update on the medical and nutritional treatment of EDs, beginning with a review of the epidemiology of EDs in children, adolescents and young adults, and concluding with a discussion of the outcome literature in these age groups.

Epidemiology

There are several statistics often quoted in the EDs literature regarding epidemiology: that the prevalence of anorexia nervosa (AN) in adolescent and young adult women is 0.5%; that 1-5% of young women have bulimia nervosa (BN); and that 5-10% of cases of EDs occur in males (Society for Adolescent Medicine, 2003; American Psychiatric Association, 2000).. It has also been said that EDs behaviors have been increasing over time, that EDs are being seen in increasingly younger ages, and that EDs are increasing in minority populations in the United States and in developing countries internationally (Society for Adolescent Medicine, 2003; American Psychiatric Association, 2000). What is the evidence to indicate the accuracy of this information and how do the statistics vary by age group?

There is clear evidence that children at increasingly younger ages are expressing concerns about their weight and participating in dieting behaviors (American Academy of Pediatrics, 2003; Krowchuk, Kreiter, Woods, Sinai and DuRant, 1998; Field, Carmago, Taylor, et al., 1999). However, there is no evidence that the numbers of cases of EDs are rising in those ages 11 years or below. In fact, the numbers of cases of true EDs in children remains small, with BN being almost non-existent in this age group and AN being limited to a relatively small group of children, who tend to be bright (hence, their precocity in having an adolescent illness) and who generally have an underlying anxiety and/or depressive disorder.

What is found in this age group that is usually not seen in those who are older, are several specific atypical EDs. These have been classified in an important article by Watkins and Lask to include several categories (Watkins and Lask, 2002): (1) Food avoidance emotional disorder (FAE), which is "a term used to describe children who have a primary emotional disorder in which food avoidance is a prominent feature;" (2) Selective eating, which describes children who "eat very few different foods and sometimes are particular about the brand of food or where the food was bought" and who have generally been this way since they were toddlers; (3) Functional dysphagia, which is characterized by "a fear of swallowing, vomiting or choking, which makes the child anxious about and resistant to eating normally, and which is often marked by a specific precipitant, such as having choked on a food or witnessing somebody else choking"; and (4) Pervasive refusal syndrome, which describes a very small subset of children with a life threatening condition who refuse to "eat, drink, walk, talk or care for themselves", "who are unwilling to communicate" and show "determined resistance to help." What distinguishes each of these atypical eating disorder from AN, BN and "eating disorder not otherwise specified" (EDNOS), is that they are not being driven by a fear of weight gain or a desire to be thin. Accordingly, treatment of these atypical EDs in children generally requires a behavioral approach, which is different from the full comprehensive approach required for AN, BN and EDNOS.

One other area of importance in children is that the diagnosis of AN differs in this age group. In addition to the obvious inability to use amenorrhea as a criterion for diagnosis in those who are premenarchal, the criterion of requiring weight loss to 15% below ideal body weight (IBW), as per the DSM IV, will also not apply to those who are not yet fully grown (American Psychiatric Association, 1994). This criterion is replaced instead by "failure to make expected weight gain during a period of growth leading to body weight <85% of that expected." When making the diagnosis, and evaluating the severity, of AN in children and early adolescents it is necessary, therefore, to construct a growth chart that plots the weights and heights throughout childhood in order to evaluate what weight and height an individual child would have been without the onset of decreased intake.

In the adolescent age group, the striking epidemiologic and diagnostic feature of EDs has been the finding that a very high percentage of teenagers with EDs have a diagnosis of EDNOS. In a study of 622 female patients presenting to an Adolescent Medicine eating disorders program between 1980 and 1995, we found that in 434 patients ages 9-19 years: 36% had a diagnosis of AN, 18% had a diagnosis of BN, 2% had a diagnosis of both AN and BN, and 41% had a diagnosis of EDNOS (Fisher, Schneider, Burns, Symons and Mandel, 2001). Of note in our study and others, the patients with EDNOS displayed the same psychiatric attributes and fear of weight gain as those who met full ED criteria and required the same intensity of treatment (Bunnell, Shenker, Nussbaum, et al., 1990). In most of the cases of EDNOS, full criteria for AN were not met because the patients had not yet had amenorrhea for three months or, more commonly, had not lost to 15% below IBW, often because they had started out significantly overweight. In some cases of EDNOS, full criteria for BN were not met because there was no binge-eating, despite very frequent vomiting, which in the author's clinical experience is a situation that occurs more commonly in adolescents than in adults.

In our study, we also found that only 2.5% of patients presenting for evaluation were male. This is different from the 5-10% range generally quoted in the literature (Carlat, Carmago and Herzog, 1997). We postulated several possible explanations for this discrepancy. It is possible that adolescent and young adult males are less likely to present for evaluation and treatment, both for psychological reasons (males being less open to treatment and more affected by the stigma of an ED diagnosis) and for physical reasons (there is no marker of amenorrhea to cause the patient and family to act as quickly). It is also likely that there are many males who have ED behaviors (such as decreased intake or vomiting) for sports-related weight control but who do not develop specific ED thinking (fear of weight gain, distorted body image). This is in contrast to the many females who develop both ED behaviors and thinking because of activities such as ballet and gymnastics. Also, there have been some studies of epidemiology that have included the diagnosis of binge eating disorder (BED), which occurs equally in males and females but is rarely seen in adolescents. Over time, however, the situation has changed. In recent years, with an increased emphasis on body shape in males, it appears that the number of adolescent and young adult males with eating disorders is rising. Unpublished data looking at adolescent patients presenting to our program between January 2006 and June 2007 revealed that 11.5% are male, more consistent with what had been previously reported in the general literature.

Our data also demonstrated that 45% of our adolescent patients were "middle class", 48% "upper class" and 7% "lower class" (Fisher, Schneider, Burns, Symons and Mandel, 2001). Although there have been some articles indicating that the classic finding of higher socioeconomic status in ED patients is not true, our data does not agree. We also found that 96% of our adolescent patients were white. Although there are indications in the literature that EDs are rising in Black and Hispanic populations, our studies in urban and suburban high schools have shown that there are major differences in weight perceptions between White and Asian adolescents on the one hand and Black and Hispanic adolescents on the other (Fisher, Pastore, Schneider, Pegler and Napolitano, 1994). It is these differences in perception that undoubtedly account for what is still a large discrepancy in ED diagnoses in different populations in the United States. On an international basis, there are both data and anecdotal evidence demonstrating increases in EDs as Western values are introduced to countries across the world (Becker, Burwell, Gilman, Herzog and Hanburg, 2002).

Treatment

There are several general treatment principles in the medical and nutritional management of children, adolescents and young adults with EDs that have received much attention in the literature and in clinical practice, along with a series of specific medical complications that also require careful attention. The general principles involve such questions as: (1) What are optimal goal weights for patients with EDs? (2) What are the most appropriate approaches to nutritional rehabilitation? (3) What are the criteria for hospital admission and discharge? (4) What is the refeeding syndrome and how is it prevented and treated? And (5) What is the role of behavior modification in treatment? The specific medical complications that require attention include: (A) Electrolyte disturbances and cardiovascular abnormalities; (B) Endocrine disorders and osteopenia / osteoporosis; and (C) Other organ system (including, neurologic, hematologic, immunologic and dermatologic) findings. Based on the discussion of medical complications comes one final question: (D) What should be included in the medical workup of the individual newly diagnosed with an ED? Each of these topics will be discussed in the next two sections:

(1) Establishing Optimal Goal Weights

From the time that the initial studies of Frisch in the 1970's demonstrated that most female patients with AN resume menses when they return to "90% of IBW," (Frisch and McArthur, 1974) it is this number that has been generally used as the treatment goal weight for most patients with AN, both female and male. While subsequent studies have shown this 90% figure for resumption of menses to be true for most patients, several issues have made the discussion more complicated over time:

A first issue is one of semantics, as the concept of "IBW" seems to inappropriately imply that there is a single best weight for each person. In reality, what has been called "IBW" for many years has really been "average body weight" for each individual's age, sex and height. This term, however, also has semantic implications since in this day and age few people want to be "average". A second issue involves the actual determination of "average body weight" since there are many growth charts and tables that have been used and these do not always agree. As a clinical short-hand, some people use the simple mnemonic of "100 pounds for 5 feet, and 5 pounds for every inch above that" for females and "106 pounds for 5 feet, and 6 pounds for every inch above that" for males to estimate average body weight in adolescents and young adults. The values calculated by this method end up being very similar to those determined by the various charts and tables and generally suffice for clinical use.

However, a third issue is the finding that the weight necessary for return of good health, including resumption of regular periods and a decreased psychological focus on weight and shape, is not determined solely by age, sex and height, but also by an individual's previous weight patterns, which in turn are influenced by eating habits, metabolism and genetics. From a clinical perspective, therefore, it is now known to be necessary to consider both "average body weight" for an individual's age, sex and height along with that person's previous maximum weight in establishing an appropriate goal weight for any individual. Finally, a fourth issue that must be considered is on-going growth in younger patients. Since girls generally gain approximately 8-10 pounds per year during early adolescence (and boys gain approximately 10-12 pounds per year during early to mid-adolescence), it is important to not establish a single goal weight for patients in this age group. Instead focusing on goal weights that return the patient to his or her growth curve, at which time normal growth and development can resume, should be the focus in the older child or young adolescent with an ED (Golden, Lanzkowsky, Schebendach, Palestro, Jacobson and Shenker, 2002).

(2) Nutritional Rehabilitation

Weight restoration is clearly one of the major components of treatment for AN, while nutritional guidance serves as an adjunctive part of treatment for BN. If one considers medical stabilization to be the key short-term treatment modality and mental health care to be the key to long-term outcome, then nutritional rehabilitation is certainly the key component of intermediate-term care for patients with EDs. In patients with AN, it is weight restoration that allows both medical stabilization and improvements in mental health to occur. There is much evidence that reversal of malnutrition is one of the prerequisites for the reversals in thinking that need to take place over time.

There are several general principles that are applied in the course of providing nutritional rehabilitation, but the details of how weight gain is accomplished varies from program to program, with no studies in the literature demonstrating the superiority of any one approach (Schebendach and Nussbaum, 1992; Rock and Curran-Celentano, 1996; Golden and Meyer, 2004). In general, hospitalized patients are expected to gain 2-4 pounds per week and out-patients are expected to gain 1-2 pounds per week, while those in partial hospitalization programs should gain somewhere in between. In all settings, patients are started on relatively small amounts of calories (generally around 1400 calories per day) to avoid the refeeding syndrome in those who are severely malnourished, as described below, and to allow for physiologic and psychologic adaptation in all patients, as described later in the chapter. Ultimately, most patients require between 2000 and 3000 calories per day for sustained weight gain.

How patients are counseled to accomplish these goals is variable. Most hospitalized patients receive their calorie intake via supervised meals and snacks; some patients require an all liquid diet, either via a naso-gastric tube or orally, and some programs rely on these approaches more than others. In the out-patient setting, some nutritionists rely on strict-calorie counts; some utilize an "exchange system" (i.e., distributing an appropriate amount of carbohydrates, protein and fat throughout the day); some provide daily or weekly menus; and some provide only the loose framework of an appropriate diet, with increases or decreases based on changes in weight over time. These same approaches are applied to patients with BN, although the main goal for these individuals is usually stabilization of eating patterns, decreasing binging/purging and maintenance of weight. As noted, there are no studies to indicate that any one in-patient or out-patient approach is preferable. In our own settings over the years, we have used all of these approaches based both on patient or family needs and personnel preference, and have not observed any major differences from a clinical perspective.

One interesting adjunct utilized in the provision of nutritional rehabilitation is the use of metabolic rate testing (Golden and Meyer, 2004). Machines are available to measure an individual's metabolism at any point in time. Patients with malnutrition generally have a low metabolism, as a way to preserve energy, and metabolism increases as weight is gained. This progress can be followed during treatment, with the initial low metabolism serving as a "proof" of the abnormality to skeptical patients, and continued low values demonstrating that there is still more to accomplish. In our setting, we find that hospitalized patients generally start out with metabolic rates that are approximately 70% of expected for age and sex; out-patients are usually at about 80%; and those patients who have resumed menses are generally at 90-100% of expected. This information can often help provide guidance for the clinicians, explanations for the family, and motivation for the patient.

(3) Hospital Admission and Discharge

Criteria for when patients with EDs should be admitted for in-patient hospitalization have been published in several versions during the past decade (Fisher, Golden, Katzman, et al., 1995; American Academy of Pediatrics, 2003). The first criterion in all versions is "<75% of IBW," indicating that under most circumstances patients are admitted to the hospital at around the time they have fallen to approximately 25% below the average body weight for their age, sex and height. Other medical, nutritional and psychological factors included in the criteria, as outlined in the version published by the Society for Adolescent Medicine, are listed in Table 1.

These factors include several physiologic abnormalities (hypotension, hypothermia, orthostatic changes) that tend to occur for most patients at about the time they have lost 75% of IBW, but whose presence may require hospitalization with lesser amounts of weight loss, and whose absence may allow out-patient treatment for those who are 25-30% below "ideal body weight." Specific definitions have been applied to the criteria of bradycardia (<50 beats/minute daytime, <45 beats per minutes night-time) and orthostatic hypotension (a decrease of 20mm Hg in systolic blood pressure and 10 mm Hg in diastolic blood pressure when going from lying to standing), but there is no evidence to indicate that these numbers must be strictly adhered to. For instance, there are patients with pulse rates in the 40's who are athletes and/or have a family history of bradycardia and who are approximately 25% below IBW who may not require immediate hospitalization.

Also included in the criteria are several that apply more commonly to BN than to AN (electrolyte disturbances, cardiac dysrhythmia, uncontrollable binging and purging), some that are related to treatment (failure of out-patient treatment, arrested growth and development), those that may indicate a more acute situation (dehydration, acute food refusal), and several specific medical complications (syncope, seizures, cardiac failure, pancreatitis, etc). Indicators of psychiatric severity, either acute (suicidal ideation, acute psychosis) or comorbid diagnoses that interfere with treatment (severe depression, obsessive compulsive disorder, severe family dysfunction) are also included in the criteria. Throughout the United States, most patients are admitted to psychiatric units, while some are admitted to medical units. This is sometimes determined by whether it is the medical or psychiatric status that is causing the need for hospitalization, but is more often determined by unit availability in the particular geographic region. There are no studies that have determined a difference between treatment on a medical unit verses a psychiatric unit, with clinical evidence indicating that both can be equally successful when they contain a dedicated program for treatment of EDs.

In contrast to admission, there are no published criteria to provide guidelines for hospital discharge. In reality, while the criteria for admission have remained essentially unchanged during the past three decades, decisions regarding discharge have changed as pressure from the insurance industry has increased over time (Kaye, Kaplan and Zucker, 1996). Throughout the 1980s patients generally remained in the hospital until they reached 90% of IBW, which was the standard that was felt to give the best chance for full recovery in subsequent out-patient treatment. Since the early 1990s patients have generally been discharged closer to 15-20% below IBW, sometimes with a day program providing the next step in care. While there is a general feeling that the shorter time of hospitalization has adversely affected outcome for many patients, and a few studies have demonstrated this effect, it has been difficult to definitely prove this finding, and it is unlikely that the financial climate will ever allow for a return to longer hospitalizations (Baran, Weltzin and Kaye, 1995; Silber and Robb, 2002).

Table 1. Indications for Hospitalization in an Adolescent With an Eating Disorder

1) Severe malnutrition (weight $\leq 75\%$ average body weight for age, sex and height)
2) Dehydration
3) Electrolyte disturbances (hypokalemia, hyponatremia, hypophosphatemia)
4) Cardiac dysrhythmia
5) Physiological instability

    a.   Severe bradycardia (heart rate <50 beats/minute daytime; <45 beats/minute at night)
    b.   Hypotension (<80/50 mm Hg)
    c.   Hypothermia (body temperature $<96^0$ F)
    d.   Orthostatic changes in pulse (>20 beats per minute) or blood pressure (>10 mm Hg)

6) Arrested growth and development
7) Failure of outpatient treatment
8) Acute food refusal
9) Uncontrollable binging and purging
10) Acute medical complications of malnutrition (e.g., syncope, seizures, cardiac failure, pancreatitis, etc.)
11) Acute psychiatric emergencies (e.g., suicidal ideation, acute psychosis)
12) Comorbid diagnosis that interferes with the treatment of the eating disorder (e.g., severe depression, obsessive compulsive disorder, severe family dysfunction)

(4) The Refeeding Syndrome

The development of medical complications, and even death, from the rapid refeeding of those who are severely malnourished was prominently discovered toward the end of World War II, with the liberation of the concentration camps in Europe. The phenomenon received attention in the EDs field in the early 1990s, with the decrease in length of stay, as discussed above, and the subsequent re-admission of more severely malnourished patients with anorexia nervosa.

The medical complications most notable in the refeeding syndrome are neurological (stupor, coma, death), cardiac (cardiac failure) and hematologic (hemolytic anemia). These complications occur secondary to the development of hypophoshatemia, which is thought to develop because of an ability to produce enough adenosine triphosphate (ATP) in depleted individuals as their previously dormant enzyme systems increase activity with the introduction of renewed nutrition (Solomon and Kirby, 1990)..

It is rare to encounter the refeeding syndrome in those who are less than 30% below IBW; it most commonly occurs in those rare patients who are greater than 40% below IBW. It occurs most often in those who are refed by an intravenous or nasogastric approach, but we have documented the onset of severe hypophosphatemia even with oral refeeding (Birmingham, Alothman and Goldner, 1996; Kohn, Golden and Shenker, 1998; Fisher, Simpser and Schneider, 2002).

Because of the refeeding syndrome, patients with EDs on in-patient units are generally refed slowly, most programs beginning with 1000-1400 calories per day and increasing 100-200 calories every 1-2 days. Phosphorus supplementation is given to those who are more severely malnourished and/or who are exhibiting low or decreasing phosphorus levels on daily laboratory testing. No specific criteria have been developed for the use of phosphorus supplementation, but there are no significant dangers to its overuse, so most in-patient programs have liberalized their use of phosphorus supplementation in recent years.

It is also worth noting that edema develops more rapidly in those who are more severely malnourished. Therefore, it is important not to provide too much fluids, either intravenously or orally, in the early stages of in-patient treatment. We have seen cases where it has taken weeks to months for acute signs of edema to dissipate and months to years for chronic signs of edema (such as ankle swelling late in the day) to resolve completely.

(5) Behavioral Modification

For the younger patient with AN, behavior modification is often one of the mainstays of treatment. In the team approach, this aspect of care is usually applied by the medical team, thus allowing the mental health team to provide psychological care without being placed in the role of an "enforcer". There are no studies looking at various behavioral approaches and their effectiveness, but it is apparent clinically that for many patients with AN, there must be an "or else" component of care in order to accomplish required changes in eating patterns and increases in weight. It is understood that a behavioral plan does not substitute for appropriate mental health care, but serves instead to provide external motivation when internal cues are absent. It is also understood that behavioral plans are used much less often for BN, since behaviors such as vomiting or laxative abuse cannot be as readily monitored as can weight changes in those with AN.

In many cases, discussing a change from one level of care to the next may serve as an effective behavioral plan. Thus the practitioner in a community setting may discuss making a referral for specialty care; or the specialist in the out-patient setting may discuss when it will be necessary for the patient to be placed in a day program or in-patient program; or the team in a medical program may discuss transfer to a psychiatric setting. When those discussions take place with adolescent patients it is necessary that parents support the plan; if they do, then the adolescent understands that it is no longer an issue of whether there will be weight gain, but only a question of where that weight gain will occur. If the patient complies, then the discussion serves as a behavioral modification approach; if the patient cannot or does not comply, then the move to the next level of care takes place. Either way, the next phase of required weight gain is accomplished. In our own practice, "weights and dates" are sometimes used to operationalize the plan (Fisher, 2006). This approach can be utilized for other behavioral plans (such as restriction of sports or other activities) as necessary in the out-patient setting. In the in-patient setting, it is more common to have several privileges on the unit (such as use of telephones and other equipment, mobility on/off the unit, increased meal choices, increased flexibility of snacks) serve as the incentive for weight increases. Although not formally studied, it is pretty clear that these behavioral approaches are necessary for successful treatment of most young patients with EDs.

Medical Complications

(A) Electrolyte Disturbances and Cardiovascular Abnormalities

Although it may seem a surprise, almost all patients with EDs are found to have normal electrolytes on laboratory testing (Fisher, 1992; Palla and Litt, 1998; Katzman, 2005). In those with AN, electrolyte disturbances are exceedingly rare; when they occur they are not due to malnutrition per se, but rather to fluid manipulation on the part of the patient. Some patients may exhibit hypernatremia as they keep themselves very dry (often so they can appear drawn and as thin as possible) while others may have hyponatremia because of water loading (sometimes done out of habit or to suppress appetite, but usually done to add pounds to the scale for weight checks). It is the latter finding that can be dangerous, as we and others have seen patients who develop hyponatremic seizures, even resulting in coma. For this reason it is important to check electrolytes in patients with AN, at the beginning of treatment, whenever there is a significant weight change, and at selected times throughout the course of treatment.

It is even more important to check electrolytes in patients with BN. Either vomiting or laxative use can cause a hypochloremic, hypokalemic metabolic alkalosis, which in turn can cause cardiac arrhythmia and sudden death. There is no clear relationship between the amount of vomiting or laxative use and the levels of potassium (K^+), chloride (Cl^-) or carbon dioxide (CO_2), but it is clear that patients who participate in both vomiting and laxative (or diuretic) use are at increased risk. On a clinical basis, when following electrolyte levels in patients with bulimia nervosa, one generally sees a rise in CO_2 first, a decrease in Cl^- second, and a decrease in K^+ third. It is crucial to respond to changes in electrolyte levels in bulimia nervosa by very close monitoring of CO_2 and Cl^- and by immediate hospitalization for the onset of hypokalemia. There is no definite protocol for when to admit to the hospital, (i.e. what levels of potassium definitely requires hospitalization – we generally use ≤ 3.0 or 3.1 mmol / L), how to treat (IV bolus vs IV drip; intensive care unit vs standard medical unit), or how long to keep patients in the hospital (we recommend allowing enough time for replenishment beyond just returning to normal electrolytes). It is known, however, that hypokalemia must be taken very seriously because among the medical causes of mortality in patients with EDs this has been the most common, and there are anecdotal reports that treating with oral potassium is not sufficient to prevent sudden death. It is thus crucial that all practitioners who treat patients with BN be aware of this potential complication and that all such patients be monitored.

The cardiovascular changes associated with AN and BN also require attention. The bradycardia and orthostatic hypotension associated with anorexia nervosa are considered evidence of cardiovascular instability and are utilized as criteria for hospitalization, but thankfully, neither symptom has been reported to lead to sudden death and both resolve with renourishment. In contrast, a prolonged QT may at times be found on the electrocardiogram; this finding, which might possibly be exacerbated by malnutrition in anorexia nervosa or more likely by hypokalemia in BN, can be a cause of sudden death and requires careful monitoring. Patients with severe malnutrition can also show evidence of a pericardial effusion on the echocardiogram, which resolves with refeeding. Ipecac, which is used as a purgative by some patients with BN, can cause an irreversible cardiomyopathy, which has led to fatality in some case reports.

(B) Endocrine Disorders and Osteopenia / Osteoporosis

In response to the state of malnutrition that develops in individuals with AN, several hormonal changes occur in order to preserve energy (Fisher, 1992; Palla and Litt, 1998; Katzman, 2005). Levels of thyroid hormone are decreased, as a way to lower the metabolism; this takes place both through a decrease in production at the hypothalamic level (leading to low levels of T_3, T_4 and TSH) and through development of the "euthyroid sick syndrome" (increased conversion of T_4 to reverse T_3 instead of T_3). On laboratory testing, T_4 levels are generally found to be at the lower limits of normal and T_3 levels are usually below normal. Treatment for this condition is simply nutritional restoration; it is important not to mistakenly give thyroid hormone to patients with AN since that will exacerbate the weight loss. The distinction between patients with AN and patients with primary thyroid disease is found in the TSH; patients with AN have low or normal TSH values, while those with primary hypothyroidism have elevated levels of TSH.

Values of LH, FSH and estradiol are also decreased in patients with AN. The amenorrhea that results, which is part of the diagnostic criteria of the illness, leads to the major long-term complication of AN, bone density findings of osteopenia and osteoporosis (Bachrach, Guido, Katzman, et al., 1990; Katzman and Zipursky, 1997; Castro, Lazaro, Pons, et al., 2000). These are measured using dual energy x-ray absorptiometry (DEXA), with osteopenia defined as $\geq$-1.0 standard deviation (SD) below the mean for age and sex and osteoporosis defined as $\geq$-2.5 SD below the mean. Under normal circumstances, bone density increases throughout the adolescent years before decreasing slowly beginning in the early to mid 20s and more rapidly after menopause. In those with AN, bone density falls during the time that the patient has amenorrhea, thus causing problems from both the lack of expected increases during the adolescent years and the on-going decreases that are similar to those that occur in menopause.

There is only one treatment, which is to return to normal eating, normal weight and regular periods; all other treatments that have been studied (including hormonal replacement, calcium and vitamin D, exercise, and bisphosphanates) have been shown to not protect the bones during the time of amenorrhea (Golden et al., 2002; Golden, 2003; Robinson, Bachrach and Katzman, 2000; Klibanski, Biller, Schoenfeld, et al., 1995; Grinspoon, Thomas, Miller, et al., 2002; Golden, Iglesias, Jacobson, Carey, Meyer, Schebendach, et al, 2005; Miller, Greico, Mulder, Grinspoon, Mickley, Yehezkel, et al., 2004). Thus, when individuals with AN return to having normal periods they will resume increasing their bone density; however, they will never be able to fully make up what was lost during the previous months or years, leaving them to enter their later years in life with a lower bone density than would have been expected based on their genetic predisposition. It is therefore important that treatment of EDs include a focus on returning to normal periods as quickly as possible. As noted, data show that this occurs generally around the return to 10% below ideal body weight, and that resumption of menses may occur immediately for some patients but may take up to 6 months for others. It is worthwhile to note that patients with bulimia nervosa may also have irregular menstrual periods, even if they are at normal weight, and that this irregularity may also have an affect on bone density, though not as severely as for those with AN.

(C) Other Medical Conditions

Almost all patients with EDs have gastrointestinal symptoms at some point during the course of the illness.[29-31] In AN there may be gastrointestinal symptoms during starvation, or more commonly, during refeeding. Symptoms can include abdominal pains, and there is often constipation, occasionally diarrhea, sometimes nausea, and rarely vomiting. Studies show prolonged gastric emptying times and decreased peristalsis. The gastrointestinal symptoms in AN may interfere with weight gain, but are almost never dangerous. Medications to provide symptomatic relief are sometimes provided but should be used sparingly. In BN, gastrointestinal symptoms are usually due to esophageal irritation. This symptom is also usually not dangerous, but the rare case of an esophageal tear can potentially occur. We carefully evaluate any patient with BN who indicates they see blood when they vomit.

Hematologic complications for patients with malnutrition include: (a) anemia, which is generally mild because the amenorrhea protects from development of iron deficiency; (b) neutropenia, which can occur with more significant weight loss; and (c) thrombocytopenia, which occurs in only the most severe cases of malnutrition. Treatment for the hematologic changes is refeeding; it is very rare for any other treatment to be required (Fisher, 1995; Pall and Litt, 1998; Katzman, 2005). Similarly, although multiple immunologic changes have been discussed in the literature, none have been found to have clinical significance or any requirement for treatment (Fisher, 1995; Palla and Litt, 1998; Katzman, 2005).

Patients with EDs rarely have pulmonary or renal complications. Neurologic complications include hyponatremic seizures, as described previously, and occasionally a peripheral neuropathy that occurs in those who lose a large amount of weight rapidly and that is responsive very quickly to refeeding. Many studies have shown that there is atrophy of brain tissue in those with EDs who lose large amounts of weight, especially if done rapidly; it is thought that these changes are reversible, but few studies have been done to demonstrate that, and there are some hints that mild neuropsychological effects of malnutrition can be long-lasting (Kingston, Szmuckler, Andrewes, Tress, Desmond, 1996).

(D) Medical Evaluation

The medical work-up recommended in the literature for patients with EDs follows directly from the discussion of medical complications (Fisher, 1992; Palla and Litt, 1998; Katzman, 2005). Laboratory tests that should be performed on all patients at presentation include a complete blood count (CBC) and metabolic panel (CMP) along with thyroid hormone studies. Patients with amenorrhea are also tested for levels of LH, FSH, estradiol and prolactin and those with amenorrhea of 6-12 months or more may undergo bone density testing. Patients with bradycardia or significant vomiting will generally have an EKG, while those who are hospitalized with severe malnutrition may also have an echocardiogram. For patients in whom the diagnosis of an ED is not completely clear, additional tests (such as an MRI of the brain or studies of the upper or lower intestinal tract) may be performed. On-going tests are performed at other points in the course of treatment for some patients, especially those with BN at risk for hypokalemia or those with AN who have not had resumption of menses despite reaching appropriate goal weight.

Outcome

Those who treat younger patients with EDs have advocated taking an aggressive approach to the nutritional and behavioral aspects of treatment with the hope that restoring the patient to normal weight as quickly as possible will result in a better outcome. While no controlled studies have compared more aggressive treatments, that include behavioral modification techniques, to slower approaches, that utilize mostly interpersonal therapy, it is instructive to compare the known outcome data for younger patients with EDs, who tend to have a more acute illness, to older patients, whose course has generally been more chronic.

The outcome literature for patients with EDs in all age group includes over 100 studies that have been performed during the past four decades (Fisher, 2003). These studies show that "approximately half of all patients do well over time with core issues of AN, whereas the rest are split between those who do reasonably well but continue to have symptoms (30% of the total) and those who do poorly (20% of the total)." In those studies where it is possible to distinguish between adolescents and adults, it appears that the younger patients do somewhat better, but not dramatically so. However, most of the studies are from psychiatric hospitals, therefore not including adolescents who are treated as either in-patients or out-patients in Adolescent Medicine settings. The few studies that have evaluated outcome in those setting have also found a somewhat better prognosis. One long-term study from Strober et al in a psychiatric setting, showed a good outcome at 6-7 years of follow-up for 50% of adolescent patients, and 75% (compared to 42% in adults) at 10-12 years (Strober, Freeman and Morrell, 1997). It can thus be concluded that adolescents with AN do have a somewhat better prognosis than adults and that an aggressive approach to treatment is therefore warranted, although success is certainly not guaranteed. For BN, the same general outcome statistics apply (50% excellent, 30% good, 20% poor) but no specific data exists for the adolescent age group (Fisher, 2002).

Case Vignette

SR is an 18 year old college freshman who presented to the Division of Adolescent Medicine because of weight loss of 20 lbs and amenorrhea for 18 months.

SR reported weighing approximately 125 lbs at a height of 66 ¾ inches in 10th and 11th grades, with normal periods and a slight desire to lose weight. During the summer after 11th grade she decided to "eat healthier" with no specific weight loss goal in mind, but over time "became obsessive about it." She lost weight throughout 12th grade, falling to 119 lbs by October, 114 lbs by January, 108 lbs by June, and 106 lbs when she entered college locally. She did not have a period throughout 12th grade and developed abdominal pains; she saw a gastroenterologist, who performed an upper endoscopy that was negative. SR denied any vomiting, bingeing or laxative / diuretic use, but did use an exercise tape for 20 minutes daily and went to a gym for 30 minutes, 3-4 days per week.

SR's family attempted a "home refeeding program" on their own during the first semester of college, without the help of a therapist or nutritionist, but when that failed and she remained at 105-106 lbs for 8 months, they brought her to the Division of Adolescent Medicine for evaluation and treatment. Her diet on admission consisted of oatmeal and milk for breakfast, a turkey and cheese sandwich for lunch, a variable amount of the family meal and desert for dinner, and a granola bar, fruit or pretzels as snacks; this was calculated to add up to approximately 1300 calories per day by the Adolescent Medicine nutritionist. SR indicated that she was never very happy in high school socially, that college is only somewhat better, and that she had a boyfriend for one year in high school, but broke up during the summer after 11th grade; she acknowledges this may have been the precipitant for her eating disorder.

At presentation, SR said she did not want to either gain or lose weight from her 105 lbs, which was calculated to be 22% below her "ideal body weight" of 134 lbs. Vital signs at evaluation were BP 116/75 and pulse 54 with an otherwise normal physical examination. Initial laboratory tests showed a normal CBC and electrolytes, normal liver and thyroid functions, along with a cholesterol of 252 mg/dl, estradiol 22 pg/ml, LH 0.4 IU/L, FSH 6.3 IU/L, and prolactin 5.9 mg/ml. A treatment plan was begun, which consisted of appointments with the Adolescent Medicine physician and nutritionist every 2-3 weeks and a therapist weekly.

The nutritionist increased SR's calories to 1800-2000 per day but she struggled for the first 6 weeks of treatment. The physician suggested that the family consider a day program admission for the summer, an idea that was not appealing to SR. In response to that suggestion, SR increased her calories as an out-patient such that her weight reached 115 lbs by the 3rd month of treatment and 120 lbs by the 6th month. Menstruation returned in the 9th month of treatment, but bone density showed osteopenia of the spine and hip.

By one year of treatment, SR has remained at 120 lbs, continues to eat well, her fears of weight gain are mostly gone, and she has had 3 consecutive normal periods. She continues to work with the nutritionist on lowering her saturated fat intake (in order to control the hyperlipidemia, which has a strong family history) while also increasing calories. She is working on getting back to her original high school weight of 125 lbs, which is a weight at which she feels comfortable and which also provides a cushion to protect against any future episodes of weight loss.

References

American Academy of Pediatrics (2003). Policy Statement: Identifying and treating eating disorders. *Pediatrics*, 111:204-11.

American Psychiatric Association (1993). Practice guidelines for eating disorders. *American Journal of Psychiatry*, 150:207.

American Psychiatric Association (1994). Diagnostic and Statistical Manual of Mental Disorders, 4th ed. Washington, DC, APA.

American Psychiatric Association (2000). Practice guidelines for the treatment of patients with eating disorders (revision). *American Journal of Psychiatry*, 157 (Suppl):1-39.

Bachrach LK, Guido D, Katzman D, et al. (1990). Decreased bone density in adolescent girls with anorexia nervosa. *Pediatrics*, 86:440-7.

Baran SA, Weltzin TE, Kaye WH (1995). Low discharge weight and outcome in anorexia nervosa. *American Journal of Psychiatry*, 152:1070-1072.

Becker AE, Burwell RA, Gilman SE, Herzog DB, Hamburg P (2002). Eating behaviors and attitudes following prolonged exposure to television among ethnic Fijian adolescent girls. *British Journal of Psychiatry,*180, 509-514.

Birmingham CL, Alothman AF, Goldner EM (1996). Anorexia nervosa: Refeeding and hypophosphatemia. *International Journal of Eating Disorders*, 20:2110-213.

Bunnell DW, Shenker IR, Nussbaum MP, et al. (1990). Subclinical versus formal eating disorders: Differentiating psychological features. *International Journal of Eating Disorders*, 9:357-62.

Carlat DJ, Camargo CA Jr, Herzog DB (1997). Eating disorders in males: a report on 135 patients. *American Journal of Psychiatry*, 154:1127-1132.

Castro J, Lazaro L, Pons F, et al. (2000). Predictors of bone mineral density reduction in adolescents with anorexia nervosa. *Journal of the American Academy of Child and Adolescent Psychiatry*, 39:1365-70.

Field AE, Camargo CA Jr, Taylor CB, et al. (1999). Overweight, weight concerns, and bulimic behaviors among girls and boys. *Journal of the American Academy of Child and Adolescent Psychiatry*, 38:754-760.

Fisher M (1992). Medical complications of anorexia and bulimia nervosa. *Adolescent Medicine: State of the Art Reviews*, 3:487-502.

Fisher M, Pastore D, Schneider M, Pegler C, Napolitano B (1994). Eating attitudes in urban and surburban adolescents. *International Journal of Eating Disorders*, 16:67-74.

Fisher M, Golden NH, Katzman DK, et al. (1995). Eating disorders in adolescents: A background paper. *Journal of Adolescent Health*, 16:420-437.

Fisher M, Schneider M, Burns J, Symons H, Mandel F (2001). Differences between adolescents and young adults of presentation to an eating disorders program. *Journal of Adolescent Health*, 28:222-227.

Fisher M, Simpser E, Schneider M (2002). Hypophosphatemia secondary to oral refeeding in anorexia nervosa. *International Journal of Eating Disorders*, 28:181-187.

Fisher M (2003). The course and outcome of eating disorders in adults and in adolescents: A review. *Adolescent Medicine: State of the Art Reviews*, 14:149-158.

Fisher M (2006). Treatment of eating disorders in children, adolescents and young adults. *Pediatrics in Review*, 27:5-15.

Frisch RE, McArthur JW (1974). Menstrual cycles: Fatness as a determinant of minimum weight for height necessary for their maintenance or onset. *Science*, 185:949.

Golden NH, Lanzkowsky L, Schebendach J, Palestro CJ, Jacobson MS, Shenker IR (2002). The effect of estrogen-progesterone treatment on bone mineral density in anorexia nervosa. *Journal of Pediatric and Adolescent Gynecology*, 15:135-143.

Golden NH (2003). Osteopenia and osteoporosis in anorexia nervosa. *Adolescent Medicine: State of the Art Reviews,* 14:97-108.

Golden N and Meyer W (2004). Nutritional rehabilitation of anorexia nervosa. Goals and dangers. *International Journal of Adolescent Medicine and Health*, 16:131-44.

Golden NH, Iglesias EA, Jacobson MS, Carey D, Meyer W, Schebendach J et al (2005). Alendronate for the treatment of osteopenia in anorexia nervosa: A randomized double-blind, placebo-controlled trial. *Journal of Clinical Endocrinology and Metabolism*, 90:3179-85.

Grinspoon S, Thomas L, Miller K, et al (2002). Effects of recombinant human IGF-I and oral contraceptive administration on bone density in anorexia nervosa. *Journal of Clinical Endocrinology and Metabolism*, 87:2883-91.

Katzman DK, Zipursky RB (1997). Adolescents with anorexia nervosa: The impact of the disorder on bones and brains. *Annals of The New York Academy of Sciences*, 817:127-37.

Katzman DK (2005). Medical complications in adolescents with anorexia nervosa: A review of the literature. *International Journal of Eating Disorders*, 37(suppl):52-59.

Kaye WH, Kaplan AS, Zucker ML (1996). Treating eating disorders patients in a managed care environment: Contemporary American issues and a Canadian response. *Psychiatric Clinics of North America*, 19:793-810.

Kingston K, Szmukler G, Andrewes D, Tress B, Desmond P (1996). Neuropsychological and structural brain changes in anorexia nervosa before and after refeeding. *Psychological Medicine*, 26:15-28.

Klibanski A, Biller BM, Schoenfeld DA, et al (1995). The effects of estrogen administration on trabecular bone loss in young women with anorexia nervosa. *Journal of Clinical Endocrinology and Metabolism*, 80:898-904.

Kohn MR, Golden NH, Shenker IR (1998). Cardiac arrest and delirium: Presentations of the refeeding syndrome in severely malnourished adolescents with anorexia nervosa. *Journal of Adolescent Health*, 22:239-243.

Krowchuk DP, Kreiter SR, Woods CR, Sinai SH, DuRant RH (1998). Problem dieting behaviors among young adolescents. *Archives of Pediatrics and Adolescent Medicine*, 152:884-888.

Miller KK, Greico KA, Mulder J, Grinspoon S, Mickley D, Yehezkel R et al. (2004). Effects of risedronate on bone density in anorexia nervosa. *Journal of Clinical Endocrinology and Metabolism*, 89:3903-6.

Palla B, Litt IF (1998). Medical complications of eating disorders in adolescents. *Pediatrics*, 81:613-623.

Robinson E, Bachrach LK, Katzman DK (2000). Use of hormone replacement therapy to reduce the risk of osteopenia in adolescent girls with anorexia nervosa. *Journal of Adolescent Health*, 26:343-8.

Rock CL, Curran-Celentano J (1996). Nutritional management of eating disorders. *Psychiatric Clinics of North America*, 19:701-713.

Schebendach J, Nussbaum MP (1992). Nutrition management in adolescents with eating disorders. *Adolescent Medicine: State of the Art Reviews*, 3:541-558.

Silber TJ, Robb AS (2002). Eating disorders and health insurance: Understanding and overcoming obstacles to treatment. *Child and Adolescent Psychiatry Clinics of North America*, 11:419-28.

Society for Adolescent Medicine (1995). Position Paper: Eating disorders in adolescents. *Journal of Adolescent Health*, 16:475-479.

Society for Adolescent Medicine (2003). Position Paper: Eating disorders in adolescents. *Journal of Adolescent Health*, 33:496-503.

Solomon SM, Kirby DF (1990). The refeeding syndrome: A review. *Journal of Parenteral and Enteral Nutrition*, 14:900-97.

Strober M, Freeman R, Morrell W (1997). The long-term course of severe anorexia nervosa in adolescents: Survival analysis of recovery, relapse and outcome predictors over 10-15 years in a prospective study. *International Journal of Eating Disorders*, 22:339-360.

Watkins B, Lask B (2002). Eating disorders in school-aged children. *Child and Adolescent Psychiatry Clinics of North America*, 11:185-199.

In: Evidence-Based Treatments for Eating Disorders   ISBN 978-1-60692-310-8
Author: Ida F. Dancyger and Victor M. Fornari   © 2009 Nova Science Publishers, Inc.

Chapter VIII

Evidence-Informed Care of Children with Eating Disorders

Sloane Madden
The Children's Hospital at Westmead
Sydney, Australia

Abstract

Eating disorders in children and adolescents are both prevalent and associated with considerable morbidity; however, the evidence base for the treatment remains weak. This chapter examines the frequency and types of eating disorder presentations seen in this age group as well as the evidence to guide their treatment. Particular emphasis is placed not only on child and adolescent specific evidence but also developmental issues and their impact on treatment presentations, treatment outcome and the use of adult treatment studies in guiding care. This chapter aims to provide clinicians with a framework for identifying and managing children and adolescents with eating disorders including where to treat, options for in and outpatient therapy and the role of medication.

Introduction

Despite increasing awareness of the occurrence of eating disorders (EDs) in children and adolescents, coupled with the understanding of high levels of morbidity and mortality associated with these disorders, the evidence base to guide the treatment and care of this group remains extremely limited. This lack of research stretches across all aspects of EDs in this age group including limited information about the prevalence and nature of EDs, the applicability of current DSM-IV and ICD-10 diagnostic criteria, treatment interventions and long-term outcomes.

This chapter will look specifically at the classic EDS, namely anorexia nervosa (AN), bulimia nervosa (BN) and related variants of these. It will not look at feeding disorders and eating difficulties seen in infants and younger children. In particular it will focus on in and out patient therapy for eating disorders in children and adolescence using the current evidence base available for this group and where necessary drawing on the adult treatment literature to address gaps in this evidence base.

One of the difficulties in reviewing the treatment literature in this age group has been the varying definitions of children and adolescents and the interchangeable use of the terms childhood onset eating disorders and early onset eating disorders. A number of criteria have been used to define these groups including age, pubertal status and menstrual status. In general childhood or early onset is defined as an ED commencing at or before 13 years of age (Peebles et al., 2006), or prior to the onset of puberty in males or menarche in females (Cooper et al., 2002). Due to the simplicity of age based cut-offs the majority of researchers are moving to this definition. Similar difficulties exist with defining adolescence with lower age limits ranging from 12 to 14 years and upper aged based cut offs ranging from 16 to 25 years. Additionally individuals aged 16 and over are frequently treated in adult based units and have been included in adult based treatment trials (Gowers et al., 2004). In this chapter children will generally refer to individuals up to the age of 12 years and adolescents as ranging from 13 to 18 years, a more narrow definition.

How Common are Eating Disorders in Children and Adolescents?

Community studies have shown lifetime prevalence rates for AN in women to range from 1.4 to 2% and with the inclusion of partial syndrome AN to be as high as 4.3% (Wade et al., 2006) and lifetime prevalence of BN to affect 4 to 7% of young women (Schmidt et al., 2007). While eating disorders are most commonly thought to have their onset in adolescence there are only a handful of epidemiological studies that have focused on adolescents and no published population based studies that have focused exclusively on children. Not only does this impact on our ability clearly describe the scale of the problem in this age group, the lack of findings make it difficult to clearly define the types of eating problems seen, particularly in children.

Three case register studies have included patients under the age of 18 years with rates of disorder varying widely between these studies. In the most recent of these studies incidence rates for AN of between 25.7 and 26.3 per 100 000 girls aged 10 to 14 years and 3.3 and 3.7 per 100 000 boys in the same age group were identified (Lucas et al., 1991 and Lucas et al., 1999). In the remaining two studies, also using the DSM IIIR diagnostic criteria but stricter weight loss criteria, incidence rates of between 4.2 and 9.2 per 100 000 girls aged 10 to 14 years (Nielsen 1990 and Joergensen 1992) were found. In all of these studies incidence rates in the 10 to 14 year old age group were approximately one third of those seen in the 15 to 19 year olds in these same studies

In their community based study of adolescent girls Lewinsohn et al., (2000) found life time prevalence rates for EDs in adolescent females were similar to those seen in adults with full syndrome AN or BN affecting 2.3% of individuals and partial syndrome AN or BN affecting 2.8% with full or partial syndrome BN not seen before 12 years of age. Interestingly when a sub-sample of adolescents were followed into early adulthood new cases of AN were extremely rare while BN continued to present at similar rates to those seen in late adolescence. Rates of EDs occurring in males in this sample were uncommon and accounted for around 1 in 20 of the total ED presentations.

Based on these findings it appears that AN is a disorder that most commonly has its onset in late adolescence with up to a quarter of all presentations first occurring in childhood. BN on the other hand is a disorder primarily presenting in late adolescence and early adulthood with only rare presentations in younger age groups. For these reasons it is not surprising that much of the research into EDs in children and adolescents has focused on AN with adolescent BN lumped in with adult-based research.

Are Eating Disorders in Children the Same as Those Seen in Adults?

Since the 1970's, epidemiological studies including clinical case series and case register studies have included individuals with childhood onset EDs, though with a few exceptions (Peebles et al., 2006, Irwin 1981 and Atkins et al., 1993) children have made up a small component of these studies and their results included in overall analyses. In almost all cases, studies including individuals with early onset EDs have looked exclusively at AN. As a result while a little is known about the incidence, onset, diagnostic characteristics and severity of illness outcomes of AN in children and adolescents (Peebles et al., 2006 and Bryant-Waugh 2000), almost nothing is known about the total spectrum of EDs in this age group.

From the small number of case series that have looked specifically at EDs in children it has been suggested that such individuals are less likely to report fear of weight gain and fatness (Lask et al., 1992), more likely to deny the severity of their illness (Fisher et al., 2001), more likely to present with non-specific somatic symptoms (Blitzer et al., 1961), more likely to be diagnosed with eating disorder not otherwise specified (EDNOS), less likely to be diagnosed with BN, more likely to be male, less likely to report vomiting or laxative abuse, to have lost weight more rapidly and to have a lower percentage ideal body weight than older individuals with EDs (Peebles et al., 2006). It is important to note that the study by Peebles et al., (2006) was the only study to include more than 100 children and the only study to compare them with older adolescents from the same cohort on multiple measures.

Developmental Considerations

As with all psychiatric disorders, ED presentations vary according to the developmental capacity of affected individuals. In EDs it must be remembered that not only are differences in psychological and social development important but that physical development is also vital to consider. These considerations have led to an ongoing debate in the literature about the applicability of current diagnostic criteria for EDs to children and younger adolescents. This is underlined by rates of EDNOS in studies of early onset EDs of between 50 and 60% (Peebles et al., 2006).

Current DSM-IV criteria for AN require patient concerns about body weight, disturbed body image and fear of weight gain. However, these criteria may not accurately reflect the clinical features in young children for several reasons. Compared with adults children have limited expressive language capacity, less ability to think in an abstract fashion and less awareness of emotions (WCEDCA 2007). Additionally the variable nature of normal growth in children undermine the utility of weight based cut offs in diagnosis and the use of amenorrhea as a marker of malnutrition. These differences may manifest in numerous ways including:

- Children may be unable to express distress in terms of body shape and weight but may instead describe somatic symptoms such as abdominal pain or discomfort once re-feeding commences
- Young children may not report fear of weight gain while at a low weight but may do so only when weight has been restored to a more healthy level
- Young children may be reluctant to confide their symptoms to adults for fear of censure
- While the presence of amenorrhea is an important diagnostic feature for AN in post-menarchal girls it may be a developmentally inappropriate criterion in young girls, in whom a history of delay in onset of puberty may be important
- The DSM-IV criteria specify that weight should be <85% of expected weight for height, however, this may lead to an underestimate of the severity of low weight in younger children in whom linear growth has also been affected (Gowers et al., 2004 and WCEDCA 2007).

In order to address these perceived deficiencies a number of groups have not only suggested modified diagnostic criteria for AN in children and adolescents but also the addition of a number of child specific diagnoses. Most prominent amongst these groups have been the Great Ormond Street (GOS) group in the UK who have not only proposed the GOS criteria for AN but also highlighted the diagnosis of Food Avoidant Emotional Disorder characterized by food avoidance in the absence of weight and shape concerns (Nicholls et al., 2000).

As with DSM-IV criteria for AN the GOS criteria focus on weight and eating abnormalities. However unlike DSM-IV, the GOS criteria allow for diagnosis to be made on the basis of behavior or psychological distortions rather than expressed psychological concerns alone. In particular the GOS criteria allows a diagnosis of AN to be made on the basis of determined food avoidance and weight loss or failure to gain weight in the absence of any physical or mental illness in addition to any two of the following: preoccupation with body weight, preoccupation with energy intake, distorted body image, fear of fatness, self-induced vomiting, extensive exercising or laxative abuse (Nicholls et al., 2000). This focus on behavior as well as reported concerns allows for diagnosis in younger children unable or unwilling to express their distress in terms of weight and shape concerns. In a review of 114 consecutive patients admitted for medical resuscitation at The Children's Hospital at Westmead, a large paediatric teaching hospital in Australia 87% of children met GOS criteria for AN while only 67% met DSM-IV criteria (Madden et al., 2005).

Food Avoidant Emotional Disorder

The term Food Avoidant Emotional Disorder (FAED) first coined in the 1980s to describe children with significant weight loss resulting from food avoidance in the absence of weight and shape concerns and underlying organic illness (Bryant-Waugh 2000 and Higgs et al., 1989). In this disorder, children frequently presented with non-specific medical complaints including abdominal pain, lethargy and nausea that were seen by the family as responsible for weight loss in addition to emotional problems, such as school avoidance, obsessional behavior or depression (Nicholls et al., 2002). Such children were reported to vehemently deny weight and shape concerns and to lack characteristic behaviors seen in AN including vomiting, exercise, laxative abuse and avoidance of high calorie foods.

Recently presented data on early onset eating disorders in Canada has highlighted the relative importance of FAED in children. In a prospective study of first presentation eating disorders in children between 8 and 12 years inclusive, latent class analysis identified 2 common presentations consistent with both AN and FAED. Over 35% of the 159 children identified fell into the FAED group. These children differed from those in the AN group in that they were less likely to be concerned about their weight or shape, did not have abnormal body image, were less likely to exercise and were more likely to have somatic complaints. Interestingly as a group they were no more likely than the AN group to have comorbid psychiatric illness or emotional distress (Pinhas et al., 2006).

While many children with FAED come to treatment because of the complications of malnutrition the lack of weight and shape concerns raises issues of late or missed diagnosis and appropriateness of current treatment interventions. In the future it will be important to clarify if this group of children are distinctly different to those with AN or whether they respond to existing treatments and face similar outcomes. In particular, is this group an early developmental presentation of AN or a distinct disorder?

In the Absence of a Strong Evidence Base for Child and Adolescent Eating Disorders is it Reasonable to Rely on Evidence in Adults?

One of the questions facing those treating children and adolescents with eating disorders is whether it is reasonable and in fact desirable to rely on adult findings in guiding treatment decisions. This is particularly relevant in the treatment of BN where treatment studies in children and adolescents are greatly outnumbered by large well run studies in adults. Similarly in AN, while there is an increasingly solid evidence base for the use of outpatient family therapy in the treatment of children and adolescents, the lack of studies in children with regard to inpatient care, individual therapy and medication management raises a similar dilemma.

Glowers and Bryant-Waugh (2004) have identified four specific issues in support of the use of adult based evidence in the treatment of children and adolescents including the similarity of AN and BN symptoms in adults and adolescents, the inclusion of older adolescents in adult treatment studies particularly for BN, the overlap between the developmental tasks of early adulthood and adolescence and the successful use of adult based psychological interventions for the treatment of children and adolescents with depression and obsessive compulsive disorder (OCD). Even if we accept such arguments it is important to be aware of the impact of differing cognitive capacity across age groups with developmentally limited communication skills, emotional expression and abstraction in children and younger adolescents when compared to adults. If treatments developed for adults are to be used in children this necessitates a preparedness to adapt such treatments to match the developmental capacities of children and adolescents being treated. This may be as simple as altering the language used to communicate with young people with EDs or involve changing the emphasis and focus of treatments to accommodate developmental realities.

Further complicating this picture are the differing physiological imperatives of children and adolescents including growth and puberty and the impact these have on the treatment priorities and goals. In particular the greater susceptibility of children and adolescents to the impacts of malnutrition requires a greater focus on intensive refeeding and preparedness for inpatient treatment earlier in the illness (Gowers et al., 2004). The impact of differing physiology in children is also relevant to medication management. Children and adolescents absorb and metabolize medications differently to adults leading to differential responses to both medication types and medication doses. This has been highlighted in the medication management of Major Depression in children and adolescents who have failed to respond to many medications that are effective in adults and been shown to develop serious side-effects not noted in adult medication trials (Hazell et al., 1995 and Mann et al., 2006)

Finally children and adolescents overwhelming live in families with parents and siblings. The nature of such relationships needs to be taken into account when planning treatment. Studies have clearly demonstrated the benefits the involvement of families treatment particularly in AN for children and adolescents (Rhodes et al., 2005), while legal requirements mandate the role of parents in consent to treatment as well as the ongoing care of children and younger adolescents.

Where to Treat

Options for treatment of EDs in children and adolescents range from specialised inpatient medical and psychiatric settings through to day-hospitals and a variety of outpatient treatments. There is little evidence to guide us as to which is the most appropriate setting with current guidelines based on consensus.

In its 2004 guidelines the National Institute of Clinical Excellence (NICE) in one of its key treatment recommendations for AN recommended specialist outpatient care as the treatment of choice for adults with AN. Interestingly despite strong evidence for the efficacy of outpatient family treatment in children and adolescents no similar recommendations were made for this younger age group.

While there are many potential advantages for managing children and adolescents in an outpatient setting and thereby allowing them to remain with their families, continue with education and maintain contact with peers many factors need to be considered in making this decision. In the case of children and adolescents it is critical to consider the availability of age appropriate treatment settings including access to educational facilities and placement with similar aged patients (NICE 2004 and APA 2006).

Admission for children and adolescents with AN is most commonly initiated because of medical concerns arising from weight loss and malnutrition. Critical indicators for admission include physiological instability including bradycardia, hypotension, hypothermia, dehydration, electrolyte abnormalities and cardiac arrhythmias. In children such changes can occur on the basis of rapid weight loss alone and as such absolute weight can not be relied on as a proxy for assessing medical risk. It is important to remember that children and adolescents are also more vulnerable to the ongoing risks of malnutrition due to its impact on puberty and growth.

Behavioral indicators for admission include severe comorbid psychiatric illness or substance abuse that prevents the initiation of outpatient care or would require admission in its own right, failure of outpatient care or a lack of appropriate supports to allow outpatient care. While motivation and eating behavior are critical in making decisions regarding admissions in adults, the presence of a motivated family often allows young people to remain in outpatient family treatment in the absence of motivation to change.

For BN outpatient care is the treatment of choice though indications for inpatient care may include severe comorbid medical complications including electrolyte abnormalities or cardiac complications arising from uncontained purging, severe comorbid psychiatric illness or severe symptoms that have failed to respond to specialised outpatient care. In such cases inpatient care to achieve containment is appropriate with referral back to outpatient care once containment has been achieved.

Treatment in the Inpatient Setting

AN is a serious psychiatric illness with severe medical morbidity and mortality and for this reason its psychological management is necessarily different to other psychiatric illnesses. In the inpatient management of children and adolescents with AN, significant malnutrition in association with medical compromise, is the rule rather than the exception. Such complications can be life threatening and dictate the need for acute medical resuscitation and monitoring, generating anxiety for both children and parents. Nutritional rehabilitation and weight restoration remain an important part of treatment for AN and are associated with decreased anorectic behavior, reduced psychological distress, improved cognitive performance, reduced morbidity and mortality. They are a prerequisite to benefiting from psychological and pharmacological interventions (Robb et al., 2002 and Halse et al., 2005).

It is the containment of this anxiety to allow resuscitation and refeeding that forms the basis of initial psychological treatment for patients with AN. The further aims of psychological intervention are; to contain eating disordered behaviors, facilitate the transition to safe eating, to develop better coping skills, and treat psychological comorbidity associated with the ED. Finally, an ED has a profound impact not only on the young person but also on their entire family. For this reason it is vital to consider and involve the patient's family in their treatment.

Managing the Ward Environment

For many decades the mainstay for promoting inpatient weight gain has been ward based behavioral treatment. Several outcome studies have demonstrated the efficacy of behavioral treatment in promoting weight gain in the short-term, though only in adult populations (Peterson et al., 1999). Despite this, behavioral programs are commonly used in child and adolescent treatment and guided by outcomes in adult treatment studies. While very strict behavioral programs have been used in the past it has been demonstrated that lenient programs produce similar gains in terms of weight and eating, lower levels of conflict and higher levels of patient satisfaction (Touyz et al., 1987).

It has been the author's experience that lenient behavioral programs with clear expectations for children and their parents are most effective in building and maintaining therapeutic alliances and managing eating disordered behaviors. In our own program parents and patients are provided with a copy of our eating disorder treatment program with explanations of treatment goals, refeeding, ward activities including school, group and physiotherapy, dining room rules, visiting hours, ward leave and appropriate interactions with other patients on the program and ward. The program works on a simple level system with progress based on medical well-being and safe eating. Progress through the level system allows more time away from the ward to practice healthy eating with family and friends. Over the years our own program has moved away from regulating all aspects of behavior to focusing on the facilitation of medical resuscitation, establishment of safe eating and containment of eating disordered behaviors.

Individual Psychotherapy in the Inpatient Setting

One of the theoretical benefits of inpatient treatment of AN is the capacity to provide intensive psychological therapy. This is appealing for several reasons including the obvious presence of cognitive distortions about eating, weight and shape, the presence of comorbid anxiety and depression and to address the developmental milestones of adolescence that have been hypothesized to have an etiological role in AN (Lock et al., 2005). For parents, in particular, the option of individual therapy is particularly attractive to address the distress and illogical thinking that have led their child becoming ill and requiring hospital. Despite this there is limited evidence to support its efficacy both during the initial period of inpatient hospitalisation and over the longer term.

Two randomized controlled trials (RCTs) have examined individual therapy in adolescents though both of these trials have involved small numbers of outpatients (Russell et al., 1987 and Robin et al., 1994). Similarly, while there have been a number of RCTs of individual therapy in adults with AN, all of these have involved outpatient treatment. Therapies have included cognitive behavioral therapy (CBT), cognitive analytic therapy (CAT) interpersonal therapy (ITP), nutritional therapy and psychodynamic psychotherapy. In all cases benefits from treatment were modest and no data is available to support their use in children and adolescents in an inpatient treatment setting (LeGrange et al., 2005).

For the reasons listed above it is difficult to recommend any particular type of individual therapy for children and adolescents whilst inpatients and difficult to recommend its use in the acutely malnourished where the effects of starvation impair the cognitive capacity for individuals to benefit from these interventions. In addition, the suggestion in the adult treatment literature of poorer outcomes from targeted ED treatments over supportive psychotherapy (McIntosh et al., 2005) indicate the need for caution in the provision of intensive eating focused psychotherapy in the inpatient setting. It has been the author's experience that non-specific supportive psychotherapy focusing on reassurance, explanation, guidance, encouragement, environmental change and catharsis is more containing and effective than specific therapies aimed at addressing weight, eating and shape concerns in severely malnourished individuals.

School and Group Therapy

The ability to keep patients busy with educational, recreational, and group therapy programs is particularly important in reducing distress, minimizing eating disordered behavior, and promoting participation in normal activities of daily living. When medically stable, ongoing school education during hospitalisation is an integral part of treatment. In the initial stages of treatment malnutrition impairs cognition, in particular attention and concentration, short term memory, cognitive processing speed, cognitive flexibility and problem solving. Research has shown that nutritional rehabilitation and weight gain reverse these cognitive deficits. Anecdotally, experienced school teachers can often flag when cognition improves providing a useful indicator of improving nutritional recovery during refeeding. With improved cognition and ability to maintain school work comes a sense of achievement and self-esteem in these children and adolescents.

Group therapy provides the opportunity to learn new coping skills, ways of relating to others and improve self-esteem. Groups can be facilitated by any member of the treating team but are generally run by occupational therapists, nurses, social workers, and psychologists.

Psychological Support of Parents and Families

When parents first present their child for treatment of AN they do so not only with anxiety about their child's well being but often with feelings of failure in their role as parents. Both in the scientific literature and in the popular press AN has been associated with family dysfunction, parental intrusiveness, over-control, and physical and sexual abuse. For these reasons early parent-professional interactions may be complex and difficult, with parents perceived as anxious and needy and professionals as critical and blaming.

In a qualitative study looking at the impact of AN on parents (Honey et al., 2006), the main priority for families was their child's physical and psychological well-being. While these are the same priorities as clinicians working with AN the importance and timing of these outcomes is often different. For clinicians, AN is a chronic illness where changes, particularly psychological changes, are a slow and gradual process and distress expected

(Steinhausen et al., 2002). For many parents, however their child's psychological distress is central and its treatment both urgent and necessary. Treatment research in children and adolescents with AN has emphasized the need to focus on safe eating, even in the face of escalating distress, rather than underlying eating disordered beliefs (Lock et al., 2005).

Hence, it is essential to meet regularly with parents to establish and build rapport, provide education about EDs, provide regular information about treatment and treatment plans and to provide regular feedback about their child's progress. In the authors' experience, regular weekly parental counseling sessions not only serve this process but allow the containment of parental anxiety and maximize the gains of inpatient treatment. Psycho-educational groups for parents and families are an efficient way of reducing parental distress and defensiveness. They also promote an understanding of the biopsychosocial complexity of the illness, encourage acceptance of change and promote a treatment alliance. Valuable insight can be gained into any cultural, individual, or family factors that influence the development and maintenance of the illness.

While strong data exists to support the efficacy of outpatient family therapy in the management of child and adolescent AN only one RCT has looked at its role in medically compromised patients in an inpatient setting (Geist et al., 2000). In this study family group psycho-education was compared with family therapy. Over a four month period both treatments were associated with weight gain with no difference in outcomes between the two groups. Interestingly neither treatment demonstrated improvements in ED psychopathology. While one could take a positive message from this trial about the importance of family involvement in the inpatient setting the absence of a control arm without family therapy makes it difficult to isolate the impact of family treatment from overall inpatient care. Additionally the lack of difference between group psycho-education and family therapy highlights the difficulty in putting the benefits of family therapy into practice whilst children and adolescents remain inpatients. A similar result was seen in an outcome trial by Halvorsen et al., (2004) that highlighted family therapy as one component of a successful multimodal inpatient treatment program. Again the failure to explore the specific impact of family therapy and the lack of a comparison treatment make it difficult to draw further conclusions from this study. The most studied of the models of family therapy, The Maudsley Model, requires that the patient be out of hospital before treatment begins (Lock et al., 2001). This makes sense as it is difficult for parents to focus on taking control of their child's eating when meals are still provided through inpatient treatment. As a precursor to family therapy inpatients with AN can be given periods of leave from hospital to practice eating with their families and successes and difficulties explored as part of routine family counseling.

Outpatient Care in Anorexia Nervosa

For the majority of children and adolescents with an ED, treatment will occur on an outpatient basis. Even for those individuals who undergo an inpatient admission the majority of care will occur on an outpatient basis. There are a number of potential advantages for children and adolescents undergoing outpatient care including ongoing contact with their families, peers and education. This is particularly relevant given the long-term nature of eating disorder symptoms with an average length of illness for many individuals of between 5 and 6 years (Steinhausen et al., 2002). Cost factors are also significant with outpatient care costing around 10% of inpatient care (Katzman et al., 2000). These factors however, need to be balanced against children and adolescents greater susceptibility to the effects of acute and chronic malnutrition and the need to carefully medically monitor them whilst in outpatient care.

The goals of outpatient care include weight restoration, or weight maintenance for those individuals who have been weight restored in inpatient care, the establishment of healthy eating, the treatment of eating disordered behaviors and psychological recovery. In order to achieve these outcomes it is necessary to combine physical treatments in particular refeeding with psychological therapy. In children and adolescents this should generally include a family based psychological intervention.

To date there have been four RCTs looking at outpatient family therapy in children and adolescents (Russell et al., 1987, Robin et al., 1994, Eisler et al., 2000, Eisler et al., 1997 and Lock et al., 2005). All four of these trials have used a form of family therapy that has focused on food, eating and weight including three that have used the Maudsley Model of Family Treatment (Russell et al., 1987, Eisler et al., 2000 and Lock et al., 2005). All four of these trials have shown positive outcomes from family therapy in terms of weight gain and reduced eating disorder pathology though only two have compared family therapy to individual therapy (Russell et al., 1987 and Robin et a., 1994). Both of these trials demonstrated improved weight outcomes when compared with individual therapy but included only small numbers of patients. Family therapy has been successful in achieving its outcomes with both underweight and weight restored patients making it optimally suited to outpatient care.

In the past family treatment has been criticized for its tendency to blame families for their child's AN. This concern stems back to Minuchin et al., (1975) description of the psychosomatic family and the role of abnormal family structure in the genesis of AN. This view is no longer widely accepted with family therapy seen as a means of utilizing family resources to treat AN.

While family therapy is successful for many children and adolescents it is not acceptable or successful for all. For many families the failure of family treatment to "appropriately" address their child's ED psychopathology is confusing and distressing. In addition the presence of comorbid psychopathology including depression or anxiety raises the issue of individual outpatient psychotherapy.

There are only two RCTs that have examined individual therapy in adolescents. The first of these trials (Russell et al., 1987) compared individual therapy with family therapy in 20 adolescents following inpatient weight restoration as part of a larger treatment trial. This study demonstrated a significant advantage for family therapy both at treatment completion and at five year follow up (Eisler et al., 1997). In the second study (LeGrange et al., 2005) individual ego-oriented therapy was compared with family therapy. In this treatment family therapy was associated with more rapid weight gain though no outcome differences were seen after 12 months.

A review of adult treatment trials has demonstrated efficacy for a number of interventions though with insufficient evidence to guide us as to an individual therapy of choice. It is worth noting that outcomes from eating disorder specific therapies such as CBT as compared to non-specific supportive clinical management were only superior in weight restored patients (Bulik et al., 2007).

Given this a number of recommendations can be made. Firstly it is important that all families be offered family treatment with the clear benefits of this approach explained. Secondly if individual therapy is to be offered it is worth considering outcomes for individual therapy seem best in weight restored individuals. Finally it is worth considering whether individual treatment can be given in a way that can work with family treatment. This is difficult as individual therapy focuses on enhancing the child's efforts to beat AN while family treatment focuses on the parents taking over responsibility for feeding and eating from their child. One potential compromise is separated family therapy where parents and children are seen separately by the same family treatment team. This approach has the potential benefit of reducing family distress and conflict without a reduction in treatment efficacy (Eisler et al., 2000). A second option is to focus individual treatment on comorbid illnesses with family therapy remaining the treatment of choice for the ED.

For individual therapy in the absence of family therapy a review of Robin et al., (1994) provides us with some guide into features that may be helpful including building ego strength, facilitating adolescent autonomy and addressing emotional blocks to eating. In cognitive behavioral terms this could include improving coping strategies to address distress and challenging negative thoughts around shape and eating. In all cases it is important to consider the important developmental tasks of adolescence including identity and independence.

Psychological Therapy in Bulimia Nervosa

To date there have been over 60 RCTs comparing behavioral interventions, medication and a combination of behavioral interventions and medication in the treatment of BN (NICE 2004). Only one of these trials however, has been carried out in an exclusively adolescent population (Schmidt et al., 2007). A small number of adult based trials have included older adolescents from 16 of years of age though small numbers have not allowed a separate analysis of treatment outcomes in this age group.

The predominant therapeutic intervention studied to date has been cognitive behavioral therapy (CBT) though other interventions have included dialectical behavioral therapy (DBT), interpersonal therapy (IPT), family therapy, guided self-help (GSH), nutritional and stress management and behavioral therapy. Psychological interventions have been carried out on both individual and group basis, and have been implemented on their own or in combination with medication interventions (Shapiro et al., 2007).

Outcomes of these studies have strongly supported the use of CBT on an individual basis for the treatment of BN with evidence for a reduction in bingeing, purging, depressive and anxiety symptoms. Some early support exists for DBT, IPT and guided self-help though CBT remains the current treatment of choice for management of BN in adults. There is some preliminary evidence to suggest the addition of medication to CBT may improve treatment outcomes though this data needs to be replicated. (Shapiro et al., 2007)

While the findings are clear in adults what does this mean for the treatment of BN in children and adolescents. To date the only study of BN in an exclusively adolescent population aged between 13 and 20 years, demonstrated that both family therapy and guided self-help (GSH) were effective in reducing bingeing and purging in adolescents though GSH produced a more rapid improvement in symptoms, was more acceptable to patients and was more cost-effective. It is important to note however, in considering the results of this study that the average age of the participants in the GSH arm was 17.4 years and in the family therapy arm was 17.9 years. While this reflects the fact that the majority of patients with BN are older adolescents or young adults it does little to guide treatment decisions in younger patients. Finally it is important to note that this study used an adult based manual for GSH rather than modifying the treatment for children and adolescents.

As the majority of children and adolescents presenting for treatment with BN are likely to be in their late teens it would seem reasonable to recommend CBT as the psychological treatment of choice. In individuals in whom this treatment is unsuccessful, unavailable or unacceptable, other options would included GSH, IPT, DBT or medication management with or without CBT. In younger adolescents or children developmental considerations and the reality of their living arrangements should raise the option of family therapy as an appropriate intervention. To date the best evidence for family therapy exists for a BN adapted version of the Maudsley model of family therapy (Schmidt et al., 2007).

The Role of Medication in Anorexia Nervosa

Current behavioral and psychotherapeutic treatments in AN have a limited evidence base for their efficacy and recovery rates from the disorder are poor both in the short and long term. It is therefore no surprise that considerable interest has been shown in the role of psychotropic medications in the management of anorexia nervosa. This material is summarized in the chapter on Pharmacological approaches to the treatment of AN.

Conclusion

Eating Disorders are being increasingly recognized in children and adolescents. Up to one third of individuals with AN will present before the age of 14 while and almost all will present before 18 years of age. While BN tends to occur in older adolescents this group still make up a significant number of eating disorder presentations. As children and adolescents are more prone to the impacts of malnutrition on their growth and development early recognition and treatment are vital. While many children and adolescents with eating disorders present with syndromes commonly seen in adults a significant minority present without body image and food concerns. In these children it is important not only to consider their expressed concerns but also their observable behavior and the impact of their malnutrition when making treatment decisions.

There is a growing body of evidence for the efficacy of outpatient treatment interventions, particularly family-based treatment. While family treatment is not the answer for all eating disorders the involvement of families in their child's care remains central to positive long-term outcomes. When faced with a child with an eating disorder it is important to recognize both the seriousness of the illness but also the positive outcomes from early intervention and close cooperation with families.

Despite the growing evidence base for the efficacy of family therapy there remains considerable gaps in the evidence base for treating children with eating disorders. Leaving aside clinical consensus there is little evidence to guide us as to the best setting for eating disorder care in children; inpatient, outpatient or day hospital and what clinical features may help guide us in such decisions. For children who are admitted to inpatient or day-hospital programs there is little evidence to guide as to the essential components and duration of such treatment and how to transition children between different levels of care. Does the lack of evidence supporting the efficacy of individual therapy and medication in children with eating disorders mean that such treatments should not be offered? How should comorbidities be treated and what happens when family treatment fails?

It is important to remember that in attempting to make such decisions and answer such questions that the lack of evidence to support the efficacy of treatment interventions in not evidence of lack of treatment effectiveness but rather a clear indicator for the need for more child and adolescent specific randomized controlled treatment trials. In the interim clinicians need to base treatment decisions on a descending hierarchy of existing evidence, expert consensus and clinical experience. The following clinical vignette highlights many of these concerns.

Sick, Sad and Grumpy

Charlotte was a nine year old girl living with her parents and two younger sisters aged 6 and 3 years. She presented to the emergency department of a large children's hospital with a nine month history of weight loss. Charlotte had lost 22lb over this period, and on admission had eaten nothing for 48 hours. Charlotte was 68lb (69% IBW) and medically unstable with a pulse rate of 38 bpm. Charlotte denied concerns about her weight and shape and was diagnosed with food avoidant emotional disorder rather than anorexia nervosa. Charlotte was admitted to a specialist eating disorder service for medical resuscitation and behavioral refeeding.

During the initial part of her admission, Charlotte continued to refuse to eat and was totally dependent on naso-gastric refeeding. She did not respond to the wards behavioral program or a modified reward program. Support and focus around eating led Charlotte to become increasingly distressed somatically focused and socially withdrawn, with associated fatigue, abdominal pain and a refusal to walk, talk and toilet herself. At this stage intervention around meal times was terminated and priority was given to maintaining Charlotte's overall level *of* functioning with regular physiotherapy sessions and engagement in the hospital school.

This vignette highlights some of the difficulties in faced by clinicians treating children and adolescents with eating disorders. Despite Charlotte's young age, her malnutrition and medical compromise necessitated her admission to hospital. Similarly despite her lack of body image concerns Charlotte was managed in the same way as other eating disorder patients, with medical resuscitation and behavioral refeeding, with the goal of a rapid transition to outpatient Maudsley family therapy. While current evidence supports such an approach there is no evidence to guide clinicians when such treatment not only fails to generate improvement but leads to a significant deterioration in symptoms. In this case a decision was made to continue with nutritional rehabilitation with naso-gastric feeding but to remove the focus from eating and to focus on improving function in other areas of Charlotte's life. With this in mind Charlotte was reintegrated to her home school and the family engaged in therapy during inpatient treatment.

Family therapy commenced at week 6 of Charlotte's admission. Despite a move away from the refeeding focus of Maudsley family therapy many features of this approach were used. Charlotte's difficulties were externalized, with her physical symptoms framed as a bully that was bossing her around and preventing her from enjoying her normal life. As in Maudsley family therapy the aim was to assist Charlotte to join her parents in the struggle back to health. Charlotte responded well to this approach and while remaining somewhat suspicious of the intentions of the therapist embraced it in her interactions with her parents.

After three weekly sessions of family therapy Charlotte began to restore her relationship with her parents. Prior to this she had become particularly close to nursing staff and told her parents that she never wanted to return home. As a result she began to request weekend leave and overnight stays from hospital, supported by nasogastric refeeding. Within one week Charlotte spontaneously began to eat reporting that she didn't remember food ever "tasting so good". A week later she announced that she felt ready to leave hospital and she was discharged within a few days. She had been admitted to hospital for a total of ten weeks.

While treatment in this case moved away from behavioral refeeding and outpatient family treatment, evidence based principals were still followed through the focus on nutritional rehabilitation and the use of many of the core therapeutic principals of successful family treatment in eating disorders, albeit on an inpatient basis. Though flexibility in our care of children with eating disorders is important an ongoing focus on the principles of evidence based care allows us to ensure effective and appropriate treatment.

References

American Psychiatric Association. (2006). Treatment of patients with eating disorders, third edition. *American Journal of Psychiatry*, 163(7 suppl), 4-54.

Atkins, D. Silber, T. (1993). Clinical Spectrum of Anorexia Nervosa in Children. *Journal of Developmental and Behavioural Pediatrics*, 14(4), 211-216.

Blitzer, J. Rollins, N. Blackwell, A. (1961). Children Who Starve Themselves: Anorexia Nervosa. *Psychosomatic Medicine*, 3(5), 369-383.

Bryant-Waugh, R. (2000). Overview of the Eating Disorders. In: Lask B, Bryant-Waugh R, editors. *Anorexia Nervosa and Related Eating Disorders in Childhood and Adolescents 2nd ed*. Hove, East Sussex: Psychology Press, pp. 27-40.

Bulik, C.M. Berkman, N.D. Brownley, K.A. Sedway, J.A. Lohr, K.N. (2007). Anorexia nervosa treatment: a systematic review of randomized controlled trials. *International Journal of Eating Disorders*, 40(4), 310-320.

Cooper, P.J., Watkins, B., Bryant-Waugh, R., Lask,. B. (2002). The nosological status of early onset anorexia nervosa. *Psychological Medicine*, 32(5), 873-880.

Eisler, I. Dare, C. Hodes, M. Russell, G. Dodge, E. Le Grange, D. (2000). Family therapy for adolescent anorexia nervosa: the results of a controlled comparison of two family interventions. *Journal of Child Psychology and Psychiatry*, 41(6), 727-736.

Eisler, I. Dare, C. Russell, G.F.M. Szmukler, G.I. LeGrange, D. Dodge, E. (1997). Family and individual therapy in anorexia nervosa: A five-year follow-up. *Archives of General Psychiatry*, 54, 1025-1030.

Fisher, M. Schneider, M. Burns, J. Symons, H. Mandel, F.S. (2001). Differences between adolescents and young adults at presentation to an eating disorders program. *Journal of Adolescent Health*, 8(3), 222-227.

Geist, R. Heinmaa, M. Stephens, D. Davis, R. Katzman, D.K. (2000) Comparison of family therapy and family group psychoeducation in adolescents with anorexia nervosa. *Canadian Journal of Psychiatry*, 45(2), 173-178.

Gowers, S., Bryant-Waugh, R. (2004) Management of child and adolescent eating disorders: the current evidence base and future directions. *Journal of Child Psychology and Psychiatry*, 45(1), 63-83.

Halse, C. Boughtwood, D. Clarke, S. Honey, A. Kohn, M. Madden, S. (2005). The illusion of food: multiple meanings of nasogastric tube feeding in the treatment of anorexia nervosa. *European Eating Disorders Review*, 13(4), 264–272.

Halvorsen, I. Andersen, A. Heyerdahl, S. (2004). Good outcome of adolescent anorexia nervosa after systemic treatment. Intermediate to long-term follow-up of a representative county-sample. *European Child and Adolescent Psychiatry*, 13, 295-306.

Hazell, P. O'Connell, D. Heathcote, D. Robertson, J. Henry, D. (1995). Efficacy of tricyclic drugs in treating child and adolescent depression: a meta-analysis. *British Medical Journal*, 310(6984), 897-901.

Higgs, J. Goodyear, I. Birch, J. (1989). Anorexia nervosa and food avoidance emotional disorder. *Archives of Disease in Childhood*, 64, 346–551.

Honey, A. Clarke, S. Halse, C. Kohn, M. Madden, S. (2006). The influence of siblings on the experience of anorexia nervosa in for adolescent girls. *European Eating Disorders Review*, 14(5), 315-322.

Irwin, M. (1981). Diagnosis of Anorexia Nervosa in Children and the Validity of DSM-III. *American Journal of Psychiatry*, 138(10), 1382-1383.

Joergensen, J. (1992). The Epidemiology of Eating Disorders in Fyn County, Denmark, 1977-1986. *Acta Psychiatrica Scandinavica*, 85, 30-34.

Katzman, D. Golden, N. Neumark-Sztainer, D. Yager, J. Strober, M. (2000). From prevention to prognosis: clinical research update on adolescent eating disorders. *Pediatric Research*, 47(6), 709-712.

Lask, B. Bryant-Waugh, R. (1992). Early-onset anorexia nervosa and related eating disorders. *Journal of Child Psychology and Psychiatry*, 33(1), 281-300.

LeGrange, D. Lock, J. (2005). The Dearth of Psychological Treatment Studies for Anorexia Nervosa. *International Journal of Eating Disorders*, 37, 79-91.

Lewinsohn, P.M., Striegel-Moore, R.H., Seeley, J.R. (2000). Epidemiology and natural course of eating disorders in young women from adolescence to young adulthood. *Journal of the American Academy of Child Adolescent Psychiatry*, 39(10), 1284-1292.

Lock, J. Agras, W.S. Bryson, S. Kraemer, H.C. (2005). A comparison of short- and long-term family therapy for adolescent anorexia nervosa. *Journal of the American Academy of Child and Adolescent Psychiatry*, 44(7), 632-639.

Lock, J. Gowers, S. (2005). Effective interventions for adolescents with anorexia nervosa. *Journal of Mental Health*, 14(6), 599-610.

Lock, J. LeGrange, D. Agras, W. Dare, C. (2001). *Treatment manual for anorexia nervosa: a family-based approach*. New York (NY): Guildford.

Lucas, A.R., Beard, C.M., O'Fallon, W.M., Kurland, L.T. (1991). 50-year trends in the incidence of anorexia nervosa in Rochester, Minn.: a population-based study. *American Journal of Psychiatry*, 148(7), 917-922.

Lucas, A.R., Crowson, C.S., O'Fallon, W.M., Melton, L.J. 3rd. (1999) The ups and downs of anorexia nervosa. *International Journal of Eating Disorders*, 26(4), 397-405.

Madden, S. Byrne, S. Rose, D. (2005). An observational study of patients admitted to the eating disorder unit at the Children's Hospital at Westmead between July 1997 and March 2004. In Bryant-Waugh R, Lask B, editors. *Proceedings of the 7th London International Eating Disorders Conference*; 2005 Apr 4-6; London, United Kingdom, pp. 86-87.

Mann, J.J. Emslie, G. Baldessarini, R.J. Beardslee, W. Fawcett, J.A. Goodwin, F.K. et al. (2006). ACNP Task Force report on SSRIs and suicidal behavior in youth. *Neuropsychopharmacology*, 31(3), 473-492.

McIntosh, V.W. Jordan, J. Carter, F.A. McKenzie, J.M. Bulik, C.M. Frampton, C.M.A. et al. (2005). Three psychotherapies for anorexia nervosa: a randomized, controlled trial. *American Journal of Psychiatry*, 162, 741-747.

Minuchin, S. Baker, L. Rosman, B.L. Liebman, R. Milman, L. Todd, T.C. (1975). A conceptual model of psychosomatic illness in children. Family organization and family therapy. *Archives of General Psychiatry*, 32(8), 1031-1038.

National Institute for Clinical Excellence. (2004) *Eating Disorders: Core interventions in the treatment and management of anorexia nervosa, bulimia nervosa and related eating Disorders: Clinical Guideline 9*. London, National Institute for Clinical Excellence. http://www.nice.org.uk/pdf/cg009niceguidance.pdf[G]

Nicholls, D. Bryant-Waugh, R. (2002). Children and young adolescents. In: Treasure, J. Schmidt, U. Van Furth, E. editors. *Handbook of Eating Disorders 2nd ed*. Chichester (United Kingdom): Wiley, pp. 415-434.

Nicholls, D. Chater, R. Lask, B. (2000). Children into DSM don't go: a comparison of classification systems for eating disorders in childhood and early adolescence. *International Journal of Eating Disorders*, 28(3), 317-324.

Nielsen, S. (1990). The Epidemiology of Anorexia Nervosa in Denmark from 1973 to 1987: A Nationwide Register Study of Psychiatric Admission. *Acta Psychiatrica Scandinavica*, 81, 507-514.

Peebles, R., Wilson, J.L., Lock, J.D. (2006). How do children with eating disorders differ from adolescents with eating disorders at initial evaluation? *Journal of Adolescent Health*, 39(6), 800-805.

Peterson, C.B. Mitchell, J.E. (1999). Psychosocial and pharmacological treatment of eating disorders: a review of research findings. *Journal of Clinical Psychology*, 55(6), 685-697.

Pinhas, L. Temple, S. Boachie, A. Katzman, D.K. Heinmaa, M. (2006). Food Avoidant Emotional Disorder: Is it time for a new diagnostic category in the DSM? In Wade T, LeGrange D, editors. *Eating Disorders Throughout the World: Exploring Similarities and Differences.* Proceedings of the 2006 International Conference on Eating Disorders; Jun 7-10; Barcelona, Spain.

Rhodes, P. Madden, S. (2005). Scientist-practitioner family therapists, post-modern medical practitioners and expert parents: second-order change in the eating disorders program, at The Children's Hospital at Westmead. *Journal of Family Therapy*, 27(2), 171 – 182.

Robb, A.S. Silber, T.J. Orrell-Valente, J.K. Valadez-Meltzer, A. Ellis, N. Dadson, M.J. et al. (2002). Supplemental nocturnal nasogastric refeeding for better short-term outcome in hospitalized adolescent girls with anorexia nervosa. *American Journal of Psychiatry*, 159, 1347–1353

Robin, A.L, Siegel, P.T. Koepke, T. Moye, A.W. Tice, S. (1994). Family therapy versus individual therapy for adolescent females with anorexia nervosa. *Journal of Developmental and Behavioral Pediatrics*, 15(2), 111-116.

Russell, G.F.M. Szmukler, G.I. Dare, C. Eisler, I. (1987). An evaluation of family therapy in anorexia nervosa and bulimia nervosa. *Archives of General Psychiatry*, 44, 1047-1056.

Schmidt, U., Lee, S., Beecham, J., Perkins, S., Treasure, J., Yi, I. et al. (2007). A randomized controlled trial of family therapy and cognitive behavior therapy guided self-care for adolescents with bulimia nervosa and related disorders. *American Journal of Psychiatry*, 164(4), 591-598.

Shapiro, J.R. Berkman, N.D. Brownley, K.A. Sedway, J.A. Lohr, K.N. Bulik, C.M. (2007). Bulimia nervosa treatment: a systematic review of randomized controlled trials. *International Journal of Eating Disorders*, 40(4), 321-336.

Steinhausen, H.C. (2002). The outcome of anorexia nervosa in the 20th century. *American Journal of Psychiatry*, 159(8), 1284-1293.

Touyz, S. Beaumont, P. Dunn, S.M. (1987). Behaviour therapy in the management of patients with anorexia nervosa. A lenient, flexible approach. *Psychotherapy and Psychosomatics*, 48(1-4), 151-156.

Wade, T.D., Bergin, J.L., Tiggemann, M., Bulik, C.M., Fairburn, C.G. (2006). Prevalence and long-term course of lifetime eating disorders in an adult Australian twin cohort. *Australian and New Zealand Journal of Psychiatry*, 40(2), 121-128.

Workgroup for Classification of Eating Disorders in Children and Adolescents (WCEDCA). (2007). Classification Child and Adolescent *Eating Disorders. International Journal of Eating Disorders,* 40(suppl), s117-122.

In: Evidence-Based Treatments for Eating Disorders   ISBN 978-1-60692-310-8
Author: Ida F. Dancyger and Victor M. Fornari   © 2009 Nova Science Publishers, Inc.

Chapter IX

Evidence-Guided Treatment for Males with Eating Disorders

Fernando Fernández-Aranda and Susana Jiménez-Murcia
University Hospital of Bellvitge and
CIBER Fisiopatología de la Obesidad y Nutrición (CIBEROBN)
Instituto Carlos III, Barcelona, Spain

Abstract

An increasing rate of males with eating disorders (EDs) has been observed during recent years, specifically bulimia nervosa (BN) and eating disorder not otherwise specified (EDNOS). Most clinical features and symptoms of men and women with EDs are similar. In this chapter, we have summarized information on similarities between male and female ED on clinical, psychopathology and therapy response. Therapy for males with ED, has received relatively little attention in the literature and most studies on therapy, have been conducted in anorexic males after undergoing non-specific inpatient-residential treatment. An extensive and updated overview of studies on therapy in males with EDs was performed. Data which have not been previously published and a description of our specific therapy program for males with EDs will be given.

Introduction

Eating disorders (EDs) are less frequent in males than in females (6-12% of cases) (Kjelsas, Bjornstrom, and Gotestam, 2004). Males make up 5-10% of people with anorexia nervosa (AN) who seek treatment (Striegel-Moore, Garvin, Dohm, and Rosenheck, 1999) and 10-15% of people with bulimia nervosa [BN] (Carlat, Camargo, and Herzog, 1997). However, an increasing rate of male ED has been observed during the last years, in Spain (Rodriguez-Cano, Beato-Fernandez, and Belmonte-Llario, 2005) as well as in other European countries (Kjelsas et al., 2004).

During the last ten years (between 1997 and 2007), in the ED Centre at the University Hospital of Bellvitge, in Barcelona (Spain), 104 males with EDs were admitted (7,1 % cases) from a total whole sample of 1.471 (males and females) ED [22,8% AN, 50,8% BN, 26,4% EDNOS], consecutively admitted patients in this period of time. If we compare these results with the male rate obtained in a previous conducted research (Alonso Ortega, Fernandez Aranda, Turon Gil, Vallejo Ruiloba, and Ramos, 1998), where the percentage of males with EDs was calculated based on number of treated attended patients between 1975-97 (3,6% of cases were male), the total number of male has now increased by more than two times.

When considering the ED subtype, during the last years, some specific diagnostic categories of males have increased more than others, namely BN and EDNOS (see Figure 1), whereas the percentage of AN has been reduced. This result is similar to recent findings in female EDs. (Machado, Machado, Goncalves, and Hoek, 2007). In these general data (1.471 ED), there were significant differences (X2. 9,814, p<.007) in ED subtype distribution, when considering the factor gender (males: 28,6% AN, 35,7 BN v 35,7% EDNOS vs. Females: 22,4%AN, 52% BN, 25,6% EDNOS). Similar diagnostic distribution among males was described in previous studies (Carlat et al., 1997).

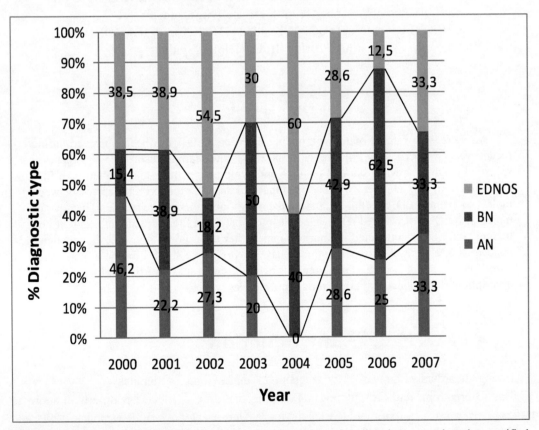

Note: AN: Anorexia nervosa, BN: Bulimia nervosa, EDNOS: Eating disorders non-otherwise specified.

Figure 1. Diagnostic distribution in males with EDs, between 2000 and 2007, at the University Hospital of Bellvitge.

Differences between Male and Female ED

Although most characteristics of men and women with EDs are similar (Andersen, 1999; Bramon-Bosch, Troop, and Treasure, 2000; DiGioacchino, Sargent, Sharpe, and Miller, 1999), even with regards to pattern of familial aggregation (Strober, Freeman, Lampert, Diamond, and Kaye, 2001) and in adolescents ED (Geist, Heinmaa, Katzman, and Stephens, 1999), in the literature we can also find gender differences (Andersen and Mickalide, 1985; Deter, Kopp, Zipfel, and Herzog, 1998; Woodside et al., 2001). Some of the discrepancies observed in the current literature are partially due to methodological gaps, lack of control groups or too small sample sizes of the clinical used samples.

Clinical and Symptomatological Differences in Males with EDs

In general, studies have indicated that the clinical manifestations in males are similar to the ones of females in terms of age of onset, weight control methods and associated ED factors (Braun, Sunday, Huang, and Halmi, 1999; Carlat et al., 1997; Keel, Klump, Leon, and Fulkerson, 1998; Olivardia, Pope, Mangweth, and Hudson, 1995). However, other studies have revealed gender specific differences on physical activity, more concern with masculine shape and more laxative use in male as compared to female ED patients (Braun et al., 1999; Carlat and Camargo, 1991; DiGioacchino et al., 1999; Fichter, Daser, and Postpischil, 1985), but also later age of onset (Grabhorn, Kopp, Gitzinger, von Wietersheim, and Kaufhold, 2003). For a review, see (Chambry, Corcos, Guilbaud, and Jeammet, 2002; Freeman, 2005; Lindblad, Lindberg, and Hjern, 2006).

As shown in Table 1, from 1.472 consecutively admitted patients, we compared clinical and symptomatological features between 104 males with EDs and 1.367 ED females. This comparison (using 0.01 level of significance, to avoid error type I), revealed significant differences by gender on higher weekly frequency of laxatives (more frequently in females, p<.01), but no significant differences were obtained on age of onset or duration of the disorder.

Regarding weight (see also Table 1), accordingly with previous reports (Andersen and Holman, 1997), females with ED wished to be thinner (p<.001) and males presented a higher lifetime maximum reached BMI, than females (p<.001). Concerns about body image is thought to be one of the key maintaining factors of EDs and is a required criterion for the diagnosis of Anorexia Nervosa (AN) and Bulimia Nervosa (BN) (Stice, 2002; Stice and Whitenton, 2002).

Females show more concerns about body dissatisfaction and drive for thinness than males, both in clinical ED samples (Joiner, Katz, and Heatherton, 2000; Kjelsas, Augestad, and Flanders, 2003), as in general population samples (Davis and Katzman, 1998; Geist et al., 1999).

Table 1. Clinical and demographic features of 104 males with EDs and 1.364 ED females consecutive patients

	ED (N= 1.468)			
	Males (N=104)		Females (N= 1.364)	
	Mean	SD	Mean	SD
Age	24,36	6,60	25,82	7,12
Age of onset	19,08	5,70	19,07	6,12
Duration of disorder	5,27	5,08	6,73	5,64
Number previous treatments	,71	,96	,94	1,20
BMI	22,58	5,72	21,95	6,14
BMI max.	28,30	6,89	25,86	5,97
BMI min.	19,03	4,31	18,29	3,35
BMI ideal	21,95	3,55	19,86	2,67
Weekly frequency of binge episodes	3,82	7,27	4,83	6,56
Weekly frequency of vomiting	5,46	9,79	5,41	7,95
Weekly frequency of laxatives	,49	2,38	3,97	13,41
Weekly frequency of diuretics	,02	,22	1,41	5,68

Note: BMI: Body Mass Index (weight/ height^2).

Many of our males with EDs were more concerned about their body shape in terms of muscularity rather than about their weight (Fernandez-Aranda et al., 2004), which is similar to the findings of many other authors (Andersen and Mickalide, 1983; Andersen et al., 1985; Benninghoven, Tadic, Kunzendorf, and Jantschek, 2007; Davis et al., 1998; Furnham, Badmin, and Sneade, 2002).

In a recent study (Nunez-Navarro et al., in press), using a case-control design, we have compared two groups of ED (60 males and 60 females) with two healthy eating comparison groups (60 males and 60 females), on several clinical and personality profiles. Regarding differences due to gender, ED women obtained higher means in two EDI-2 subscales ("drive for thinness", p<0.0005 and "body dissatisfaction", p<0.0005) than males with EDs, but a similar trend was also observed in healthy eating controls by gender. This result may reflect just socio-cultural gender differences, as the differential pattern is similar to the one between males and females in the healthy non ED population.

Regarding motivation to change (assessed by lineal scale, described elsewhere (Casasnovas et al., 2007), and taking into account the initial 104 males with EDs, when compared with 1.367 ED females, males were less motivated for therapy than females. Basically, males were less concerned about their ED (p<.001), and showed low subjective need for therapy (p<.001) and lower wish to be treated (p<.001). These results are in concordance with a previous study (Woodside et al., 2004).

Table 2. Eating psychopathology in Eating disorder patients and healthy controls by gender (adapted from Nunez-Navarro et al., in press)

| | Mean (SE) | | | | ANCOVA Principal effects: Mean differences (95% C.I.) | |
| | Controls | | Cases | | | |
	Males (N=60)	Females (N=60)	Males (N=60)	Females (N=60)	Sex	Diagnose
EDI-2: Drive for thinness	1.9 (0.8)	5.2 (0.8)	9.3 (0.7)	13.5 (0.7)	3.8 (2.2; 5.3)*	7.9 (6.3; 9.4)*
EDI-2: Body dissatisfaction	2.9 (1.0)	6.8 (1.0)	10.9 (0.9)	16.7 (0.9)	4.9 (3.0; 6.8)*	9.0 (7.2; 10.8)*
EDI-2: Interoceptive awareness	1.6 (0.7)	2.3 (0.8)	7.5 (0.7)	11.3 (0.7)	2.2 (0.8; 3.7)	7.5 (6.1; 8.9)*
EDI-2: Bulimia	0.4 (0.6)	1.0 (0.6)	5.0 (0.6)	6.4 (0.6)	1.0 (-0.2; 2.2)	5.0 (3.9; 6.2)*
EDI-2: Interpersonal distrust	3.0 (0.5)	1.9 (0.6)	6.1 (0.5)	5.9 (0.5)	-0.6 (-1.7; 0.4)	3.6 (2.5; 4.6)*
EDI-2: Ineffectiveness	1.7 (0.8)	2.0 (0.8)	8.5 (0.7)	11.8 (0.7)	1.8 (0.2; 3.3)	8.3 (6.9; 9.8)*
EDI-2: Maturity fears	4.8 (0.7)	4.7 (0.8)	9.4 (0.7)	8.4 (0.7)	-0.5 (-1.9; 0.9)	4.2 (2.8; 5.5)*
EDI-2: Perfectionism	4.3 (0.6)	3.3 (0.6)	4.5 (0.5)	6.0 (0.5)	0.2 (-0.9; 1.4)	1.5 (0.4; 2.6)
EDI-2: Impulse regulation	2.1 (0.8)	1.3 (0.8)	6.4 (0.7)	8.3 (0.7)	0.5 (-0.9; 2.0)	5.6 (4.2; 7.0)*
EDI-2: Asceticism	2.4 (0.6)	1.9 (0.6)	6.2 (0.5)	7.0 (0.5)	0.2 (-0.9; 1.3)	4.4 (3.4; 5.5)*
EDI-2: Social insecurity	2.7 (0.6)	2.3 (0.7)	7.3 (0.6)	8.4 (0.6)	0.4 (-0.9; 1.6)	5.4 (4.2; 6.6)*
EDI-2: Total score	27.8 (5.4)	32.7 (5.6)	81.6 (4.9)	103.7 (4.9)	13.5 (3.0; 24.0)	62.4 (52.3; 72.6)*

[1]Sex factor: difference obtained for females-males. [1]Diagnose factor: difference obtained for cases-controls.

*The parameter is significant at 0.002 level. EDI: Eating Disorder Inventory.

Psychopathological Differences in Males with EDs

In general terms, ED men have been described to have more general psychopathology and co-morbidity than ED females (Bean, Maddocks, Timmel, and Weltzin, 2005). In several comparative studies, males with EDs have shown: higher alcohol dependence (Striegel-Moore et al., 1999; Woodside et al., 2001) and higher levels of co-morbidity on Axis I (Weltzin et al., 2007a) or Axis II (Striegel-Moore et al., 1999).

In the previously mentioned study (Nunez-Navarro et al., in press), males with EDs showed lower general psychopathology (measured by SCL90R) than ED females, and especially in somatization, depression and anxiety subscales.

Table 3. General psychopathology in Eating disorder patients and healthy controls by gender (adapted from Nunez-Navarro et al., in press)

	Mean (SE) Controls Males (N=60)	Females (N=60)	Cases Males (N=60)	Females (N=60)	ANCOVA Principal effects: Mean differences (95% C.I.) Sex	Diagnose
SCL-90-R: GSI score	0.6 (0.1)	0.7 (0.1)	1.4 (0.1)	1.8 (0.1)	0.3 (0.1; 0.5)*	0.9 (0.8; 1.1)*
SCL-90-R: PSDI score	1.5 (0.1)	1.5 (0.1)	2.1 (0.1)	2.4 (0.1)	0.2 (0.0; 0.3)	0.8 (0.7; 0.9)*
SCL-90-R: PST score	30.7 (2.7)	39.7 (2.7)	55.3 (2.6)	65.0 (2.6)	9.3 (4.0; 14.6)*	24.9 (19.7; 30.1)*

1Sex factor: difference obtained for females-males. 1Diagnose factor: difference obtained for cases-controls.
*The parameter is significant at 0.002 level.

Personality and Males with EDs

The few studies assessing personality in men with EDs have shown that male AN patients exhibited lower scores on harm avoidance, reward dependence, and co-operativeness and higher scores on novelty seeking than females with AN (Fassino et al., 2001; Woodside et al., 2004). As regards to BN, another study (Joiner et al., 2000) demonstrated higher levels of perfectionism and interpersonal distrust in males in comparison to females. In contrast, other studies (Alvarez-Moya et al., 2007; Fernandez-Aranda et al., 2004; Strober et al., 2006) were not able to find substantial gender differences in personality traits in ED patients (males vs. females). When diagnostic ED subgroups were examined, considerably few gender-specific differences on personality traits were found (Woodside et al., 2004).

Pre-Morbid Obesity and Males with EDs

Compared to females with EDs, a few studies have demonstrated that males tend to have higher levels of weight problems prior to the onset of their ED (Carlat et al., 1991; Robinson and Holden, 1986). They report generally being further away from their ideal weight than female ED patients (Carlat et al., 1997; Fernandez-Aranda et al., 2004). These observations are interesting because we have previously indicated that men might have certain defenses from EDs due to their low occurrence of dieting and more positive body image. Nevertheless, males who are in fact obese may possibly have a negative view of their bodies and might therefore feel an elevated pressure to lose weight. Therefore their environmental stressors appear to be similar to the ones of women who are vulnerable to EDs. Accordingly, in a previous study (Carlat et al., 1991; Fernandez-Aranda et al., 2004), it was found that males gave a history of pre-morbid overweight or obesity more frequently (45% vs. 15%, p<038), and basically in those with BN.

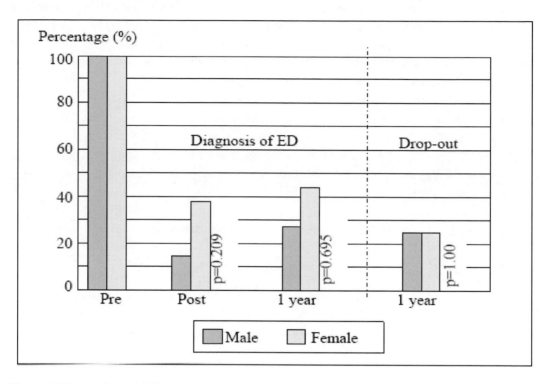

Figure 2. Diagnostic variability at 1 year follow-up and drop-out in males with EDs (N=19) and females (N=19), after following an outpatient CBT group therapy (adapted from Fernández-Aranda, in press).

Therapy and Males with EDs

To date, although most literature connecting gender to EDs has focused on a symptomatology and psychopathological level, there is a lack of published studies examining the specific therapy of males with EDs.

Some of the first descriptions of therapy in males appeared in publications at the beginning of 1970's. Some of the first reports that were published at that time, most of them single case studies or series of cases, described those atypical ED disorders and the therapeutic approaches used.

Bruch (Bruch, 1971) described nine registered inpatient treated AN males, at the New York State Psychiatry Institute, observed between 1944 and 1969. The therapy was evaluated as successful in some of the cases, after using psychotherapy, nutritional measures and additional medication.

Roussounis at the Alexandra Hospital (Roussounis and Savage, 1971) described a 11 year old boy with AN. He was treated as an inpatient with a combination of drug therapy (chlorpromazine -Largactil) and gradually increasing food and weight, with successful results after 90 days. Furthermore, Crisp and colleagues (Crisp and Toms, 1972) described the clinical picture and therapy outcome of 13 AN males. They concluded that males with EDs carried a worse prognosis than the parallel female population.

Later on, additional series on AN males were published using psychotherapeutic and medical measures (Buvat et al., 1983; Galletly and James, 1979; Goebel, 1976; Larsen and Skovgard, 1977), however the results were poor.

The therapy for bulimia in males has received relatively little attention in the literature. It was not until the middle 80's, when some of the first descriptions of treated male BN cases were published (Andersen, 1984; Mitchell and Goff, 1984).

The few case-control studies where therapy with males with EDs was specifically analyzed, obtained heterogeneous results (Andersen et al., 1997; Weltzin et al., 2005). Bean et al. (Bean et al., 2005), compared the effectiveness of a residential therapy in ED (154 females and 27 males), and obtained that although females present more psychopathology symptoms at the beginning of treatment, they make better progress than males in reducing these symptoms over time.

Table 4. Overview of the literature on therapy outcome in males with EDs

Author	Year	Sample	Setting	Follow-up (years)	Results
Burns	1985	27 AN males	Inpatient	8	Outcome ED males = ED females
Crisp	1986	36 AN males 100 AN females	Inpatient	8	Outcome ED males = ED females
Woodside	1994	15 ED males 334 ED females	Hospital Day	-	Outcome ED males = ED females
Deter	1998	10 AN males 84 AN females	Residential	12	ED males better outcome than ED females
Oyebode	1998	13 AN males 13 AN females	--	9,2	ED males poorer outcome than ED females
Grabhorm	2003	20 ED males 764 ED females	Residential	2,5	Outcome ED males = ED females
Bean	2005	27 ED males 154 ED females	Residential	-	ED females better outcome than ED males
Strober	2006	14 AN males 85 AN males	Inpatient-residential	1	ED males better outcome than ED females
Lindblad	2006	61 AN males 748 AN females general population	Inpatient	-	ED males better outcome than ED females
Weltzin	2007	59 AN males 30 BN males 16 EDNOS males	Residential	1	Outcome ED males = ED females
Fernandez-Aranda	In press	19 BN males 19 BN females	Outpatient	1	Outcome ED males = ED females

Note: AN: Anorexia nervosa, BN: Bulimia nervosa, EDNOS: Eating disorders non-otherwise specified.

As shown in table 4, to date, several non-specifics therapeutic approaches for males with EDs have been tested, in comparison with the improvements observed in ED female counterparts. Their setting ranged from residential or inpatient therapy (Bean et al., 2005; Crisp, Burns, and Bhat, 1986; Deter et al., 1998; Strober et al., 2006; Weltzin, Weisensel, Cornelia-Carlson, and Bean, 2007b), to hospital day (Woodside and Kaplan, 1994). Therefore, most studies dealing with therapy, were conducted in males with AN, after having successful non-specific inpatient-residential treatment. The therapy for males with BN or EDNOS is still rather unknown (Weltzin et al., 2007b).

In summary, men with EDs, especially AN, after a non-specific therapy appear to have similar outcome than females. However, there is some uncertainty about the outcome of the bulimic disorders. To date, there is also a lack of specific therapy approaches for males with EDs, and especially outpatient programs.

Recently, we have published a pilot study that compared the short-middle term response to an specific outpatient cognitive-behavioural therapy (CBT) group intervention in male BN, and we have compared their results with those obtained in female counterparts after using a similar approach (Fernandez-Aranda et al., in press). Males appear to have similar outcome than females, even after one year follow-up.

Regarding randomized trials, as reported in a recent meta-analytical studies, conducted by the North Carolina Group, to date no controlled trials exists on differential efficacy of pharmacotherapy or psychotherapy interventions for AN by sex (Bulik, Berkman, Brownley, Sedway, and Lohr, 2007). Similar lack of studies was obtained, when considered BN controlled trials (Shapiro et al., 2007). Regarding binge eating disorder (BED), a meta-analytic review study has shown (Brownley, Berkman, Sedway, Lohr, and Bulik, 2007) that, although in spite of including also male cases in BED controlled trials (of the 680 individuals enrolled in the 12 drug or medication plus behavioral intervention trials, less than 10% were men), no studies explicitly tested differential therapies by sex.

Outcome and Males with EDs

One of the first references (see table 4), came from Burns and colleagues (Burns and Crisp, 1985), who published data on 27 males with AN, that have been followed up over a mean of 8 years, and their outcome was also assessed. When compared with outcome in female patients with similar initial pictures, they found that poor relationship with parents during childhood, absence of normal adolescent sexual behavior, long duration of illness, previous treatment and greater weight loss during illness were strongly predictive of a poor outcome. They have found similarity in outcome pattern between the male and female patients.

Similar results were obtained in a later study conducted by the same group (Crisp et al., 1986), where 36 consecutively referred male anorectics were compared with those of a similar series of 100 female cases. Overall, the same background and presentation factors in both sexes predict similar outcomes.

Deter et al. (Deter et al., 1998) analyzed possible differences in the disease course of male and female patients. Total assessment after a mean of 12 years revealed that the male had a better prognosis than the female patients. Male anorectics were in better physical condition than their female counterparts at the time of follow-up. Male patients had a more favorable course regarding psychosocial integration but a similar course as female patients regarding ED symptoms.

The few case-control studies where the effect of gender on the prognosis has been analyzed have shown a similar course and outcome in males with EDs when compared with those results obtained in ED females (Andersen et al., 1997; Deter et al., 1998; Eliot and Baker, 2001; Muise, Stein, and Arbess, 2003; Saccomani, Savoini, Cirrincione, Vercellino, and Ravera, 1998), whereas others referred to better outcome (Deter et al., 1998; Lindblad et al., 2006; Strober et al., 2006) or even poorer outcome in males (Oyebode et al., 1988).

Similarly to ED females, better outcome was found to be associated to less initial severity of ED symptoms, higher BMI at the admission and lower frequency of obsessive-compulsive behaviors (Strober et al., 2006; Weltzin et al., 2007a).

Regarding randomized trials , as reported in a recent meta-analytical study (Berkman, Lohr, and Bulik, 2007), looking across all three disorders (AN, BN , BED), no studies yielded information on gender and therapy outcome. Very few studies included males and even if they did, males were underrepresented.

Our Own Experience Treating Males with EDs

At the Eating Disorders Unit (University Hospital of Bellvitge), well-known and internationally recognized ED center in Spain, several types of therapies are being applied, from psychological therapy (CBT oriented) to combination with drug therapy. The treatment is carried out in several optional settings: from outpatient, day hospital and residential therapy, to internet based self-management. A broad spectrum of ED patients are being treated, from AN and BN, to EDNOS and BED. Since 2001, we have developed and applied a specific therapy program, CBT oriented, for males with EDs (both individual and group therapy). The CBT program for males is based on the cognitive model postulated by Fairburn and colleagues (Fairburn, Marcus, and Wilson, 1993; Fairburn, 1997). The group intervention consists of 19 weekly outpatient sessions (90 minutes each) with a total of 8-10 patients per group. Men and women are treated in separate groups. The group is directed by a psychologist and a co-therapist (one male and one female).

As in the case of females (Fernandez-Aranda et al., 1998; Fernandez et al., 1998), the topics to be addressed in the group included: nutritional patterns and monitoring of meal plans, strategies for decreasing bingeing and purging behaviour, cognitive restructuring, problem solving strategies and relapse prevention. With males several topics were more emphasized than with females, such as: difficulties with dealing with stress, interpersonal relationships and shyness (many times as a consequence of the negative experience of being criticized for previous obesity or overweight), cognitive style and underlying irrational believes (e.g. muscularity, fear of gaining weight and becoming obese again), hyperactivity, autonomy from family and homosexuality in some cases.

In group therapy with males with EDs, two therapeutic factors have a crucial relevance (even more than in females): universality (other male patients have similar problem) and overcoming resistance to change. An intensive work about the patients' own motivational factors, even during the sessions, to encourage the participation of all group members, will be conducted. Successful and encouraging results were obtained, even after one-year follow-up, with this type of specific program (Fernandez-Aranda et al., in press) – see Figure 2-.

Moreover, according to our own experience, we propose eight to nine patients per group as the ideal number of patients and to consider as exclusion criteria those patients with severe eating or medical problems, psychiatric instability (e.g. suicidality), and/or severe personality disorder.

In order to promote group cohesion, variables such as homogeneity (e.g. similar age and duration of the disorder, closed group), and number of participants will have to be taken into account.

Conclusion

In summary, an increasing rate of male ED has been observed during the last few years, mainly in BN and EDNOS. Although males seem to use laxatives with less frequency, have less preoccupation with thinness, and are less motivated for a therapy, most clinical features and symptoms of men and women with EDs are similar. Many of males with EDs are more concerned about their body shape in terms of muscularity rather than about their weight. Furthermore, males seem to have lower general psychopathology than females and no substantial gender differences in personality traits were found.

The therapy for males with EDs, especially for BN, has received relatively little attention in the literature. Most studies dealing with therapy, were conducted in males with AN after having successful non-specific inpatient-residential treatment, showing similar outcome rates to the ones of females. However, there is uncertainty about the outcome of the bulimic disorders, the results of specific therapy approaches for males with EDs, and especially outpatient programs.

There is a lack of evidence in the literature (particularly controlled trials) that explicitly tested differential therapies by sex. Future outcome studies should explicitly emphasize the factor gender. Furthermore, we recommend that specific programs for males with EDs should be developed.

Case Report

A 26 years old man, technician in telecommunications, developed the complete clinical picture of bulimia nervosa (purging subtype), according to the DSM-IV criteria (American Psychiatric Association, 1994), since he was 18 years old. The ED started after extreme diet behavior to lose weight. The patient described current 3-4 weekly binge-vomiting episodes, mainly late afternoon, and irregular eating patterns. No abuse of laxatives or diuretics was described. Weekly consume of drug, when he was 17-18 years old. At the first interview, the patient had a body weight of 68 Kg (1.74 meters, BMI 22.5) and still presented overconcern with his body shape in terms of muscularity rather than about their weight. After having premorbid obesity (maximal body weight of 121 Kg- BMI 36.7, when he was 17 years old), he has an intense fear of becoming fat again.

The patient was the younger of two children (all boys). He still lived with his family and reported no relationship problems with them. In partnership, since he was 20 years old. No other psychiatric illnesses were described by the patient or his relatives. 19 weekly outpatient cognitive-behavioural group sessions (group therapy for males with ED's) plus 4 follow-up sessions (at 1, 3, 6 and 12 months) were conducted. The main goals of the therapy were: to increase her motivation, to complete a behavioral analysis, to normalize eating habits, to learn behavioral techniques such as coping with stress and solving problems (in spite of escaping from them by binging) and to analyze and learn restructuring of irrational beliefs on weight, shape and food. After the therapy, a reduction of eating symptoms was observed and maintained after a follow-up.

References

Alonso Ortega, P., Fernandez Aranda, F., Turon Gil, J., Vallejo Ruiloba, J., and Ramos, M. J. (1998). Trastornos de la alimentacion en varones: analisis comparativo de los pacientes ingresados en el periodo 1975-1997. *Anales de Psiquiatria,* 14, 295-300.

Alvarez-Moya, E. M., Jimenez-Murcia, S., Granero, R., Vallejo, J., Krug, I., Bulik, C. M., and Fernandez-Aranda, F. (2007). Comparison of personality risk factors in bulimia nervosa and pathological gambling. *Comprehensive Psychiatry,* 48, 452-7.

Andersen, A. E. (1984). Anorexia nervosa and bulimia in adolescent males. *Pediatric Annals,* 13, 901-4, 907.

Andersen, A. E. (1999). Gender-related aspects of eating disorders: a guide to practice. *Journal of Gender Specific Medicine,* 2, 47-54.

Andersen, A. E., and Holman, J. E. (1997). Males with eating disorders: challenges for treatment and research. *Psychopharmacological Bulletin,* 33, 391-7.

Andersen, A. E., and Mickalide, A. D. (1983). Anorexia nervosa in the male: an underdiagnosed disorder. *Psychosomatics,* 24, 1066-75.

Andersen, A. E., and Mickalide, A. D. (1985). Anorexia nervosa and bulimia. Their differential diagnoses in 24 males referred to an eating and weight disorders clinic. *Bulletin of the Menninger Clinic,* 49, 227-35.

Bean, P., Maddocks, M. B., Timmel, P., and Weltzin, T. (2005). Gender differences in the progression of co-morbid psychopathology symptoms of eating disordered patients. *Eating and Weight Disorders,* 10, 168-74.

Benninghoven, D., Tadic, V., Kunzendorf, S., and Jantschek, G. (2007). Koerperbilder maennlicher patienten mit essstoerungen. *Psychotherapie Psychosomatik Medizinische Psychologie,* 57, 120-127.

Berkman, N. D., Lohr, K. N., and Bulik, C. M. (2007). Outcomes of eating disorders: a systematic review of the literature. *International Journal of Eating Disorders,* 40, 293-309.

Bramon-Bosch, E., Troop, N. A., and Treasure, J. L. (2000). Eating disorders in males: A comparison with female patients. *European Eating Disorders Review,* 8, 321-328.

Braun, D. L., Sunday, S. R., Huang, A., and Halmi, K. A. (1999). More males seek treatment for eating disorders. *International Journal of Eating Disorders,* 25, 415-424.

Brownley, K. A., Berkman, N. D., Sedway, J. A., Lohr, K. N., and Bulik, C. M. (2007). Binge eating disorder treatment: a systematic review of randomized controlled trials. *International Journal of Eating Disorders,* 40, 337-48.

Bruch, H. (1971). Anorexia nervosa in the male. *Psychosomatic Medicine,* 33, 31-47.

Bulik, C. M., Berkman, N. D., Brownley, K. A., Sedway, J. A., and Lohr, K. N. (2007). Anorexia nervosa treatment: a systematic review of randomized controlled trials. *International Journal of Eating Disorders,* 40, 310-20.

Burns, T., and Crisp, A. H. (1985). Factors affecting prognosis in male anorexics. *Journal of Psychiatric Research,* 19, 323-8.

Buvat, J., Lemaire, A., Ardaens, K., Buvat-Herbaut, M., Racadot, A., and Fossati, P. (1983). [Profile of gonadal hormones in 8 cases of male anorexia nervosa studied before and during weight gain]. *Annals of Endocrinology (Paris),* 44, 229-34.

Carlat, D. J., and Camargo, C. A., Jr. (1991). Review of bulimia nervosa in males. *American Journal of Psychiatry,* 148, 831-43.

Carlat, D. J., Camargo, C. A., Jr., and Herzog, D. B. (1997). Eating disorders in males: a report on 135 patients. *American Journal of Psychiatry,* 154, 1127-32.

Casasnovas, C., Fernandez-Aranda, F., Granero, R., Krug, I., Jimenez-Murcia, S., Bulik, C. M., and Vallejo-Ruiloba, J. (2007). Motivation to change in eating disorders: clinical and therapeutic implications. *European Eating Disorders Review,* 15, 449-56.

Crisp, A. H., Burns, T., and Bhat, A. V. (1986). Primary anorexia nervosa in the male and female: a comparison of clinical features and prognosis. *British Journal of Medical Psychology,* 59 (Pt 2), 123-32.

Crisp, A. H., and Toms, D. A. (1972). Primary anorexia nervosa or weight phobia in the male: report on 13 cases. *British Medical Journal,* 1, 334-8.

Chambry, J., Corcos, M., Guilbaud, O., and Jeammet, P. (2002). [Masculine anorexia nervosa: realities and perspectives]. *Annales de Medecine Interne (Paris),* 153, 1S61-7.

Davis, C., and Katzman, M. A. (1998). Chinese men and women in the United States and Hong Kong: body and self-esteem ratings as a prelude to dieting and exercise. *International Journal of Eating Disorders,* 23, 99-102.

Deter, H. C., Kopp, W., Zipfel, S., and Herzog, W. (1998). [Male anorexia nervosa patients in long-term follow-up]. *Nervenarzt,* 69, 419-26.

DiGioacchino, R. F., Sargent, R. G., Sharpe, P. A., and Miller, P. (1999). Gender differences among those exhibiting characteristics of binge eating disorder. *Eating and Weight Disorders,* 4, 76-80.

Eliot, A. O., and Baker, C. W. (2001). Eating disordered adolescent males. *Adolescence,* 36, 535-543.

Fassino, S., Abbate-Daga, G., Leombruni, P., Amianto, F., Rovera, G., and Rovera, G. G. (2001). Temperament and character in italian men with anorexia nervosa: a controlled study with the temperament and character inventory. *Journal of Nervous and Mental Diseases,* 189, 788-94.

Fernandez-Aranda, F., Aitken, A., Badia, A., Gimenez, L., Collier, D., and Treasure, J. (2004). Personality and psychopathological traits of males with an eating disorder. *European Eating Disorders Review,* 12, 367-374.

Fernandez-Aranda, F., Bel, M., Jimenez, S., Vinuales, M., Turon, J., and Vallejo, J. (1998). Outpatient group therapy for anorexia nervosa: a preliminary study. *Eating and Weight Disorders,* 3, 1-6.

Fernandez-Aranda, F., Krug, I., Jimenez-Murcia, S., Granero, R., Nunez-Navarro, A., Penelo, A., Solano, R., and Treasure, J. (in press). Male eating disorders and therapy: A controlled pilot study with one year follow-up. *Behavior Therapy and Experimental Psychiatry.*

Fernandez, F., Sanchez, I., Turon, J. V., Jimenez, S., Alonso, P., and Vallejo, J. (1998). [Psychoeducative ambulatory group in bulimia nervosa. Evaluation of a short-term approach]. *Actas Luso Españolas de Neurología, Psiquiatría y Ciencias Afines,* 26, 23-8.

Fichter, M. M., Daser, C., and Postpischil, F. (1985). Anorexic syndromes in the male. *Journal of Psychiatric Research,* 19, 305-13.

Freeman, A. C. (2005). Eating disorders in males: A review. *South African Psychiatry Review,* 8, 58-64.

Furnham, A., Badmin, N., and Sneade, I. (2002). Body image dissatisfaction: gender differences in eating attitudes, self-esteem, and reasons for exercise. *The Journal of Psychology,* 136, 581-96.

Galletly, C., and James, B. (1979). Anorexia nervosa in a male: comment and illustration. *The New Zealand Medical Journal,* 89, 171-3.

Geist, R., Heinmaa, M., Katzman, D., and Stephens, D. (1999). A comparison of male and female adolescents referred to an eating disorder program. *The Canadian Journal of Psychiatry,* 44, 374-8.

Goebel, F. D. (1976). [Anorexia nervosa in the male]. *MMW Munchener Medizinische Wochenschrift,* 118, 1557-8.

Grabhorn, R., Kopp, W., Gitzinger, I., von Wietersheim, J., and Kaufhold, J. (2003). [Differences between female and male patients with eating disorders--results of a multicenter study on eating disorders (MZ-Ess)]. *Psychotherapie Psychosomatik Medizinische Psychologie,* 53, 15-22.

Joiner, T. E., Jr., Katz, J., and Heatherton, T. F. (2000). Personality features differentiate late adolescent females and males with chronic bulimic symptoms. *International Journal of Eating Disorders,* 27, 191-7.

Keel, P. K., Klump, K. L., Leon, G. R., and Fulkerson, J. A. (1998). Disordered eating in adolescent males from a school-based sample. *International Journal of Eating Disorders,* 23, 125-32.

Kjelsas, E., Augestad, L. B., and Flanders, D. (2003). Screening of males with eating disorders. *Eating and Weight Disorders,* 8, 304-10.

Kjelsas, E., Bjornstrom, C., and Gotestam, K. G. (2004). Prevalence of eating disorders in female and male adolescents (14-15 years). *Eating Behaviours,* 5, 13-25.

Larsen, J. K., and Skovgard, B. (1977). [Anorexia nervosa. Behavior therapy in a male patient]. *Ugeskr Laeger,* 140, 18-9.

Lindblad, F., Lindberg, L., and Hjern, A. (2006). Anorexia nervosa in young men: A cohort study. *International Journal of Eating Disorders, 39*, 662-6.

Machado, P. P., Machado, B. C., Goncalves, S., and Hoek, H. W. (2007). The prevalence of eating disorders not otherwise specified. *International Journal of Eating Disorders, 40*, 212-7.

Mitchell, J. E., and Goff, G. (1984). Bulimia in male patients. *Psychosomatics, 25*, 909-13.

Muise, A. M., Stein, D. G., and Arbess, G. (2003). Eating disorders in adolescent boys: a review of the adolescent and young adult literature. *Journal of Adolescent Health, 33*, 427-35.

Nunez-Navarro, A., Aguera, Z. P., Araguz, N., Collier, D., Gorwood, P., Granero, R., Jiménez-Murcia, S., Karwautz, A., Krug, I., Moragas, L., Penelo, E., S., S., Treasure, J., and Fernández-Aranda, F. (in press). *Personality and psychopathological traits in eating disorder males: A case-control study.*

Olivardia, R., Pope, H. G., Jr., Mangweth, B., and Hudson, J. I. (1995). Eating disorders in college men. *American Journal of Psychiatry, 152*, 1279-85.

Robinson, P. H., and Holden, N. L. (1986). Bulimia nervosa in the male: a report of nine cases. *Psychological Medicine, 16*, 795-803.

Rodriguez-Cano, T., Beato-Fernandez, L., and Belmonte-Llario, A. (2005). New contributions to the prevalence of eating disorders in Spanish adolescents: Detection of false negatives. *European Psychiatry, 20*, 173-178.

Roussounis, S. H., and Savage, T. S. (1971). Anorexia nervosa in a prepubertal male. *Proceedings of the Royal Society of Medicine, 64*, 666-7.

Saccomani, L., Savoini, M., Cirrincione, M., Vercellino, F., and Ravera, G. (1998). Long-term outcome of children and adolescents with anorexia nervosa: study of comorbidity. *Journal of Psychosomatic Research, 44*, 565-71.

Shapiro, J. R., Berkman, N. D., Brownley, K. A., Sedway, J. A., Lohr, K. N., and Bulik, C. M. (2007). Bulimia nervosa treatment: a systematic review of randomized controlled trials. *International Journal of Eating Disorders, 40*, 321-36.

Stice, E. (2002). Risk and maintenance factors for eating pathology: a meta-analytic review. *Psychological Bulletin, 128*, 825-48.

Stice, E., and Whitenton, K. (2002). Risk factors for body dissatisfaction in adolescent girls: a longitudinal investigation. *Development Psychology, 38*, 669-78.

Striegel-Moore, R. H., Garvin, V., Dohm, F. A., and Rosenheck, R. A. (1999). Eating disorders in a national sample of hospitalized female and male veterans: detection rates and psychiatric comorbidity. *International Journal of Eating Disorders, 25*, 405-14.

Strober, M., Freeman, R., Lampert, C., Diamond, J., and Kaye, W. (2001). Males with anorexia nervosa: a controlled study of eating disorders in first-degree relatives. *International Journal of Eating Disorders, 29*, 263-9.

Strober, M., Freeman, R., Lampert, C., Diamond, J., Teplinsky, C., and DeAntonio, M. (2006). Are there gender differences in core symptoms, temperament, and short-term prospective outcome in anorexia nervosa? *International Journal of Eating Disorders, 39*, 570-5.

Weltzin, T., Cornella-Carlson, T., Weisensel, N., Timmel, P., Hallinan, P., and Bean, P. (2007a). The combined presence of obsessive compulsive behaviors in males and females with eating disorders account for longer lengths of stay and more severe eating disorder symptoms. *Eating and Weight Disorders,* 12, 176-82.

Weltzin, T. E., Weisensel, N., Cornelia-Carlson, T., and Bean, P. (2007b). Improvements in the severity of eating disorder symptoms and weight changes in a large population of males undergoing treatment for eating disorders. *Best Practices in Mental Health: An International Journal,* 3, 52-65.

Weltzin, T. E., Weisensel, N., Franczyk, D., Burnett, K., Klitz, C., and Bean, P. (2005). Eating disorders in men: Update. *Journal of Men's Health and Gender,* 2, 186-193.

Woodside, D. B., Bulik, C. M., Thornton, L., Klump, K. L., Tozzi, F., Fichter, M. M., Halmi, K. A., Kaplan, A. S., Strober, M., Devlin, B., Bacanu, S. A., Ganjei, K., Crow, S., Mitchell, J., Rotondo, A., Mauri, M., Cassano, G., Keel, P., Berrettini, W. H., and Kaye, W. H. (2004). Personality in men with eating disorders. *Journal of Psychosomatic Research,* 57, 273-8.

Woodside, D. B., Garfinkel, P. E., Lin, E., Goering, P., Kaplan, A. S., Goldbloom, D. S., and Kennedy, S. H. (2001). Comparisons of men with full or partial eating disorders, men without eating disorders, and women with eating disorders in the community. *American Journal of Psychiatry,* 158, 570-4.

Woodside, D. B., and Kaplan, A. S. (1994). Day hospital treatment in males with eating disorders: Response and comparison to females. *Journal of Psychosomatic Research,* 38, 471-475.

In: Evidence-Based Treatments for Eating Disorders
Author: Ida F. Dancyger and Victor M. Fornari

ISBN 978-1-60692-310-8
© 2009 Nova Science Publishers, Inc.

Chapter X

Treatment Resistance: Persuasion, Perceived Coercion and Compulsion

Angela S. Guarda and Janelle W. Coughlin
The Johns Hopkins School of Medicine
Baltimore, Maryland, USA

Abstract

Ambivalence towards treatment and treatment resistance are characteristic of eating disorders, particularly anorexia nervosa. Because attempts at normalizing weight and eating patterns threaten the ego-syntonic nature of dieting behavior, patients with anorexia nervosa rarely enter treatment of their own accord. Instead, some degree of pressure, or coercion, ranging from gentle persuasion to legal certification, is often applied to oblige resistant patients into treatment. Coercion is controversial however, and there is limited research to guide practitioners on the ethics and clinical management of treatment refusal. This chapter will discuss ambivalence and treatment resistance as core phenomenological features of eating disorders with emphasis on anorexia nervosa. The literature on treatment refusal, including competency and capacity to consent to treatment, perceived coercion about the admission process and compulsory treatment will be reviewed as well as empirical evidence regarding the therapeutic value and role, if any, of coercive interventions, ranging from mere persuasion to the extreme of compulsory inpatient treatment. Finally, the chapter will close with a case study, a suggested approach for managing treatment resistance and a discussion of directions for future clinical research.

Introduction

Eating disorders and anorexia nervosa in particular, are behavioral conditions characterized by denial of illness, ambivalence towards treatment and treatment resistance. Refusal of treatment raises significant ethical dilemmas for clinicians, family members, educators and employers given the high mortality of anorexia nervosa (Hoek, 2006; Millar et al., 2005). In health care practice, conflicts arise between the principle of patient autonomy, or right to self-govern, and the principles of beneficence (duty to act in the best interest of patients) and nonmaleficence (duty not to harm patients). Paternalistic acts, which restrict patients' freedom to self-govern, are typically justified only when a patient's capacity to consent to treatment is impaired and the act ensures good or prevents harm. Eating disorders present specific challenges in determining: i) whether patients have the capacity to make treatment decisions, ii) under what instances paternalistic acts are clinically justified and iii) to what extent and how these acts should be implemented when deemed appropriate.

Ambivalence Towards Treatment Is a Symptom of Eating Disorders

In anorexia nervosa, "motivated eating restraint" (Schmidt and Treasure, 2006) fuels an overvalued fear of fatness. Dieting is pursued beyond the bounds of reason and to the exclusion of other socially and developmentally appropriate activities (McHugh and Slavney, 1998). Since dieting is strongly ego-syntonic in both bulimia and in anorexia nervosa, attempts at normalizing eating behavior are experienced as uncomfortable. In anorexia nervosa, treatment avoidance is in essence a symptom of the condition, making it unlike refusal of medical intervention in other illnesses (Tiller, Schmidt, and Treasure, 1993). When patients seek treatment they do so to obtain temporary relief from unpleasant physical, psychological and social consequences of their behavior, however they do not want to give the behavior up in its entirety. This situation results in a fundamental conflict between the goals of patient and those of the provider and places clinicians in the position of constantly attempting to persuade reluctant patients to change their behavior. As a result, the experience of working with patients with eating disorders can feel exhausting and frustrating to both the novice therapist and the seasoned clinician.

Because they seek treatment on their own terms, patients with anorexia nervosa act more like clients than patients. They have been found to favor interventions that allow them to talk about, rather than to change what they do (Newton, 1993) and may shop around for the treatment that feels best rather than the one that is best for them (McHugh et al., 1998). In keeping with these observations, most patients are precontemplative or contemplative rather than in the action stage in terms of their readiness to change, especially with respect to altering their restricting behavior (Hasler, Delsignore, Milos, Buddeberg, and Schnyder, 2004).

Although ultimately recovery must be willed and owned by the patient, most patients initiate treatment following pressure by others. Clinical experience and anecdotal patient reports suggest that motivation for treatment in eating disorders increases with mastery over behavior change. Thus, denial of illness and avoidance of treatment are one of the main obstacles to therapeutic engagement for many patients who might otherwise have a reasonable prognosis.

Eating Disorders are Motivated Behavioral Disorders

Eating disorders and substance abuse share phenomenological similarities. Both are driven behavioral disorders characterized by ambivalence towards treatment, increasing salience of drug/food stimuli, narrowing of the behavioral repertoire, escalation of the disordered behavior over time despite increasingly negative consequences, and frequent relapse (Davis and Claridge, 1998). Affected individuals describe loss of voluntary control over their eating disordered or substance use behaviors, however this loss of control is not complete and it is state-dependent (Hyman, 2007). Recovery requires consistent, long-term behavior change by patients' with waxing and waning rationality and insight. As a result, the clinician's role is akin to that of a trainer, repeatedly encouraging the practice of healthy behaviors and the blocking of conditioned maladaptive behavior patterns.

Trait-related multigenic vulnerability modulated by environmental risk factors contributes to the etiology of both eating and substance use disorders. Once established however, these conditions are sustained by both conditioned learning and by state-related pathophysiological changes (Faris et al., 2006; Kaye, 2007; McHugh et al., 1998). In anorexia nervosa for example, restrictive eating is sustained by starvation-induced prolonged gastrointestinal transit times, early satiety and abdominal pain (Waldholtz and Andersen, 1990; Kamal et al., 1991). Starvation also increases preoccupation with food, ritualized eating behaviors and depressive symptomatology (Keys, Brozek, Henschel, Mickelsen, and Longstreet Taylor, 1950; Meehan, Loeb, Roberto, and Attia, 2006). In bulimia nervosa, self-induced vomiting leads to decreased gastric emptying, blunted postprandial cholecystokinin release (Devlin et al., 1997) and vagal changes that may facilitate the binge-purge cycle (Faris et al., 2006). Reversing these pathophysiological changes is necessary for recovery (Hyman, 2007; McHugh et al., 1998).

Common neural pathways have been implicated in both addiction and in feeding (Kelley and Berridge, 2002) and dopaminergic brain pathways involved in natural rewards (e.g. food and sex) may be usurped by drugs of abuse and dysregulated in eating disorders (Hyman, 2005; Volkow and Li, 2005; Kaye, 2007). In animals, restricting food intake amplifies the reward of both food and of drugs of abuse (Levine and Billington, 2004; Carr and Papadouka, 1994) while chronic exercise decreases mu-opioid sensitivity (Smith and Lyle, 2006), suggesting that opioidergic dysregulation may be involved in the escalating patterns of exercise observed in anorexia nervosa.

Data on Coercive Treatment for Substance Abuse

The preponderance of data from the substance abuse field suggests that the outcome of legally coerced addiction treatment provided in lieu of alternative consequences (e.g. jail, loss of driving license, loss of child custody, loss of job) can motivate reluctant patients to accept treatment, has outcomes equal to or superior to voluntary treatment, and is more cost-effective in the long-term (Miller and Flaherty, 2000). Furthermore, no empirical study has demonstrated the harm or ineffectiveness of using such leverage. Besides legal leverage, family pressure can play an important role in motivating patients to change substance use behavior and to engage in treatment (Fernandez, Begley, and Marlatt, 2006; Copello, Templeton, and Velleman, 2006). Empirical data is limited; however professionally-guided, family-based interventions for alcohol and substance abuse match or improve on the outcome of individual interventions. Flexible approaches incorporating motivational techniques have been gaining popularity and some evidence suggests they are effective in engaging unmotivated substance abusers into treatment (Meyers, Smith, and Lash, 2003; Meyers, Miller, Hill, and Tonigan, 1998). Similar approaches may have value for the treatment of eating disorders given the phenomenological parallels between these behavioral conditions.

Competence to Refuse Treatment in Anorexia Nervosa

In anorexia nervosa, a central ethical and legal question is whether the disorder impairs an individual's capacity to make a rational and free choice regarding acceptance or refusal of treatment. Legal definitions of informed consent require that patients: (i) are given adequate information to make informed decisions about risks and benefits of treatment, (ii) make treatment decisions voluntarily and (iii) are competent to make these decisions (Simon, 1992). Competence (typically a legal term) is task-specific and implies the cognitive capacity (typically a clinical term) to make an informed rational decision. It does not, however, require that patients make a rational choice.

Incompetence to refuse treatment in anorexia nervosa has been described as "subtle" (Gutheil and Bursztajn, 1986) because patients are rarely grossly incompetent. They usually recognize that their beliefs are not shared by others and demonstrate good reasoning in most areas. Although usually able to appreciate the need for others with the same disorder to receive treatment, they demonstrate a subjective defect in self-evaluation, appearing unable to recognize their own need for weight restoration. They provide seemingly rational and articulate explanations for their treatment refusal, arguing they are different in some fundamental way from other patients with the same disorder and need not gain weight or eat certain foods. Although neither actively psychotic nor suicidal, their behavior (self-starvation) contradicts their denial of suicidal intent (Appelbaum and Rumpf, 1998).

Although some have argued that select chronic treatment resistant patients may be competent to refuse treatment even when their life is in danger (Draper, 1998; Gans and Gunn, Jr., 2003; Draper, 2000), a more convincing argument can be made that in life-threatening anorexia nervosa, patients are usually incompetent to make treatment decisions involving their own eating and weight as a result of their starved state and lack the ability to choose freely and to fully appreciate their risk of death (Appelbaum et al., 1998; Gutheil et al., 1986; Kluge, 1991). This state-dependent, lack of capacity is supported by clinical evidence that once weight-restored, many involuntarily treated patients retrospectively view their treatment as justified (Watson, Bowers, and Andersen, 2000). Consistent with the view that patients' reality testing is impaired while acutely ill, a recent study found that 20% of patients with anorexia nervosa reported a dominant belief related to fear of weight gain that fell in the delusional category based on the Brown Assessment of Beliefs Scale (Steinglass, Eisen, Attia, Mayer, and Walsh, 2007).

Evidence suggests that tests of competence may fail to identify individuals with anorexia nervosa whose capacity is impaired (Gutheil et al., 1986; Tan, Hope, Stewart, and Fitzpatrick, 2003). The most rigorously validated standardized test of competence used in psychiatric populations, the MacCAT-T, is modeled after the legal criteria for capacity including understanding, reasoning, and appreciation of illness and treatment options (Grisso *et al*, 1997). In a small study by Tan and colleagues utilizing the MacCAT-T (Tan, Hope, and Stewart, 2003a), patients with anorexia nervosa all scored in the normal range, although qualitative interviews exploring beliefs, attitudes and values surrounding treatment revealed difficulties in reasoning arising from the ego-syntonic characteristic of the disorder. Beliefs fell into three general themes: (i) a relative unimportance of the risk of death compared with anorexia, (ii) an overvalued importance of the anorexia relative to other life roles and (iii) ambivalence towards treatment and recovery (Tan, Hope, and Stewart, 2003b; Tan et al., 2003a). The authors conclude that anorexia nervosa challenges current conceptions of legal capacity and competence to refuse treatment because it affects patient values, values that arise from the state of having anorexia nervosa and are therefore not independent of the illness.

Coercive Treatment and the Adolescent Patient

Treatment of the adolescent patient with anorexia nervosa is more paternalistic and coercive by definition. Minors are usually considered incompetent to make treatment decisions and consent is typically obtained from a parent or legal guardian. Consistent with being less free to refuse treatment, hospitalized adolescents with eating disorders report higher levels of perceived coercion surrounding their admission compared to adult patients (Guarda et al., 2007). Nonetheless, treatment outcome for adolescent anorexia nervosa is superior to that for adult patients. Perhaps adolescent anorexia nervosa is a milder self-limited disorder or the physiological, psychological and social sustaining factors are not yet established (Fairburn, 2005); however, a third possibility is that family involvement in treatment helps contain eating disordered behavior by promoting the practice of healthier eating behavior and blocking habitual conditioned eating disordered response patterns. If so, then the efficacy of family therapy in the treatment of adolescent anorexia nervosa (Robin, Siegel, Koepke, Moye, and Tice, 1994; Russell, Szmukler, Dare, and Eisler, 1987) may hinge more on parental compliance with treatment recommendations than on patient motivation for treatment. Conversely, when parents are more aligned with their ill children than with care providers they may reinforce treatment resistance (Fornari, Dancyger, Schneider et al., 2001). Consistent with this hypothesis, a strong therapeutic alliance between parents and clinical provider predicted lower drop out and higher total weight gain in an outpatient family therapy intervention for adolescent anorexia nervosa (Pereira, Lock, and Oggins, 2006).

Formal or informal family education is a component of most outpatient and inpatient interventions for adolescent anorexia nervosa. Parents model communication with their child based on the behavior of the treating team. This includes empathically stigmatizing and enforcing consequences for eating disordered behavior, encouraging and reinforcing healthy behavior and cognitions and increasing patient autonomy as behavior normalizes. In a small study of adolescents' perceptions of treatment decisions, although patients with anorexia nervosa complained that clinical decisions were made unilaterally by parents or by clinicians against their will, they denied desiring more freedom to refuse treatment. When asked why they did not want more autonomy they reported they would want to refuse what was best for them if they had the choice (Tan and Fegert, 2004). This incongruity between what patients know is best for them and their desire to avoid treatment illustrates a characteristic dilemma faced by patients with anorexia nervosa.

Family Therapy and the Adult Patient

Research on family involvement in treatment for adult patients with anorexia nervosa or bulimia is scant. Many adult patients are functionally impaired and dependent on their families both financially and emotionally. Although a small study suggests that family therapy is less effective than individual therapy for adults with anorexia nervosa (Russell et al., 1987), it is unclear whether the focus of the family intervention included use of behavioral contingencies and the types of leverage (housing, money, tuition) that have been found effective in substance abusing adults (Miller et al., 2000).

Voluntary Treatment and Perceived Coercion

Pressure imposed by family, friends, employers, educators or clinicians is a component of most voluntary psychiatric admissions for anorexia nervosa. Social persuasion can take various forms including, coaxing, begging, bargaining, selective information or ultimatums. At the extreme, some patients agree to hospitalization only under threat of involuntary certification. Whereas coercion is a powerful and evocative term, empathic support and persuasion are features common to all effective psychotherapeutic interventions (Frank, 1961). The boundary between persuasion and perceived coercion is not always distinct however and lies to some extent "in the eye of the beholder".

Amongst 139 eating disorder patients admitted to a behavioral specialty program, perceived coercion regarding hospital admission was more prominent in patients with anorexia nervosa than in those with bulimia, consistent with anorexia nervosa's more ego-syntonic nature (Guarda et al., 2007). Furthermore, although one-third of the 139 patients reported that they did not believe they needed to be admitted, within two weeks 40% of these converted to endorsing a need to be hospitalized. This study was not adequately powered to examine associations between conversion in belief about need for hospitalization and behavioral (e.g., weight gain) or cognitive (e.g., change in drive for thinness) outcomes, however, conversion in belief regarding need for treatment is consistent with the clinical observation that as patients change their behavior and engage therapeutically with the treatment team their motivation to change improves. Judicious, thoughtful use of coercive leverage may help engage those patients who would otherwise avoid clinical intervention.

At least one study suggests that stage of change based on Prochaska's transtheoretical model of change (Prochaska, 1995) is predictive of treatment response in eating disorder outpatients (Geller, 2006), however a second study found that the prognostic value of stage of change was related to self-referral status (Hasler et al., 2004). This finding suggests that amongst those patients who avoid treatment altogether, stage of change has less predictive value with respect to potential treatment outcome. Furthermore, although various markers of illness severity have been associated with risk of drop-out from inpatient behavioral programs (Kahn and Pike, 2001; Woodside, Carter, and Blackmore, 2004), unpublished data from our group suggests that perceived coercion and readiness to change at admission are not predictive of early dropout amongst underweight eating disorder patients.

Involuntary Treatment

There is uncertainty and confusion on behalf of clinicians and the courts about the applicability of involuntary treatment to anorexia nervosa (Gutheil et al., 1986; Ramsay, Ward, Treasure, and Russell, 1999; Appelbaum et al., 1998). Despite the high lethality of this disorder, involuntary treatment remains controversial and is employed rarely by few treatment centers, and this is true internationally. In Israel, the Mental Health Act restricts consideration for compulsory treatment to the category of psychotic disorders, thereby excluding anorexia nervosa (Melamed, Mester, Margolin, and Kalian, 2003; Mitrany and Melamed, 2005), while in the United Kingdom the majority of involuntary commitments to a behavioral specialty unit are instituted only after voluntary inpatients express a desire to leave the hospital so that patients who avoid treatment altogether are unlikely to be compulsorily detained (Ramsay et al., 1999).

In the United States, only a handful of eating disorder specialty programs treat civilly-committed patients (Appelbaum et al., 1998). In the absence of local access to such a unit, patients with anorexia nervosa are occasionally committed to general psychiatric units or are treated in medical inpatient settings. Attempts at treatment in these alternate settings are usually limited to medical stabilization since a specialized treatment team and a critical patient volume is needed to implement a behavioral protocol capable of weight restoring the majority of patients.

Research on the outcome of involuntary treatment for anorexia nervosa is limited, however case-control studies of involuntary vs. voluntary inpatients treated in specialty programs suggest that discharge BMI is equivalent for both groups (Ramsay et al., 1999; Griffiths, Beumont, Russell, Touyz, and Moore, 1997; Watson et al., 2000). Higher long-term mortality for involuntary cases in one study suggests this group may be more treatment refractory (Ramsay et al, 1999), although their worse long-term prognosis may be explained by higher case severity. Indeed, longer illness duration, higher number of prior admissions, and or lower admission BMI have all been elevated in involuntary cases (Ramsay et al, 1999; Griffiths et al, 1997). History of self-mutilating behavior (Brunner, Parzer, and Resch, 2005,Ramsay, 1999) or of reported abuse (Ramsay et al, 1999), psychiatric comorbidity and greater likelihood of experiencing the refeeding syndrome during treatment (Carney, Crim, Wakefield, Tait, and Touyz, 2006; Carney, Tait, Wakefield, Ingvarson, and Touyz, 2005;

Carney, Tait, Richardson, and Touyz, 2007; Carney, Tait, and Touyz, 2007) have also been more commonly reported amongst involuntary patients.

Empirical data indicating harm from involuntary treatment is absent, and when it is effective, involuntary treatment is often met with gratitude on behalf of patients and families (Tiller et al., 1993). In a large U.K. questionnaire survey of patients hospitalized for an eating disorder, 50% of those who reported being hospitalized against their will retrospectively described the compulsory order as "a good thing" (Newton et al. 1993). Similarly, in a U.S. study of 66 involuntarily admitted patients, many endorsed a need for treatment by the time of discharge and none lodged a formal or informal complaint about the inappropriateness of their admission, although it appears unlikely the majority would have accessed treatment but for their involuntary status (Watson et al., 2000). A survey of the perceived acceptability of compulsory treatment for anorexia nervosa among the general public suggests its acceptability is more closely linked to the likelihood of a favorable outcome than to a patient's emotional reaction to the detention (Newton, Patel, Shah, and Sturmey, 2005). In sum, a strong argument can be made that when treatment has a reasonable likelihood of improving prognosis, commitment should be considered in severe cases of anorexia nervosa (Appelbaum et al., 1998; Watson et al., 2000; Ramsay et al., 1999). Determining which patients will benefit from imposed treatment and to what extent remains a challenge.

Acutely ill patients with anorexia nervosa have difficulty imagining their lives without the disorder and describe their anorexia as integral to their identity (Stein and Corte, 2007; Tan et al., 2003b). The following case report illustrates how involuntary treatment and pressure for admission by others can result in favorable short-term treatment response, conversion in patient's belief regarding perceived need for treatment and formation of a therapeutic alliance despite the adversarial nature of the admissions process.

Case report: A 41-year-old nursing student was admitted to a behavioral eating disorders inpatient unit at a BMI of 11.7 with a 27 year history of chronic life-threatening anorexia nervosa. She reported over 22 prior hospitalizations to at least four different behavioral eating disorder programs, a psychiatric state hospital and several medical units. During all of these she had gained little if any weight. Over 15 of these admissions were precipitated by medical emergencies, including electrolyte imbalances, delirium or seizures attributed to her eating disorder. Minimum lifetime BMI was 9.0 at age 38. On physical exam she was hypothermic and bradycardic, had marked lower extremity edema with skin breakdown, cachexia and osteoporosis. She was edentulous from vomiting. She endorsed marked fear of fatness, had poor insight and impaired judgment insisting she did not need inpatient treatment. She maintained she would never recover and repeatedly stated "I am my eating disorder".

She was brought to the hospital by her father under an ultimatum that she would need to be evaluated or could no longer live in his house. She agreed to voluntary admission only after the admitting officer told her he would certify her involuntarily if she refused to sign in. Once on the unit she immediately requested to leave the hospital and was certified. She subsequently became agitated requiring seclusion over the first weekend of her stay. She intermittently exhibited multiple behavioral problems and poor compliance with the treatment protocol including: hoarding food in her room, vomiting into a newspaper and was often argumentative with staff. Nonetheless, she participated in group therapy, engaged with peers and was able to provide positive feedback to other patients regarding their need for treatment.

Her weight gain was slower than average, however she reached a BMI of 17 prior to transition to partial hospital. She refused to attend the partial program and was subsequently discharged against medical advice.

In a thank you letter received several months after her discharge she wrote " ... I just wanted to thank you and the eating disorder team for your kind attention, guidance, patience, and understanding given to me during my recent stay...Even though as you well know I at times presented considerable resistance to your treatment, the constant and concerted efforts of the staff helped me to face and tackle many of the obstacles that have been keeping me sick for years. When I came to you I was totally hopeless in anyone's attempt to help me get better and I was determined to prove to you that I was beyond help. Now that I am home and am doing relatively well I can see how much progress I have made. I never thought I would admit you have an excellent program that essentially saved my life. You were able to provide me with a healthier mind and body while teaching me to be less fearful of food and helping me to develop more controlled eating behavior patterns. ...There is absolutely no question in my mind that I am much better off now than when I was admitted on the brink of death. Thank you for not giving up on me, keeping me safe, and allowing me the opportunity to live a much healthier life where I may follow my dreams to become a nurse. I will never forget the experience and education I gained from the program and will recommend it to anyone who may need help and I know you will be there for me if I should ever need you again. I now understand the "method to your madness". Once again I would like to express my sincere gratitude for all you have given back to me".

Four years later, although still chronically underweight, she has maintained her discharge BMI, is working as a critical care nurse, and has not been rehospitalized. Her father reports she is doing the best she has in years.

The Spectrum of Coercion: From Persuasion to Compulsion

Because the legal process is, by nature, adversarial and can delay and interfere with the formation of a therapeutic alliance (Geist, Katzman, and Colangelo, 1996), the least restrictive therapeutic intervention for the individual patient should always be attempted first in keeping with the principle of autonomy (Melamed et al., 2003). When other attempts fail, when a patient's life is at risk and when there is reasonable confidence that the treatment will be beneficial, involuntary treatment should be considered (Russell, 2001).

Treatment setting is important, with higher likelihood of benefit in specialty programs experienced in managing treatment resistant patients than on a general psychiatric or medical unit. Similarly, feeding method may influence outcome. Oral feeding is safer than enteral or parenteral feeding and may be associated with lower relapse risk. Although preferable, oral feeding may be ineffective in achieving consistent weight gain outside of a behavioral specialty unit experienced in implementing behavioral and group therapy techniques with treatment resistant cases.

When the decision is taken to pursue legal commitment, involvement of family in the commitment hearing is recommended. Given the adversarial nature of the legal commitment process, therapeutic progress can be undermined if the family is not aligned with the treatment team or opposes commitment. At the hearing, parents or the spouse of an adult patient can supply collateral history to the judge about recent behavior that may be crucial to the assessment of competence. The family member's presence also helps convey the message that both the family and the clinical team are committed to the patient's recovery and need for treatment. Civil commitment may be preferable to the appointment of a family member as the legal guardian since it relieves the family from being the decision maker in compelling treatment and frees the family to take on a more supportive role in assisting the patient to follow the clinical team's recommendations. In this sense commitment may paradoxically alleviate adversarial tension between patient and family, allowing the formation of a more collaborative recovery-oriented alliance. Family involvement is likely to remain important not only during hospitalization and weight restoration but throughout the early stages of relapse prevention.

Although ethical issues concerning compulsory treatment of anorexia nervosa have engendered considerable discussion amongst clinicians and academicians (Draper, 2003; Giordano, 2003; Hebert and Weingarten, 1991; Williams, Pieri, and Sims, 1998), much less has been written regarding the more ubiquitous issue of treatment resistance. Since treatment resistance is endemic to anorexia nervosa, ethical decision-making pervades the treatment of this condition (MacDonald, 2002). Goldner (Goldner, M., Birmingham, and Smye, 1997; Goldner, 1989) has outlined a series of useful recommendations aimed at preventing or diminishing treatment resistance. These recommendations include amongst others: identifying reasons for refusal, carefully explaining treatment recommendations, avoiding battle and scare tactics and conceptualizing resistance as an evolutionary process.

A Rational Approach to Countering Treatment Resistance. Patient Role Induction, Family Involvement, Persuasion and Conversion

Successful treatment must win the cooperation of the patient over time in order to achieve conversion from seeing dieting as the ideal to stigmatizing it as a negative behavior (Guarda and Heinberg, 2003). For chronic patients who have been ill for years, recovery must also address impairment in psychosocial function and assist patients in achieving mastery and self-confidence in other areas of their life. Role induction, formation of a therapeutic alliance and empathic persuasion are three important elements of effective treatment.

Role induction includes countering demoralization, instilling hope and covering expectations for participation in treatment and for clinical progress. Explicit discussion of target dates for the achievement of measurable treatment goals (e.g. change in frequency of eating disorder behaviors or expected weight gain per week) and contingency plans should these targets not be met (e.g. hospitalization or more intensive treatment), are best reviewed at the outset of treatment. Frankness on behalf of the clinician can help earn a patient's trust by conveying commitment to the patients' recovery and refusal to settle for a view of the eating disorder as a chronic illness. Treatment should respect patient autonomy and clinicians should always express empathy and concern, however a caring yet paternalistic stance or "confrontation with a smile" (McHugh et al., 1998) may help engage patients.

Motivational interviewing strategies (Vitousek, Watson, and Wilson, 1998) are very useful but may be insufficient to engage those patients with anorexia nervosa whose judgment is severely impaired. In these cases, judicious and sensitive use of leverage may help patients progress in treatment. Involving family from the outset is preferable. This can be done by routinely requesting that patients bring a close family member to the initial evaluation. Family participation should be presented as an expected and routine part of treatment. In patients who have life-threatening anorexia there is an argument to be made that this should be a requirement of treatment since the patient's competence is at issue. Interviewing the family member briefly can provide useful collateral information and including family in a final review of treatment recommendations reinforces treatment goals and expectations. Relatives may request guidance from clinicians regarding how to support the patient or in deciding what leverage they might consider applying to help contain the patient's eating disordered behavior. Examples of leverage may include financial support for college for a child who is refusing treatment, involvement of school officials, limiting access to a gym or use of the car or a cell phone, as well as positive incentives for weight gain and normalized eating behavior.

The threat of leverage may be sufficient to contain a patient's behavior. However, if a decision is taken to leverage treatment it should always be framed by a firm yet empathic therapeutic stance with the explicit understanding that the plan will be re-evaluated in the setting of progress towards therapeutic goals. Importantly, continued coercive pressure is not justified in the absence of clinical progress and consultation should be sought from other experts regarding treatment alternatives should this occur. Care is needed to assess countertransference and to avoid the extremes of nihilistic passive care or of heroic yet futile aggressive intervention. When treatment reaches an extended impasse it may be therapeutic to discuss termination and referral to another provider if noncompliance and lack of progress persist. For many patients who have established a therapeutic alliance with their treating clinician the threat of termination can be a strong motivator for change.

Conclusion

The issue of competency to refuse treatment and coercive treatment of eating disorders has been understudied and practical guidelines are scarce. Nonetheless, there is a reasonable argument to be made for the use of coercion in an "honest, transparent and open manner" (Carney et al., 2007) given that ambivalence towards treatment is "part and parcel" of anorexia nervosa (Ramsay et al., 1999). Meanwhile, there is an urgent need for clinical research examining competence, outcome of involuntary treatment and patient views of treatment. Furthermore, development and empirical assessment of professionally-guided family interventions aimed at engaging adult treatment resistant patients and preventing relapse should be encouraged. Future research should also compare the long-term outcome of patients who report feeling coerced into admission yet who convert to recognizing they needed intensive treatment to those who fail to convert and to self-referred patients. Data on the outcome of involuntary treatment of anorexia nervosa on general psychiatric or medical units or following enteral or parenteral refeeding is altogether lacking with the exception of anecdotal case reports (Lanceley and Travers, 1993; Geist et al., 1996). There is a need for comparative studies examining these alternate treatment settings and refeeding interventions since behavioral specialty units are often inaccessible due to geographic, insurance or other financial limitations.

References

Appelbaum, P. S. and Rumpf, T. (1998). Civil commitment of the anorexic patient. *General Hospital Psychiatry, 20,* 225-230.

Carney, T., Crim, D., Wakefield, A., Tait, D., and Touyz, S. (2006). Reflections on coercion in the treatment of severe anorexia nervosa. *The Israel Journal of Psychiatry and Related Sciences, 43,* 159-165.

Carney, T., Tait, D., Richardson, A., and Touyz, S. (2007). Why (and when) clinicians compel treatment of anorexia nervosa patients. *European Eating Disorders Review,16,* 199-206.

Carney, T., Tait, D., and Touyz, S. (2007). Coercion is coercion? Reflections on trends in the use of compulsion in treating anorexia nervosa. *Australasian Psychiatry: Bulletin of Royal Australian and New Zealand College of Psychiatrists, 15,* 390-395.

Carney, T., Tait, D., Wakefield, A., Ingvarson, M., and Touyz, S. (2005). Coercion in the treatment of anorexia nervosa: clinical, ethical and legal implications. *Medical Law Review, 24,* 21-40.

Carr, K. D. and Papadouka, V. (1994). The role of multiple opioid receptors in the potentiation of reward by food restriction. *Brain Research, 639,* 253-260.

Copello, A. G., Templeton, L., and Velleman, R. (2006). Family interventions for drug and alcohol misuse: is there a best practice? *Current Opinion in Psychiatry, 19,* 271-276.

Davis, C. and Claridge, G. (1998). The eating disorders as addiction: a psychobiological perspective. *Addictive Behaviors, 23,* 463-475.

Devlin, M. J., Walsh, B. T., Guss, J. L., Kissileff, H. R., Liddle, R. A., and Petkova, E. (1997). Postprandial cholecystokinin release and gastric emptying in patients with bulimia nervosa. *American Journal of Clinical Nutrition, 65,* 114-120.

Draper, H. (2003). Anorexia nervosa and refusal of naso-gastric treatment: a reply to Simona Giordano. *Bioethics, 17,* 279-289.

Draper, H. (1998). Treating anorexics without consent: some reservations. *Journal of Medical Ethics, 24,* 5-7.

Draper, H. (2000). Anorexia nervosa and respecting a refusal of life-prolonging therapy: a limited justification. *Bioethics, 14,* 120-133.

Fairburn, C. G. (2005). Evidence-based treatment of anorexia nervosa. *International Journal of Eating Disorders, 37 Suppl,* S26-S30.

Faris, P. L., Eckert, E. D., Kim, S. W., Meller, W. H., Pardo, J. V., Goodale, R. L. et al. (2006). Evidence for a vagal pathophysiology for bulimia nervosa and the accompanying depressive symptoms. *Journal of Affective Disorders, 92,* 79-90.

Fernandez, A. C., Begley, E. A., and Marlatt, G. A. (2006). Family and peer interventions for adults: past approaches and future directions. *Psychology of Addictive Behaviors, 20,* 207-213.

Fornari, V., Dancyger, I., Schneider, M., Fisher, M., Goodman, B., and McCall, A. (2001). Parental medical neglect in the treatment of adolescents with anorexia nervosa. *International Journal of Eating Disorders*, 29, 358-362.

Frank, J. D. (1961). *Persuasion and healing: A comparative study of psychotherapy.* Baltimore: The Johns Hopkins University Press.

Gans, M. and Gunn, W. B., Jr. (2003). End stage anorexia: criteria for competence to refuse treatment. *International Journal of Law and Psychiatry, 26,* 677-695.

Geist, R., Katzman, D. K., and Colangelo, J. J. (1996). The Consent to Treatment Act and an adolescent with anorexia nervosa. *Health Law Canada, 16,* 110-114.

Geller, J. (2006). Mechanisms of action in the process of change: helping eating disorder clients make meaningful shifts in their lives. *Clinical Child Psychology and Psychiatry, 11,* 225-237.

Giordano, S. (2003). Anorexia nervosa and refusal of naso-gastric treatment: a response to Heather Draper. *Bioethics, 17,* 261-278.

Goldner, M., Birmingham, C. L., and Smye, V. (1997). Addressing treatment refusal in Anorexia Nervosa: Clinical, Ethical, and Legal Considerations. In D.M.Garner and P. E. Garfinkel (Eds.), *Handbook of Treatment for Eating Disorders* (pp. 450-461). New York, London: The Guilford Press.

Goldner, E. (1989). Treatment refusal in anorexia nervosa. *International Journal of Eating Disorders, 8,* 297-306.

Griffiths, R. A., Beumont, P. J., Russell, J., Touyz, S. W., and Moore, G. (1997). The use of guardianship legislation for anorexia nervosa: a report of 15 cases. *Australian and New Zealand Journal of Psychiatry, 31,* 525-531.

Guarda, A. S. and Heinberg, L. J. (2003). Inpatient and partial hospital approaches to the treatment of anorexia nervosa and bulimia nervosa. In Thompson J.K. (Ed.), *Handbook of Eating Disorders and Obesity* (pp. 297-320). New York: Wiley.

Guarda, A. S., Pinto, A. M., Coughlin, J. W., Hussain, S., Haug, N. A., and Heinberg, L. J. (2007). Perceived coercion and change in perceived need for admission in patients hospitalized for eating disorders. *American Journal of Psychiatry, 164,* 108-114.

Gutheil, T. G. and Bursztajn, H. (1986). Clinicians' guidelines for assessing and presenting subtle forms of patient incompetence in legal settings. *American Journal of Psychiatry, 143,* 1020-1023.

Hasler, G., Delsignore, A., Milos, G., Buddeberg, C., and Schnyder, U. (2004). Application of Prochaska's transtheoretical model of change to patients with eating disorders. *Journal of Psychosomatic Research, 57,* 67-72.

Hebert, P. C. and Weingarten, M. A. (1991). The ethics of forced feeding in anorexia nervosa. *Canadian Medical Association Journal, 144,* 141-144.

Hoek, H. W. (2006). Incidence, prevalence and mortality of anorexia nervosa and other eating disorders. *Current Opinions in Psychiatry, 19,* 389-394.

Hyman, S. E. (2005). Addiction: a disease of learning and memory. *American Journal of Psychiatry, 162,* 1414-1422.

Hyman, S. E. (2007). The neurobiology of addiction: implications for voluntary control of behavior. *American Journal of Bioethics, 7,* 8-11.

Kahn, C. and Pike, K. M. (2001). In search of predictors of dropout from inpatient treatment for anorexia nervosa. *International Journal of Eating Disorders, 30,* 237-244.

Kamal, N., Chami, T., Andersen, A., Rosell, F. A., Schuster, M. M., and Whitehead, W. E. (1991). Delayed gastrointestinal transit times in anorexia nervosa and bulimia nervosa. *Gastroenterology, 101,* 1320-1324.

Kaye, W. (2007). Neurobiology of anorexia and bulimia nervosa. *Physiology and Behavior, 94,* 121-135.

Kelley, A. E. and Berridge, K. C. (2002). The neuroscience of natural rewards: relevance to addictive drugs. *Journal of Neuroscience, 22,* 3306-3311.

Keys, A., Brozek, J., Henschel, A., Mickelsen, O., and Longstreet Taylor, H. (1950). *The Biology of Human Starvation.* Minneapolis, MN: The University of Minnesota Press.

Kluge, E. H. (1991). The ethics of forced feeding in anorexia nervosa: a response to Hebert and Weingarten. *Canadian Medical Association Journal, 144,* 1121-1124.

Lanceley, C. and Travers, R. (1993). Anorexia nervosa: forced feeding and the law. *British Journal of Psychiatry, 163,* 835.

Levine, A. S. and Billington, C. J. (2004). Opioids as agents of reward-related feeding: a consideration of the evidence. Physiology and Behavior, *82,* 57-61.

MacDonald, C. (2002). Treatment resistance in anorexia nervosa and the pervasiveness of ethics in clinical decision making. *Canadian Journal of Psychiatry, 47,* 267-270.

McHugh, P. R. and Slavney, P. R. (1998). The Perspectives of Psychiatry. second, 151-209. Johns Hopkins University Press, Baltimore, MD. Ref Type: Serial (Book,Monograph)

Meehan, K. G., Loeb, K. L., Roberto, C. A., and Attia, E. (2006). Mood change during weight restoration in patients with anorexia nervosa. *International Journal of Eating Disorders, 39,* 587-589.

Melamed, Y., Mester, R., Margolin, J., and Kalian, M. (2003). Involuntary treatment of anorexia nervosa. *International Journal of Law and Psychiatry, 26,* 617-626.

Meyers, R. J., Miller, W. R., Hill, D. E., and Tonigan, J. S. (1998). Community reinforcement and family training (CRAFT): engaging unmotivated drug users in treatment. *Journal of Substance Abuse, 10,* 291-308.

Meyers, R. J., Smith, J. E., and Lash, D. N. (2003). The Community Reinforcement Approach. *Recent Developments in Alcoholism, 16,* 183-195.

Millar, H. R., Wardell, F., Vyvyan, J. P., Naji, S. A., Prescott, G. J., and Eagles, J. M. (2005). Anorexia nervosa mortality in Northeast Scotland, 1965-1999. *American Journal of Psychiatry, 162,* 753-757.

Miller, N. S. and Flaherty, J. A. (2000). Effectiveness of coerced addiction treatment (alternative consequences): a review of the clinical research. *Journal of Substance Abuse Treatment, 18,* 9-16.

Mitrany, E. and Melamed, Y. (2005). Compulsory treatment of anorexia nervosa. *Israel Journal of Psychiatry and Related Sciences, 42,* 185-190.

Newton, J. T., Robinson, P. and Hartley, P. (1993). Treatment for eating disorders in the United Kingdom. Part II. Experiences of treatment: A survey of members of the Eating Disorders Association. *Eating Disorders Review 1,* 10-21.

Newton, J. T., Patel, H., Shah, S., and Sturmey, P. (2005). Perceptions of the use of compulsory detention in treatment of people with eating disorders. *Psychological Reports, 96,* 701-706.

Pereira, T., Lock, J., and Oggins, J. (2006). Role of therapeutic alliance in family therapy for adolescent anorexia nervosa. *International Journal of Eating Disorders, 39,* 677-684.

Prochaska, J. O. (1995). Why do we behave the way we do? *Canadian Journal of Cardiology, 11 Suppl A,* 20A-25A.

Ramsay, R., Ward, A., Treasure, J., and Russell, G. F. (1999). Compulsory treatment in anorexia nervosa. Short-term benefits and long-term mortality. *British Journal of Psychiatry, 175,* 147-153.

Robin, A. L., Siegel, P. T., Koepke, T., Moye, A. W., and Tice, S. (1994). Family therapy versus individual therapy for adolescent females with anorexia nervosa. *Journal of Developmental and Behavioral Pediatrics, 15,* 111-116.

Russell, G. F. (2001). Involuntary treatment in anorexia nervosa. *Psychiatric Clinics of North America, 24,* 337-349.

Russell, G. F., Szmukler, G. I., Dare, C., and Eisler, I. (1987). An evaluation of family therapy in anorexia nervosa and bulimia nervosa. *Archives of General Psychiatry, 44,* 1047-1056.

Schmidt, U. and Treasure, J. (2006). Anorexia nervosa: valued and visible. A cognitive-interpersonal maintenance model and its implications for research and practice. *British Journal of Clinical Psychology, 45,* 343-366.

Simon, R. I. (1992). *Psychiatry and law for clinicians.* Washington: American Psychiatric Press, Inc.

Smith, M. A. and Lyle, M. A. (2006). Chronic exercise decreases sensitivity to mu opioids in female rats: correlation with exercise output. *Pharmacology, Biochemistry, and Behavior, 85,* 12-22.

Stein, K. F. and Corte, C. (2007). Identity impairment and the eating disorders: content and organization of the self-concept in women with anorexia nervosa and bulimia nervosa. *European Eating Disorders Review, 15,* 58-69.

Steinglass, J. E., Eisen, J. L., Attia, E., Mayer, L., and Walsh, B. T. (2007). Is anorexia nervosa a delusional disorder? An assessment of eating beliefs in anorexia nervosa. *Journal of Psychiatric Practice, 13,* 65-71.

Tan, J., Hope, T., and Stewart, A. (2003a). Competence to refuse treatment in anorexia nervosa. *International Journal of Law and Psychiatry, 26,* 697-707.

Tan, J. O. and Fegert, J. M. (2004). Capacity and competence in child and adolescent psychiatry. *Health Care Analysis, 12,* 285-294.

Tan, J. O., Hope, T., and Stewart, A. (2003b). Anorexia nervosa and personal identity: The accounts of patients and their parents. *International Journal of Law and Psychiatry, 26,* 533-548.

Tan, J. O., Hope, T., Stewart, A., and Fitzpatrick, R. (2003). Control and compulsory treatment in anorexia nervosa: the views of patients and parents. *International Journal of Law and Psychiatry, 26,* 627-645.

Tiller, J., Schmidt, U., and Treasure, J. (1993). Compulsory treatment for anorexia nervosa: compassion or coercion? *British Journal of Psychiatry, 162,* 679-680.

Vitousek, K., Watson, S., and Wilson, G. T. (1998). Enhancing motivation for change in treatment-resistant eating disorders. *Clinical Psychology Review, 18,* 391-420.

Volkow, N. and Li, T. K. (2005). The neuroscience of addiction. *Nature Neuroscience, 8,* 1429-1430.

Waldholtz, B. D. and Andersen, A. E. (1990). Gastrointestinal symptoms in anorexia nervosa. A prospective study. *Gastroenterology, 98,* 1415-1419.

Watson, T. L., Bowers, W. A., and Andersen, A. E. (2000). Involuntary treatment of eating disorders. *American Journal of Psychiatry, 157,* 1806-1810.

Williams, C. J., Pieri, L., and Sims, A. (1998). Does palliative care have a role in treatment of anorexia nervosa? We should strive to keep patients alive. *British Medical Journal, 317,* 195-196.

Woodside, D. B., Carter, J. C., and Blackmore, E. (2004). Predictors of premature termination of inpatient treatment for anorexia nervosa. *American Journal of Psychiatry, 161,* 2277-2281.

In: Evidence-Based Treatments for Eating Disorders
Author: Ida F. Dancyger and Victor M. Fornari

ISBN 978-1-60692-310-8
© 2009 Nova Science Publishers, Inc.

Chapter XI

Cognitive Behavioral Therapy for Anorexia Nervosa

Kathleen M. Pike and Marisa A. Yamano
Temple University, Japan

Abstract

Cognitive behavioral therapy (CBT) represents one of the most influential theories and therapies in the treatment of eating disorders. Over the course of the past twenty-five years, several adaptations of CBT for bulimia nervosa (BN), anorexia nervosa (AN), and binge eating disorder (BED) have been developed and evaluated. The empirical foundation for CBT in the treatment of eating disorders is especially strong for BN. In the case of AN, the emerging data base indicates that CBT has the potential to be an effective psychotherapy, particularly for individuals with weight-restored AN. This chapter provides an overview of the empirical research of CBT for AN, core theoretical principles of CBT for AN, and a discussion of the essential features of CBT for AN in clinical practice. Further investigations of CBT for AN are necessary to advance an evidence-based practice in AN treatment.

Introduction

Cognitive behavioral therapy (CBT) is one of the most important and influential theories of mental health and illness informing clinical practice today. Developed and elaborated by A.T. Beck and colleagues (e.g., Beck, 1976; Beck, Rush, Shaw, and Emery, 1979; Hawton, Salkovskis, Kirk, and Clark, 1989; Beck, Freeman, et al., 1990; Young, 1990; Hollon and Beck, 1993; J.S. Beck 1995, 2005), numerous applications and adaptations of CBT exist to address a wide range of disorders, including eating disorders. This chapter provides an overview of the application of CBT to the treatment of Anorexia Nervosa (AN). It includes a review of the empirical research, a discussion of core conceptual principles and essential principles of clinical practice of CBT for AN (CBT-AN). It concludes with recommendations for future directions.

Empirical Support for CBT for Anorexia Nervosa (CBT-AN)

Within the eating disorders field, CBT for bulimia nervosa (BN) enjoys the most extensive empirical evidence, with dozens of studies documenting its efficacy. Across a wide range of treatment settings, and compared to a wide range of alternative psychotherapies and medications, CBT shows consistent efficacy and is thus widely considered the treatment of choice for BN (NICE, 2004; Annenberg, 2005). The empirical database for CBT for AN (CBT-AN) is more limited but initial investigations suggest support for its use in outpatient treatment, particularly for weight restored individuals.

The first study to provide empirical evidence for CBT-AN was a year-long, post-hospital study evaluating CBT-AN for weight restored adults (Pike, Walsh, Vitousek, Wilson, and Bauer, 2003). Results from this clinical trial showed that 77% of the CBT-AN group (N=18) achieved an intermediate or better outcome. In terms of clinical pathology, as well as dropout and relapse rates, the CBT-AN group fared significantly better than the comparison group (N=15) that received supportive nutritional counseling. This study established a foothold in the field of treatment for adult AN by providing the first empirical evidence of efficacy for any psychological intervention in the treatment of weight restored AN. However, the sample size was small and the question remained whether CBT-AN was more effective than other psychotherapy interventions given that the comparison treatment in this study was supportive nutritional counseling. Thus, Carter, McFarlane, Bewell and colleagues (2007) conducted a one-year, non-randomized trial comparing CBT-AN to "Maintenance Treatment as Usual" (MTAU) to assess whether CBT-AN is more efficacious than standard psychotherapy interventions offered in the community for adults with weight-restored AN. In most cases, MTAU consisted of individual psychotherapy with a therapist in the community. Because these data are based on a non-randomized assignment of treatment condition they must be viewed as preliminary; however, they offer further support for CBT-AN, suggesting that it is more effective than MTAU. Specifically, 67.5% of the women in the CBT-AN treatment condition (N=46) were able to keep their weight above a BMI of 17.5 m/kg^2 without developing bulimic symptoms compared to only 34.4% in the MTAU group (N=42).

In terms of acute treatment, a recent controlled clinical trial examined the efficacy of CBT-AN for individuals with non-weight restored AN, and the data suggest that CBT-AN may be as effective as non-specific supportive clinical management (NSCM) but not better (McIntosh, Jordon, Carter, et al., 2005). In this study, CBT-AN was compared to Interpersonal Psychotherapy (IPT) and NSCM for non-weight restored adults in a 20-session outpatient treatment. The intent-to-treat analyses showed that IPT was the least effective intervention and significantly less effective than NSCM. The efficacy of CBT-AN fell between IPT and NSCM and was not significantly different from either (McIntosh, Jordon, Carter, et al., 2005). The drop out rate and the degree of ongoing eating pathology in all groups was high, suggesting that additional components of intervention and/or longer duration of treatment are necessary. The findings from this study challenge us to consider the different treatment needs of individuals with AN during the weight restoration phase of treatment as compared to maintenance and follow-up treatment. Clearly replication studies and studies with larger sample sizes are necessary to further advance an evidence-based approach to treatment for AN.

Formulation of CBT for Eating Disorders

The application of CBT to eating disorders is well articulated (Fairburn, Marcus, and Wilson; 1993; Garner, Vitousek and Pike, 1997; Marcus, 1997; Pike, Roberto, and Marcus, 2007). At its core, the CBT model of eating disorders conceptualizes these disorders as the confluence of cognitive disturbances overvaluing weight, shape and appearance coupled with behavioral disturbances in weight and dietary regulation. Individuals with low-self esteem are vulnerable to the ubiquitous and pernicious messages regarding feminine beauty ideals and the mythology that achieving such ideals will relieve feelings of low self-esteem and self-loathing. As individuals internalize these beliefs, they develop a set of dysfunctional ideas that overvalue eating, shape and weight. These cognitive beliefs translate into behavioral strategies aimed at attaining beauty ideals that are unrealistic or achieved only by engaging in extreme eating and weight control behaviors. In the case of BN, BED, and bulimic AN, the extreme efforts to restrict intake backfire, resulting in loss of control and binge eating. In the case of restrictive AN, severe emaciation sets in.

In addition to the attitudinal and behavioral problems directly linked to eating, weight and shape, individuals with AN struggle with issues of motivation, affect regulation, extreme perfectionism, and interpersonal problems, and CBT-AN focuses much care and attention on these issues. Because at its core CBT is not content-specific (i.e., the fundamental principles of CBT apply across a wide spectrum of disorders), the broad application of CBT described in theoretical and clinical writings provide thoughtful, well-articulated discussions of how to understand and approach these issues from a CBT perspective.

Five Core Conceptual Principles of CBT-AN

1. *Self-worth is over-determined by body weight and shape for individuals with AN.* Across all the eating disorders, weight and shape play a disproportionate role in determining self-worth. Clinical features in the diagnostic criteria for AN include attitudinal and behavioral disturbances related to body weight, shape and appearance. For individuals with AN, the excessive importance of body shape and weight reflects not only a beauty ideal but also an extreme need to rigidly achieve control. If successful, individuals with AN experience an enhanced sense of self-worth and esteem, albeit resulting in a wide range of other significant symptoms and co-morbid clinical problems.

For many individuals with AN, the importance of weight and shape in determining self-worth is so extreme that it typically appears irrational to loved ones and can even appear almost psychotic. For example Sarah,[*] a 17 year old high school senior who struggled with AN for five years, described ambitious academic and professional goals despite the fact that her body mass index (BMI) was barely 15 m/kg^2 and she suffered from primary amenorrhea. In addition to these core symptoms, she was prone to depressive symptoms at this low weight and was isolated socially. She was able to identify many reasons to gain weight, including being able to pursue the university experience that she had always dreamed of; however, she was not able to stay committed to weight gain during outpatient therapy and co-morbid medical and psychological symptoms increased during her last year of high school. Following high school graduation, she was readmitted to an inpatient eating disorders program for the third time and was not able to enroll in college as planned. During this hospitalization Sarah decided that she would gain and maintain a low-normal weight despite her body weight and shape concerns so that she could pursue her education. As is typical for many individuals with AN, Sarah continued to overvalue weight and shape and decided to gain weight not because she wanted to but because she no longer wanted to miss out on the many things that were increasingly difficult or impossible due to her AN.

2. *The overvaluation and overcontrol of weight and shape characteristic of individuals with AN reflects the desire to compensate for low self-esteem.* According to the CBT model of eating disorders, low self-esteem increases the vulnerability of individuals to pursue and maintain beliefs that attaining thinness will increase self-esteem to compensate for subjectively experienced deficits. A set of rigid rules that governs behaviors in pursuit of thinness becomes the central organizing principle for individuals with AN (Pike, Loeb, Vitousek, 1996). Ironically, empirical data indicate that self-esteem actually increases with weight gain (Geller et al., 2000), but for individuals with AN, rigid control over weight and shape and pursuit of extreme thinness prevails.

The issues of control and low self-esteem are often masked at first glance by the apparent sense of esteem garnered by the eating disorder. However, the centrality of low self-esteem in the etiology and maintenance of AN becomes readily apparent when individuals enter treatments that include weight restoration and maintenance as a primary goal. Andrea, a 15 year old girl who had AN for two years, was brought to treatment by her parents upon the recommendation of the school guidance counselor. She appeared to have positive relationships with her family and friends and was popular at school. Andrea claimed that everything was great and she did not appreciate the disruption to her routine and activities caused by various medical and psychotherapy appointments associated with her AN. Although Andrea reported feeling content with her life, and although many dimensions of Andrea's life actually appeared to be going well, it became evident that Andrea's AN was centrally connected to profound issues of low self-esteem and social anxiety. Andrea was intensely concerned about what others thought of her and she struggled greatly with social anxiety. School parties and social events were a great strain for her, and the only way that she managed to function in such situations was to commit to organized participation such as clean-up or set-up for an event. Andrea excelled at her school work but the awards and public recognition never seemed to satisfy her anxiety and fears about not being accepted socially.

---

[*] All clinical material represents composite cases where details and names have been changed to respect patient confidentiality.

As she engaged more fully in recovery, she described feeling unworthy of the recognition of her academic success. She reported that school achievement came easily to her so the real challenge was restoring her weight and maintaining it, something that she only had brief periods of success with over the course of several years of treatment. One of the most significant milestones in her recovery occurred when she opted to limit her studying for a science test so that she could join some friends for an evening out. She discovered that her performance was barely affected and she also discovered that her relationships with her friends and family improved as she loosened her rigid and perfectionistic goals.

3. *The overcontrol of weight and food intake characteristic of AN also reflects significant interpersonal stress and deficits in affect regulation.* In CBT-AN, significant focus is placed on interpersonal issues and self-regulation, with particular emphasis on affect regulation (Pike et al.,1996; Garner et al., 1997; Marcus, 1997). Empirical evidence suggests that difficulties in interpersonal functioning and affect regulation are significant in the onset of AN (Fairburn et al., 1999; Karwauth et al., 2001; Pike et al., 2007). It is also likely that such problems are further exacerbated as the eating disorder endures. Once an individual develops AN, all relationships and decisions are made with the preservation of the eating disorder in mind. Behaviors such as dietary restriction, extreme exercise, binge eating and purging, the use of laxatives or diuretics, and other compensatory efforts, over time become routine coping strategies that may serve to create distance in relationships and make difficult emotional states more tolerable. Although such strategies fail to resolve the underlying interpersonal or emotional problems, they offer temporary relief for as long as the individuals can sustain the effort. Thus it is with desperate persistence that individuals with AN redouble their efforts. CBT-AN strives to identify the relationship between the behavioral patterns of the eating disorder and their connection to interpersonal difficulties and affect regulation. CBT-AN explores the ways in which the eating disordered behavior fails to provide deeper resolution to these interpersonal and emotional issues and works with individuals to foster healthier, more adaptive strategies of functioning.

Carly was a 22 year old woman with AN who reported an exacerbation of her symptoms when she ran into difficulties with her roommates as university. Carly went to a large high school and managed to get by emotionally and socially but reported that at high school graduation when everyone else was overcome with emotion, she did not feel particularly connected to any of her high school classmates and had no desire to stay in touch with anyone when they all departed for university. When she arrived at university, she continued to be emotionally distant despite efforts by her roommates whose overtures actually created feelings of anxiety for Carly. She did not know how to manage the emotions she was feeling and resorted to isolating herself emotionally and binge eating and purging when the social and interpersonal problems became overwhelming. Carly described retreating from her relationships with her roommates because she felt too anxious and uncomfortable if they got too close emotionally, regardless of whether the emotions were positive or negative.

In therapy, Carly often described feeling bored, her affect was flat, and her connection with her therapist was fragile. It was only with long-term CBT-AN treatment focused on affect regulation that Carly was able to recognize the pattern of retreat that occured when her feelings threatened to overwhelm her. Identifying the cognitive and behavioral patterns that reinforced the social isolation and emotional avoidance were essential in beginning to change her affect regulation and relatedness. With practice, Carly was able to the challenge cognitive distortions and learn more adaptive behavioral strategies so that she could more effectively regulate her affect and build more engaged relationships. As she did so, her eating disorder symptoms and social relationships improved steadily.

4. *AN is a multidetermined eating disorder and the complexity of etiology and maintenance of the disorder needs to be recognized and addressed in treatment.* AN is multidetermined with genetic, biological, sociocultural, familial, and developmental factors that render individuals vulnerable (Pike, Devlin, Loeb, 2003; Jacobi et al., 2004; Pike et al., 2007). Due to the complex etiology of AN, effective therapy must acknowledge the range of potential contributing factors and have the capacity to provide an integrated understanding. In addition to recognizing AN as multi-determined, fundamental to all CBT approaches is the importance of distinguishing factors that maintain eating pathology from the etiological factors of the disorder. In general, CBT approaches begin with a therapeutic focus on the dysfunctional attitudes and beliefs associated with maintenance patterns of the disorder and progress to more distal factors in treatment (Fairburn, Marcus, Wilson, 1993; Pike, Devlin, Loeb, 2003).

Given that the list of factors associated with increased risk for AN is long, no two individuals report exactly the same etiological course. Elizabeth reported that she intended to diet to lose 2 kilograms for a gymnastics competition but that the weight loss got "out of control." Prior to this weight loss "everything was fine." Upon further exploration, Elizabeth reported that she had been involved with a gymnastics team for many years and that she had aspirations to compete in the junior Olympics. In the year preceding the onset of her eating disorder, her parents arranged for her to train with a more competitive team that was coached by former Olympians. Shortly after joining this more elite team, and upon the recommendation of her coaches, Elizabeth tried to lose weight to help improve her performance.

In contrast, Fiona reported a very complicated social and developmental history prior to the onset of her AN. Her father died when she was eight years old. Prior to her father's death, she was very close to him, and they spent a lot of time camping together. Her mother fell into a major depression and started drinking excessively after Fiona's father died. Fiona tried desperately to help lift her mother from depression but to no avail. When Fiona was 12 years old, her mother married a man who moved into their home and set up a home office across from Fiona's bedroom. It was not long after his arrival that he began abusing Fiona sexually. When Fiona told her mother, her mother did not believe Fiona and told her that if she continued to make such accusations she would have to go live with her paternal grandparents. Shortly thereafter, Fiona's mother became pregnant and Fiona increasingly withdrew from family life although her performance at school remained stable. With the arrival of the newborn half-sibling, Fiona's school performance declined and her weight plummeted.

Although the developmental factors associated with the course for Elizabeth's and Fiona's eating disorders were quite different, from a CBT perspective, the unifying starting point is determining what the cognitive, behavioral, and emotional factors are that maintain the pattern of the extreme restriction associated with AN. Through careful inquiry, the goal is to make explicit the ways in which certain thoughts and behaviors reinforce each other for the purpose of regulating affect, and achieving control and enhanced self-esteem through AN.

Typically, CBT will begin with a focus on these maintenance factors and over time explore the ways in which the maintenance and precipitating factors are related. Almost always there are some continuities and some distinctions to be drawn between how and why the eating disorder began compared to how and why it is maintained.

5. *CBT recognizes the symptoms of AN not simply as symbolic representations of underlying problems but also as essential problems in their own right that have significant clinical implications requiring focused attention.* It is a fundamental tenet of CBT-AN that eating disorder symptoms have a direct impact on cognitive, emotional and behavioral functioning and therefore CBT-AN begins treatment with a focus on resolution of these attitudes and behaviors. Low weight, restrictive eating, and compensatory behaviors are therapeutic priorities given that they directly affect the emotional, behavioral, and cognitive functioning of the individual (Pike, Carter, Olmsted, 2004). Thus, CBT-AN begins with a focus on overt and specific eating disorders symptoms with the goal of expanding breadth and depth as necessary and appropriate to promote meaningful and lasting change.

When Michelle began treatment, she reported difficulty concentrating, restless sleep, and frequent episodes of hypersensitivity and crying. She also described exercising excessively and compulsively despite increasing pain in one of her knees. In addition to these immediate symptoms she reported a significant history of trauma and loss from when she was a young child and two siblings were killed in an automobile accident from which she was the sole survivor. Although her trauma history had profound psychological significance and impact on Michelle's functioning, from a CBT perspective, the strategy is typically to begin with the more proximal and immediate symptoms and then work back to the more distal factors. In this case, CBT focused on weight gain and the cognitive, behavioral and emotional factors maintaining the current pattern of excessive restriction and exercise with the explicit goal of gaining weight and normalizing eating to reduce the cognitive, mood and physical symptoms that Michelle found distressing. By focusing on these personally significant and immediately tangible symptoms, Michelle was able to increase her motivation for recovery because as the core symptoms of the eating disorder improved so did these other aspects. With time, as the acute symptoms of her AN resolved and as the cognitive, mood, and physical health symptoms improved, Michelle was in a much stronger state of mental and physical health to address the psychological meaning and impact of the earlier trauma.

Ten Essential Principles of Clinical Practice for CBT-AN

1. CBT-AN requires a sound therapeutic relationship between the client and therapist. The importance of the therapeutic relationship is perhaps universal to all psychotherapy; but in the practice of CBT-AN, therapists run the risk of focusing on the content of the CBT interventions at the expense of the relationship, especially when first learning how to work from a CBT-AN model. Failing to attend to the relationship will have significant potential negative effects. Data from psychotherapy studies consistently document that the patient-therapist alliance mediates treatment outcome (Garner, Rockert, Garner, Davis, Olmsted, and Eagle, 1993; Orlinsky, Grawe, and Parks, 1994), as do the non-specific qualities such as warmth, empathy, respect and openness (Truax and Mitchell, 1971; Thompson and Williams, 1987). Although the patient-therapist relationship does not have the same role that it has in psychoanalytic psychotherapy, a good therapeutic relationship is nonetheless an essential ingredient to successful CBT-AN.

In addition to these non-specific aspects of the relationship, when working from within a CBT-AN model, therapists need to feel comfortable being relatively active during psychotherapy sessions. Especially in the beginning of a course of CBT-AN, therapists play an important role in providing direction and structure to the session itself. Throughout the course of therapy, CBT-AN therapists strive to align with individuals and convey the essential qualities of warmth, genuineness, and acceptance balanced with technical competence in CBT and knowledge about the phenomenology of eating disorders (Garner and Bemis,1982; Wilson and Pike, 2001). It is a delicate balance. CBT-AN therapists strive to suspend judgment, and provide clients with accurate empathy, understanding, and acceptance. Concomitantly, they challenge faulty thinking and beliefs of clients without undermining the client's perception of reality, and at a pace that is therapeutically appropriate.

Of course, the therapeutic relationship also depends on client characteristics and the ability of clients to engage in treatment. The success of CBT-AN depends largely on the active participation and collaboration of the client in therapy (Wilson and Pike, 2001). In general, individuals with BN and BED seek treatment on their own initiative and are generally motivated to achieve recovery. In contrast, individuals with AN are often brought to treatment by other family members, and their investment in building a collaborative therapeutic relationship may be quite low initially. In addition to motivation, the client's capacity to engage in an honest and trusting relationship with a therapist will have a significant impact on the course of treatment. Even for those individuals who seek treatment on their own initiative, various interpersonal difficulties, and character pathology, particularly borderline pathology, can greatly stress the therapeutic relationship (Pike, Loeb, Vitousek; 1996). In these cases, explicit attention must be paid to the therapeutic relationship and applications and extensions of CBT described by Marsha Linehan in her work on Dialectical Behavioral Therapy (DBT) can be extremely helpful (Linehan, 1993).

Sound therapeutic relationships have many variations of personality, and a strong, healthy therapeutic alliance will be characterized by strong positive connections that can withstand the tension and conflict that may be part of therapy. The essential issue is that the range of feelings experienced are acknowledged and understood by therapists. In general, from a CBT perspective, if the therapeutic relationship is strong and working well, the therapist and client will not necessarily spend a significant amount of time focused explicitly on the relationship; however, it is essential that CBT therapists monitor the quality of the relationship at all times. Betty was a 27 year old woman with a 10 year history of AN who presented for outpatient CBT following inpatient treatment for acute care and weight restoration. Betty was extremely friendly and compliant in sessions. She agreed with all the therapist suggestions and always promised to pursue the behavioral challenges between sessions. However, upon return to her subsequent session, she would invariably report that she didn't get a chance to do as they had planned and had difficulty getting the foods ready for the challenges they had planned. In another case, Mary openly disagreed with therapist recommendations and challenged the CBT model. Although at first glance it might have appeared that the therapeutic relationship was stronger with Betty, in actual practice, the therapist felt that the therapeutic relationship with Mary was stronger. Mary was able to engage in more honest and open discussion about profoundly meaningful issues than Betty who opted to superficially comply with recommendations but did not actually grapple with the core issues that were associated with the maintenance of her eating disorder. The therapist addressed these issues with Betty who began to assert herself, timidly at first, to be more candid and engaged in the therapeutic relationship.

2. *The therapeutic relationship in CBT emphasizes collaboration.* The centrality of collaboration in the recovery process is a hallmark feature of CBT-AN. This means that the therapist and client share responsibility for determining the focus of therapy sessions and setting the pace for recovery. In the first phase of CBT-AN, therapists may play a more active role in setting the agenda for a session and focusing the therapy work both in the session and between sessions. However, by the end of the course of treatment, the goal of CBT-AN is for the client to learn the skills necessary for her to "become her own therapist." Thus, even from the start, it is important that the therapist and client collaboratively build the agenda for a session and work together to modify aims for each session as needed. Similarly, CBT-AN frequently entails experimenting with challenges and change outside the therapeutic hour. The focus and pace of treatment will largely be driven by the client's motivation, the degree of distress associated with particular problems, and the practical consideration of how amenable to change a particular problem is. All these factors are discussed explicitly with clients as appropriate throughout the course of treatment.

In the example above, one of the fundamental errors that occurred in the work between the therapist and Betty in the initial sessions was that the therapist was working unilaterally on what she thought was important without Betty's full engagement. The therapist took the lead in formulating an understanding of the maintenance of Betty's eating disorder, and the therapist did nearly all the work in focusing sessions, setting agendas, and establishing treatment goals. Once the therapist recognized this imbalance she attempted to rectify it by increasing the focus on the relationship and the importance of collaboration in the therapeutic work of CBT-AN. With time and with the therapist's assistance in focusing on the quality of the relationship, Betty gradually grew more comfortable asserting herself and participating actively in building a more collaborative relationship.

3. *CBT-AN begins with a focus on the present.* One of the particular defining features of CBT-AN is that therapy begins in the "here-and-now." CBT-AN focuses less on how the eating disorder developed and more on why it continues, especially in the early stages of treatment. CBT-AN recognizes eating disorders as complex developmental disorders that often have distant but meaningful origins, and from a CBT-AN perspective, it is important to conduct a thorough developmental history when beginning treatment. However, whereas other psychotherapies place greater emphasis on uncovering and exploring antecedent developmental experiences to achieve recovery, CBT-AN begins with primary focus on identifying maintenance factors that help account for a client's unsuccessful struggle, oftentimes for years, to resolve her eating disorder today.

There are at least two primary and related assumptions that account for this focus. First, by the time an individual presents for treatment, the eating disorder has often taken on a life of its own. Therefore, the CBT-AN assumption is that focusing on what maintains the eating disorder will have greater potential for resolving the eating disordered pathology compared to focusing on the developmental antecedents. Of course, certain factors (e.g., perfectionism or depression) may contribute to both the etiology and the maintenance of an eating disorder but the primary therapeutic focus will be on their relevance to the perpetuation of the eating disturbance based on the rationale that achieving some resolution of these symptoms relatively rapidly has the practical implication of relieving stress and increasing self-efficacy. Thus, the second and related assumption is that this progress will help fuel motivation and increase momentum for further change.

In the case of Jill, the focus on the present served to relieve Jill of worries about "placing blame" for her eating disorder. Whereas in past therapies, she had spent much time exploring developmental experiences associated with her eating pathology with little impact on her current eating symptoms, CBT – AN gave her a new focus and freed her up to distinguish between etiological factors and maintenance. This was especially useful since Jill was 12 years old when she developed her AN and 22 years old when she presented for CBT treatment.

4. CBT-AN begins with a focus on the eating disorder symptoms. When individuals with AN present for treatment, most often they also are struggling with a number of related emotional, psychological and interpersonal issues. Depression and anxiety are common co-morbid conditions, and interpersonal conflicts and complex developmental life experiences are not unusual (Garner, Vitousek, Pike, 1997; Fairburn, Doll, Welch, 1999; Karwautz et al., 2001; Pike et al., 2007). With such a complex presentation, it is essential that psychotherapy focus treatment in an organized way to avoid the risk of superficially covering too many topics but never reaching the depth necessary to achieve improvement or resolution on any of the issues.

Because the eating disorder has frequently taken on a life of its own by the time someone presents for treatment, many of the factors maintaining the eating disorder are entrenched and automatic, both behaviorally and cognitively. The intensive focus on daily functioning takes people off "auto-pilot" and catalyzes people to become more cognizant of the thoughts and behaviors that are integral to perpetuating the self-destructive cycles of the eating disorder. Once greater awareness is achieved, the goal of CBT-AN is to help individuals challenge dysfunctional beliefs and thoughts so that they can experiment with changing behavior. Conversely, CBT-AN also promotes behavioral experimentation and change with the expectation that modifying behavior will also serve as a catalyst for modifying dysfunctional thoughts. Many of the initial CBT interventions focus on behavioral assessment, experimentation, and change because the assumption is that the difficulties encountered in this realm will inform us of the cognitive and emotional factors at play.

Susan was a 20 year old woman with AN that began when she was approximately 14 years old. She had been in therapy for most of that time and described gaining some understanding of her very complicated family history which tended to be the focus of treatment in previous therapies. However, the core eating pathology remained largely unchanged. In CBT-AN, the focus on the current eating pathology challenged Susan to make explicit the assumptions she made regarding eating, weight and shape and their relationship to her sense of self and self-esteem. By keeping the focus at the start of therapy closely tied to the eating pathology, Susan was able to make significant strides in understanding what the core thoughts and behaviors were that maintained her eating disorder for so many years. She was also challenged early on to experiment behaviorally with changes in food choices, social behaviors related to eating, and exercise activities. Although Susan found this very challenging, she and her therapist developed a list of behavioral changes that would need to occur for Susan to feel that she had recovered from her eating disorder. They delineated a list that identified the many small steps that it would take to attain the larger goal. For example, Susan acknowledged that in order to recover from her AN she needed to eat foods that had fat. Having acknowledged this broad goal, she and her therapist went through her daily eating routines and discussed each food that she is currently eating and explored ways to increase fat intake (e.g., low-fat or regular fat yogurt instead of no-fat; low-fat or regular fat milk instead of non-fat, etc.). Together they identified many specific and small steps that would increase Susan's fat intake and then they graded them from most approachable to most challenging. Once the list was established, Susan and her therapist used it to gradually and steadily support Susan's experimentation with this aspect of her eating. This behavioral change is an essential component of CBT, but equally essential is the therapeutic work of discussing, exploring, and understanding the cognitive and emotional issues that arise in the course of the behavioral experimentation. By discussing the thoughts and feelings that emerged, Susan and her therapist were better able to understand the cognitive and emotional components that were central to maintaining her AN and thus were able to explore the alternative cognitive beliefs and strategies for regulating emotions in more adaptive ways.

5. *CBT-AN attends to client motivation, continuously and explicitly exploring and clarifying client goals to determine focus and pace of treatment.* CBT is a collaborative psychotherapy both in terms of overall process and in terms of goal setting. In order for therapists and clients to share a truly collaborative relationship, therapy needs to address openly and honestly each client's goals and motivations. Although it might seem self-evident that a client is motivated to resolve her eating disorder by virtue of the fact that she is in treatment, this is often not the case. Most notably, many individuals with AN lack motivation for recovery when they first present for treatment, with a large percentage of individuals with AN participating in therapy only under duress. In these cases, the lack of motivation for recovery is readily apparent.

Especially at the start of therapy, cultivating motivation for treatment is core to CBT-AN. Data suggest that therapy outcome improves when motivation is carefully assessed and interventions are matched to a person's stage of motivation (Proschaska and DiClemente, 1983; Miller and Rollnick, 1991; Proschaska, DiClemente, and Norcross, 1992). Within the field of eating disorders, specific strategies for assessing and enhancing motivation have been articulated by Vitousek and colleagues (Vitousek, Watson, and Wilson, 1998). In the initial stages of CBT-AN, a significant focus is placed on articulating the mixed feelings that individuals are likely to have regarding recovery and addressing the issues that interfere with the individual's capacity to commit to recovery. CBT-AN focuses on uncovering a client's values and goals and exploring whether she can achieve them without the high costs associated with the maintenance of the eating disorder. Exploring client goals and values also entails addressing incompatible goals and fears regarding the meaning and implications of resolving (losing) the eating disorder (Orimoto and Vitousek, 1992).

As mentioned above, Susan and her therapist worked in a very focused and strategic manner to develop behavioral challenges to help break down the rigid rules governing Susan's restrictive eating and exercise. In the course of developing the behavioral challenges, Susan's ambivalence about recovery from her eating disorder became clearly evident as is typical for virtually all individuals with AN. The goal of CBT-AN is to pursue as thoroughly and explicitly as possible the client's thoughts, behaviors, and feelings that work to maintain the eating pathology. With Susan, it became clear that she was invested in an excessively thin ideal and despite clear competences in other areas of her life, she struggled greatly with self-doubt and low self-esteem. Thus, she and her therapist in each session reviewed benefits and costs associated with maintaining her AN, and her therapist encouraged her to experiment with challenging the beliefs that the only source of self-esteem for Susan lay in her AN. Over time, Susan was able to recognize that her eating disorder provided short-term relief from anxiety but that the cost was that she was also becoming less confident in other areas of her life. For example, Susan recognized that her social interactions became strained because she would change plans, isolate herself, or withdraw in situations with family and friends when meals were involved. She recognized that at one level, she was frequently opting to "indulge" her eating disorder at the cost of relationships that mattered to her. She became a less reliable friend and sister, which was painful for her and served to motivate her to challenge the rules that maintained her eating disorder. These understandings served as sources of motivation for her as she slowly chipped away at the rigid rules of the eating disorder.

6. *The cognitive and behavioral focus of CBT is intimately linked to the emotional world of the client.* One of the most problematic misunderstandings of CBT is the mistaken assumption that CBT does not address feelings. Distilled down to its simplest principles, CBT focuses on the link between cognitions, behaviors and feelings. It is unfortunate that its name fails to acknowledge the emotional or affective component integral to the work of CBT; however, the omission of affect in the title in no way reflects its omission in the conduct of the therapy. Good CBT cannot be carried out without regard for the emotional and affective dimensions of an individual's experience.

The inclusion of cognitive and behavior in the name CBT reflects the premise that cognitions and behaviors have a direct impact on one's emotional world and that in order to feel better we need to address the problematic thoughts and behaviors that perpetuate psychological problems. If CBT fails to focus on material that is emotionally significant and potent, it will fail to achieve significant success. However, from a CBT perspective, emotional catharsis is not typically sufficient for achieving lasting change. Thus, in CBT, emotional expression and experience are integral to setting the pace and the targets, and by focusing on the cognitions and behaviors that are linked to the emotional issues, CBT strives to improve psychological symptoms and emotional health in general.

Angela was typical of young women with AN in that her emotional world was very private and protected. When she began CBT-AN, she was compliant with the cognitive and behavioral work but demonstrated a notable poverty of emotional expressiveness. The presence of alexithymia is not unusual in AN, and it is essential that CBT-AN therapists work with clients to develop emotional language and expression of emotion that links cognitions, behavior and feelings in a meaningful manner. With Angela, this work started at the most basic level of generating vocabulary for describing a range of emotional experience and working in session to simulate certain interpersonal situations that would evoke emotional experiences in a safe environment so that they could be better understood and explored.

As Angela gained weight, she became more expressive emotionally, but it was several months into therapy when she and her therapist knew that Angela had a break through. Angela entered the session, and began by saying that she wanted to discuss a problem she was having with her mom. Previously Angela had been overly compliant and emotionally withdrawn from her relationship with her mom but the day prior to this session Angela described taking the risk of talking to her mom about how angry she felt about the way her mom intruded on her relationships with her friends. Angela reported that her mom was defensive at first and that it was not until Angela fully expressed her anger that her mom truly began to listen. The problem was that when Angela's mom tried to apologize and connect to Angela emotionally, Angela said that she felt "a freeze come over her" and that she felt "like a statue." She realized that she felt "panicked" by the thought of being close to her mom but did not know why she had such strong feelings of this sort. This served as the starting point for many subsequent sessions that focused on interpersonal issues, their role in setting the context in which her eating disorder thrived, and the changes necessary to resolve her eating disorder fully.

7. *CBT-AN adheres to an explicit structure and duration.* At the beginning of each CBT-AN session, clients and therapists set an explicit agenda for that session. Setting the agenda is a collaborative process: clients bring material from the course of the week that they would like to address in the session and CBT therapists contribute to the agenda setting based on information that clients provide and observations of where clients are in the course of therapy. The CBT therapist's recommendations will be guided by an understanding of the CBT model for eating disorders and experience, with possible next steps that could help an individual move forward in the resolution of the eating disorder.

In the early stages of therapy, CBT therapists need to introduce clients to a number of concepts, psycho-educational components and cognitive and behavioral interventions. There is a relatively logical and natural sequence to follow in building a coherent and shared understanding of the principles and course of CBT with clients. In the manual-based treatments, a clear, stepwise sequence provides a "standard course" although in actual practice, the sequence is rarely so clear or straightforward. The essential element is that CBT therapists collaboratively build a shared understanding of the assumptions, concepts, psycho-educational components, and change strategies with clients, and that these components of CBT be introduced in a meaningful and logical sequence for each client. Thus, especially in the early stages of CBT, it is important that therapists contribute to setting the session agenda in a way that both connects to the client's clinical status and expands the client's understanding of CBT.

Once the client and therapist agree on the session agenda, the assumption is that they will work on these issues through the course of the session. If the focus of the therapy sessions veers significantly from the agreed-upon agenda, therapist and clients will decide whether to revise the session agenda or redirect the session back to the agreed-upon focus. Of course, important and interesting issues arise during the course of the session, and it is possible that the client and therapist will collaboratively agree to revise the agenda for the session. Alternatively, the issue may become the focus of another session. Either way, the essential point is that the therapist and client collaboratively agree on the focus of the session and then see it through. CBT sessions are structured in this way based on the rationale that failure to focus intensively and intentionally on particular issues will perpetuate cycles of avoidance and negative reinforcements that serve to maintain the psychological, behavioral and emotional problems of the eating disorder.

Just as the beginning of the session has an explicit agenda-setting component, time is allocated at the closure of sessions to summarize the issues covered in the session and to discuss the work that clients can do between sessions. Therapists typically take responsibility for the process of summarizing sessions in the early stages of treatment, but as with other aspects of treatment, over the course of time clients increasingly assume responsibility for this piece of the work.

In addition to following an explicit session structure, the duration of CBT-AN is often time-limited, and the course of therapy is structured more explicitly than in open-ended psychotherapy. CBT-AN treatment programs utilized in clinical research studies represent time-limited treatments. In the CBT-AN manual by Pike, Carter, and Olmsted (2004), treatment includes 50 sessions over the course of 1 year. The intervention conducted by McIntosh and colleagues (McIntosh et al., 2005) included 20 sessions over a minimum of 20 weeks. Of course, these psychotherapy protocols are time-limited in part because it is necessary to standardize the duration of care when conducting a controlled clinical trial. However, this is not the only reason why the CBT protocols are time-limited. Increasingly, psychotherapy research demonstrates that initial gains in treatment strongly predict treatment outcome (Wilson and Pike, 2001). In addition, much has been written about the clinical utility of limiting the course of therapy as a means of heightening focus and motivation. Clearly, in general clinical practice, it is not necessary to set fixed time limits; however, it is very useful in clinical practice to set assessment and review points to evaluate the efficacy of treatment. By building these checkpoints into the therapy, both the therapist and client will share a heightened awareness of the purpose of treatment and its efficacy.

8. CBT-AN relies on active engagement in treatment outside the therapy session. Many CBT therapists use the term "homework" to describe the between-session work of therapy but this term has certain negative connotations so may be best avoided. Homework is a term most commonly associated with school, and as a function of their school experience, many individuals think of homework as "extra," "unnecessary," and "irrelevant." Moreover, not only is homework superfluous, but it is often described with negative attributions such as "useless," "boring," and "difficult."

From a CBT perspective, the between-session work is as important as the work accomplished in session, and a synergy occurs when both components of treatment are maximized. Given the intensive focus on the here-and-now in CBT, much can be learned from carefully monitoring and experimenting with assumptions and routines of daily living. In the case of AN, the cognitive and behavioral disturbances and the pernicious cycles of the eating disorders are an integral part of daily life. To the extent that individuals experiment and extend the work of their CBT sessions to their daily living the potency of treatment is greatly enhanced.

Just as the psychotherapy session of CBT-AN follows a particular structure, so too, the work that individuals engage in between sessions reflects a logical and thoughtful sequence that appropriately challenges individuals to grow and change. Work outside of therapy aims to bring awareness of cognitive factors that maintain the eating disorder and challenge the client to experiment with behavior change within a supportive, therapeutic environment. Between-session work for AN may include self-monitoring of food intake as well as of social and emotional experiences in the context of the eating disorder, addressing interpersonal issues, and engaging in exercises that challenge dysfunctional cognitions and behaviors. In order for clients to invest in this work and perceive it to be valuable, it must be integrally connected to the focus of the psychotherapy sessions. One of the primary responsibilities of the CBT therapist is to empower and support clients as they engage in the process of experimentation and discovery between sessions.

During psychotherapy sessions Michelle appeared to be fully engage in therapy but she failed to engage in the work between sessions. Although this is not unusual at the beginning of CBT, it is essential that therapists address lack of engagement between sessions as it occurs. When Michelle's therapist explored Michelle's lack of commitment to the behavioral challenges and exercises, Michelle's ambivalence regarding recovery became much more evident. It also became evident to her therapist that the tasks reflected the therapist's goals but not Michelle's goals. Thus, the focus of CBT shifted back to an exploration of treatment goals and motivation, and Michelle and her therapist worked extensively on issues of trust and collaboration in their relationship so that the therapy process had real integrity. Michelle recognized that her engagement in therapy had been largely to placate her parents and keep her therapist happy so she had been keeping her "real thoughts to herself." The issues of motivation became the central and explicit focus of therapy, and as Michelle shared the intense conflicts she felt about recovery, she made slow and somewhat fitful but real progress in recovery from her AN.

9. An important component of CBT-AN is psycho-education. With all the media attention focused on eating disorders, one might expect that individuals with eating disorders would have sound and accurate knowledge about their problems. In fact, many individuals with eating disorders do know a lot about health and nutrition and eating pathology; however, they typically have many gaps and distortions in their knowledge base as well. Some of the primary psycho-educational topics addressed in the early stages of CBT for eating disorders are: the naturalistic course of illness, nutritional education, psychological and physiological effects of starvation, medical risks associated with eating disorders, and the ineffectiveness of compensatory behaviors to achieve weight loss. Data from the hallmark study conducted by Keys and colleagues at the University of Minnesota during World War II (Keys, Brozek, Henschel, Mickelsen, and Taylor, 1950) are utilized to underscore many of the deleterious consequences of starvation and distinguish the symptoms of starvation from the symptoms unique to AN.

10. CBT-AN has certain "non-negotiable" principles. Underlying every relationship is a social contract of assumptions, rules and agreements related to the interested parties. Most often, this social contract is implicit and "understood." In contrast, in the course of initiating CBT-AN, it is important that certain critical principles be made explicit. In particular, it is useful to establish either an oral agreement or preferably a written contract that explicitly stipulates the few but critical situations that have the potential to change the focus and confidentiality of treatment. The non-negotiable parameters address situations of imminent danger to self and others consistent with the fundamental ethical obligations of therapists in general. In the case of CBT-AN, it is useful to articulate explicitly the situations that will abrogate patient confidentiality and cause the therapist to redirect the focus of treatment or end treatment. In particular, the contract needs to articulate: 1) procedures for monitoring weight and managing weight loss; 2) an explicit statement regarding when outpatient treatment would be considered not viable due to weight loss or deterioration of clinical condition; and 3) when involuntary inpatient care would be pursued.

Ann is a 26 year old woman who recovered from her eating disorder approximately nine years ago. She recently contacted her CBT therapist to report that she had graduated from college and was engaged to be married. One of the primary reasons that Ann wrote to her therapist and requested to meet for a session was because nine years ago, when Ann ended treatment with her therapist, she was enraged because her therapist recommended that Ann be hospitalized due to failure to achieve significant weight restoration in outpatient treatment. Ann's parents hospitalized Ann against her will, and Ann's hospitalization was characterized by anger and opposition to recovery. After a prolonged hospitalization, Ann did gain weight and when she was discharged from the hospital she refused to resume treatment with her outpatient therapist. In her follow-up meeting with her therapist nine years later, Ann expressed gratitude to her therapist for refusing to negotiate with her about more outpatient therapy, and in retrospect Ann feels that her hospitalization was an essential part of her ability to break with her eating disorder. At the time she was furious but with time she expressed how important it was to her that she knew that she and her therapist had agreed on certain limits because without such limits she wonders if she would still be alive today.

Conclusion

Clinical research on treatment for AN is limited due to the complexity and relatively low prevalence of the disorder. Initial studies of CBT-AN suggest that it may be an effective psychotherapy in the treatment of AN; however, the data are limited and much more research is necessary. Three specific issues need to be addressed in future investigations.

First, the role of CBT-AN at different stages of treatment of AN needs further exploration. Each stage of treatment requires the prioritization of different factors. Before resolution of AN may be possible, issues of motivation need to be addressed. In the acute phase of care, once treatment begins, weight gain needs to be prioritized. As treatment progresses, the psychological and emotional issues need to be addressed and explored to achieve recovery beyond weight gain. Ultimately, issues of maintenance of recovery are critical given the typically high rates of relapse associated with AN. The particular role and efficacy of CBT-AN at each of these stages of care should be explored further.

Another extremely important priority for CBT-AN is the question of whether it has a role in treatment of adolescent AN. Studies of early onset, short duration AN indicate that family therapy is an effective intervention at this stage of care (Locke and LeGrange, 2001). However, it may be that CBT-AN also has a role to play in this stage of care, but it has not yet been scientifically evaluated. In fact, the field lacks empirical evidence to support any individual treatment approach for adolescents. This gap in our knowledge base has significant implications because in clinical practice, individual therapy is still commonly utilized, either as the primary intervention or as part of an overall treatment program. Such treatment should be informed by an evidence base, and thus, it is appropriate to evaluate whether CBT-AN may play a role in this stage of care.

Finally, given the complexity and severity of AN, it is clear that no one intervention will be sufficient or even effective for all stages of care and for all symptoms of AN. Thus, future investigations that explore combinations of treatment and sequencing of care will be of great value. This will require significant research funding for multi-site trials that support collaboration across clinical research centers so that future studies bring together necessary professional expertise and sufficiently large clinical samples.

Anorexia nervosa is a profoundly debilitating and life-threatening disorder that has challenged and largely stumped the professional community. Achieving major breakthroughs in treatment will require persistent and collaborative efforts. This clinical research agenda is essential so that more fully elaborated, evidence based approaches to AN treatment are established to guide clinical care and thereby reduce the suffering and loss of life that is associated with AN.

References

Annenberg. (2005). *Treating and preventing adolescent mental health disorders: What we know and what we don't know*. Edited by Evans, D., Foa, E., Gur, R., Hendin, H., O'Brien, C., Sligman, M., Walsh, B.T. Oxford: University Press.

Beck, A. T. (1976). *Cognitive therapy and the emotional disorders*. New York: International University Press.

Beck, A. T., Freeman, A., and Associates. (1990). *Cognitive therapy for the personality disorders*. New York: Guilford Press.

Beck, A. T., Rush, A. J., Shaw, B. F., and Emery, G. (1979). *Cognitive therapy for depression*. New York: Guilford Press.

Beck, J. S. (1995). *Cognitive therapy: Basics and beyond*. New York: Guilford Press.

Carter, J., McFarlane, T., Bewell, C., Crosby, R., Olmsted, M., Woodside, D.B., and Kaplan, A. (April, 2007). Maintenance treatment for anorexia nervosa: Cognitive behavior therapy versus treatment as usual. *International Conference on Eating Disorders*, Pittsburgh.

Fairburn, C.G. (1985). Cognitive-behavioral treatment for bulimia. In D.M. Garner and P.E. Garfinkel (Eds.), *Handbook of psychotherapy for anorexia nervosa and bulimia*. New York: Guilford Press.

Fairburn, C.G., Doll, H.A., Welch, S.L. (1999). Risk factors for anorexia nervosa: Three integrated case-control comparisons. *Archives of General Psychiatry, 56*, 468-476.

Fairburn, C.G., Marcus, M. D., and Wilson, G. W. (1993). Cognitive-behavioral therapy for binge eating and bulimia nervosa. In C. G. Fairburn and G. T. Wilson (Eds.), *Binge eating: Nature, assessment, and treatment* (pp. 361-404). New York: Guilford Press.

Garner, D.M., and Bemis, K.M. (1982). Anorexia nervosa: A cognitive-behavioral approach to AN. *Cognitive Therapy and Research, 6*, 123-150.

Garner, D.M., Vitousek, K., and Pike, K.M. (1997). Cognitive behavioral therapy for anorexia nervosa. In D.M. Garner and P.E. Garfinkel (Eds.), *Handbook of treatment for eating disorders*. (pp. 94-144). New York: Guilford Press.

Garner, D.M., Rockert, W., Garner, M.V., Davis, R., Olmsted, M.P., and Eagle, M. (1993). Comparison of cognitive-behavioral and supportive expressive therapy for bulimia nervosa. *American Journal of Psychiatry, 150*, 37-46.

Geller, J., Srikameswaran, S., Cockell, S.J., and Zaitsoff, S.L. (2000). The assessment of shape and weight-based self-esteem in adolescents. *International Journal of Eating Disorders, 28*, 339-345.

Hawton, K., Salkovskis, P. M., Kirk, J., and Clark, D. M. (1989). *Cognitive behavioral therapy for psychiatric problems*. New York: Oxford University Press.

Hollon, S. D., and Beck, A. T. (1994). Cognitive and cognitive-behavioral therapies. In A. E. Bergin and S. L. Garfield (Eds.), *Handbook of psychotherapy and behavior change* (4th ed., pp. 428-466). New York: Wiley.

Jacobi, C., Hayward, C., de Zwaan, M., Kraemer, H., and Agras, S. (2004). Coming to terms with risk factors for eating disorders: An application of risk terminology and suggestions for a general taxonomy. *Psychological Bulletin, 130*, 19-65.

Karwautz, A., Hesketh, S., Hu, X., Zhao, J., Sham, P., Collier, D.A., et al. (2001). Individual-specific risk factors for anorexia nervosa: A pilot study using a discordant sister-pair design. *Psychological Medicine, 31*, 317-329.

Keys, A., Brozek, J., Henschel, A., Mickelsen, O., and Taylor, H.L. (1950). *The biology of human starvation* (Vols. 1 and 2). Minneapolis: University of Minnesota Press.

Linehan, M. M., (1993). *Cognitive-behavioral treatment of borderline personality disorder*. New York: Guilford Press.

Lock, J., and Le Grange, D. (2001). Can family-based treatment of anorexia nervosa be manualized? *Journal of Psychotherapy Practice and Research, 10*, 253-261.

Marcus, M.D. (1997). Adapting treatment for patients with binge-eating disorder. In D.M. Garner and P.E. Garfinkel (Eds.), *Handbook of treatment for eating disorders* (2nd ed., pp. 484-493). New York: Guilford Press.

McIntosh, V.V.W., Jordan, J., Carter, F.A., Luty, S.E., McKenzie, J.M., Bulik, C.M., Frampton, C.M.A., and Joyce, P.R. (2005). Three psychotherapies for anorexia nervosa: A randomized controlled trial. *American Journal of Psychiatry, 162*, 741-747.

Miller, W.R., and Rollnick, S. (1991). *Motivational interviewing: Preparing people for change*. New York: Guilford Press.

Orimoto, L., and Vitousek, K., (1992). Anorexia nervosa and bulimia nervosa. In P. W. Wilson (Ed.), *Principles and practices of relapse prevention* (pp. 85-127). New York: Guilford Press.

Orlinsky, D.E., Grawe, K., and Parks, B.K. (1994). Process and outcome in psychotherapy: Noch einmal. In A. E. Bergin and S. L. Garfield (Eds.), *Handbook of psychotherapy and behavior change* (4th ed., pp. 270-376). New York: Wiley.

Pike, K.M., Carter, J., and Olmsted, M. (2004, unpublished). *Cognitive behavioral therapy manual for anorexia nervosa*.

Pike, K.M., Devlin, M.J., and Loeb, K. (2003). Cognitive behavioral therapy in the treatment of anorexia nervosa, bulimia nervosa, and binge eating disorder. In J. K. Thompson (Ed.), *Handbook of eating disorders and obesity*. New York: Wiley.

Pike, K.M., Hilbert, A., Wilfrey, D.E., Fairburn, C.G., Dohm, F.A., Walsh, B.T., and Striegel-Moore, R. (2007). Toward an understanding of risk factors for anorexia nervosa: A case-control study. *Psychological Medicine*.

Pike, K.M., Loeb, K., and Vitousek, K. (1996). Cognitive-behavioral therapy for anorexia nervosa and bulimia nervosa. In J. K. Thompson (Ed.), *Body image: Eating disorders and obesity* (pp. 253-302). Washington, DC: American Psychological Association.

Pike, K.M., Roberto, C., and Marcus, M. (2007). Evidence based and innovative psychological treatments for eating disorders. In G.O. Gabbard (Ed.), *Treatments of DSM-IV-TR Psychiatric Disorders*.

Pike, K.M., Walsh, B.T., Vitousek, K., Wilson, G.T., and Bauer, J. (2003). Cognitive behavioral therapy in the post-hospital treatment of anorexia nervosa. *American Journal of Psychiatry, 160 (11)*, 2046-2049.

Proschaska, J., and DiClemente, C. (1983). Stages and processes of self-changing of smoking: Toward an integrative model of change. *Journal of Consulting and Clinical Psychology, 51*, 390-395.

Proschaska, J., DiClemente, C., and Norcross, J. (1992). In search of how people change. *American Psychologist, 49*, 1102-1114.

Thompson, J.K., and Williams, D.E. (1987). An interpersonally based cognitive behavioral psychotherapy. In M. Herson, R.M. Eisler, and P.M. Miller (Eds.), *Progress in behavior modification* (Vol. 21, pp. 230-258). New York: Sage.

Traux, C.B., and Mitchell, K.M. (1971). Research on certain therapist interpersonal skills in relation to process and outcome. In A.E. Bergin and S.L. Garfield (Eds.), *Handbook of psychotherapy and behavior change: An empirical analysis* (pp. 299-344). New York: Wiley.

Vitousek, K.B., Watson, S., and Wilson, G.T. (1998). Enhancing motivation in eating disorders. *Clinical Psychology Review, 18*, 476-498.

Wilson, G.T., and Pike, K.M. (2001). Eating disorders. In D.H. Barlow (Ed.), *Clinical handbook of psychological disorders* (3rd ed., pp. 332-375). New York: Guilford Press.

Young, J.E. (1990). Schema-focused cognitive therapy for personality disorders. In A. Beck and A. Freeman (Eds.), *Cognitive therapy for personality disorders*. New York: Guilford Press.

In: Evidence-Based Treatments for Eating Disorders   ISBN 978-1-60692-310-8
Author: Ida F. Dancyger and Victor M. Fornari   © 2009 Nova Science Publishers, Inc.

Chapter XII

Cognitive Behavioral Therapy for Bulimia Nervosa

Devra Lynn Braun
Weill Cornell Medical College
New York, New York,USA

Abstract

Cognitive behavioral therapy (CBT) has been widely endorsed as the initial treatment of choice for bulimia nervosa (BN). According to the cognitive behavioral model on which the treatment is based, BN develops and is perpetuated as a result of a vicious cycle of interrelated cognitions and behaviors associated with low self-esteem, extreme concerns about shape and weight, strict dieting, binge eating and self-induced vomiting.

While CBT specifically tailored for the treatment of BN (CBT-BN) is generally considered the single most effective current treatment, fewer than half of subjects assigned to CBT-BN in most studies are abstinent from binge eating and purging by the time treatment concludes. Recent advances in our understanding of brain processes and of the pathogenesis of eating disorders have inspired the modification and expansion of the original CBT-BN model. This chapter describes the evolution of a more individualized, broadened CBT-BN treatment protocol and provides practical information about how to implement it clinically.

Introduction

Cognitive Behavioral Therapy for Bulimia Nervosa: An Evidence-Based Psychotherapy

Cognitive behavioral therapy (CBT) is widely recognized as the treatment of choice for bulimia nervosa (BN) (Mitchell, Agras and Wonderlich, 2007; Wilson and Pike, 2001; NICE,

2004; American Psychiatric Association Practice Guideline, 2006) based on nearly three decades of outcomes research (Shapiro, Berkman, Brownley, Sedway, Lohr and Bulik, 2007).

CBT specifically tailored for the treatment of BN (Fairburn, 1981) was developed by Fairburn shortly after BN was introduced in the medical literature in 1979 (Russell, 1979). According to the model, the development and perpetuation of BN is due to a vicious feedback cycle of interrelated cognitions and behaviors associated with low self-esteem, extreme concerns about shape and weight, strict dieting, binge eating and self-induced vomiting (illustrated in Figure 1, below).

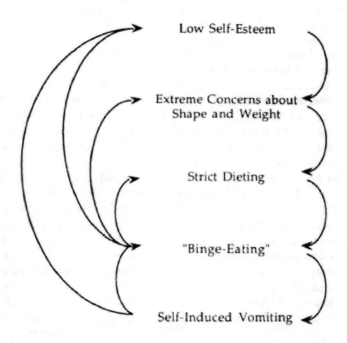

Cognitive-Behavioral Treatment

Low Self-Esteem

Extreme Concerns about Shape and Weight

Strict Dieting

"Binge-Eating"

Self-Induced Vomiting

The cognitive view of the maintenance of bulimia nervosa.

From "Cognitive-behavioral therapy for binge eating and bulimia nervosa: a comprehensive treatment manual" by Fairburn CG, Marcus MD, Wilson GT. (1993). In *Binge Eating: Nature, assessment and treatment*. Fairburn CG, Wilson GT, Eds. New York: Guilford Press, p 369. Reprinted by permission of CG Fairburn.

Fairburn's update of the above model (Fairburn, 2008) acknowledges important additional or alternative triggers including:

Negative affects and mood changes triggered by external events
Interpersonal conflict and loss are important triggering events
Maladaptive cognitive-affective chain reactions resulting from:
        perfectionism and dichotomous thinking;
        overvaluation of the importance of control of weight and diet
        Poor emotion regulation skills

Figure 1. Fairburn's Cognitive-Behavioral Model for the Development and Maintenance of Bulimia Nervosa.

Fairburn and the group at Oxford University used this model as the basis for a manualized, theory-driven CBT for adult outpatients diagnosed with BN (Fairburn, 1985). This manual has been widely utilized by both researchers (Fairburn et al., 1991; Fairburn, Norman, Welsh, O'Connor, Doll and Peveler, 1995) and clinicians (Fairburn, Marcus and Wilson, 1993; Fairburn, 1985).

In 2004, manualized individual CBT-BN was the first non-pharmacological therapy to be recommended by the U.K.'s National Institute for Clinical Excellence (NICE) as the initial treatment of choice for a psychiatric disorder (Wilson, Grilo and Vitousek, 2007; NICE, 2004). NICE recommended offering 16 to 20 sessions of CBT-BN to most adults presenting with BN (NICE, 2004).

In recent years, eating disorder treatment outcome studies have benefited from progressive methodological advances. Studies have increased in size and statistical power (NICE, 2004); and treatments, diagnostic instruments, and outcome measures have been better standardized. In addition, longer-term follow-up data have accumulated (Agras, Walsh, Fairburn, Wilson and Kraemer, 2000; Cooper and Steere, 1995; Fairburn et al., 1995; Shapiro et al., 2007).

General Advantages of CBT-BN

- Effectiveness in treating core bulimia-related symptoms (Agras et al., 2000; Hay, Bacaltchuk and Stefano, 2004; Shapiro et al., 2007);
- Beneficial influence on a spectrum of associated attitudes including concerns about shape and weight, dietary restraint, self-directedness and self-esteem (Agras, et al., 2000; Anderson, Joyce, Carter, McIntosh and Bulik, 2002; Shapiro et al., 2007; Wilfley and Cohen, 1997);
- Rapid onset of action: significant changes are commonly noted within a few weeks of beginning treatment (Wilson, Fairburn, Agras, Walsh, Kraemer, 2002; Wilson, Vitousek and Loeb, 2000);
- Durable effect: improvement is generally maintained at 6 and 12 month follow-up (Agras et al., 2000; Fairburn et al. 1995);
- Brief duration and cost-effectiveness: Manualized treatment usually involves 18 to 20 sessions over a four to five month period (Fairburn, et al., 1993; Fairburn, 2008);
- Comparable or superior efficacy to medication alone, with better long-term maintenance of change (Jacobi, Dahme and Dittmann, 2002; Pyle, Mitchell, Eckert, Hatsukami, Pomeroy and Zimmerman, 1990; Walsh, Hadigan, Devlin, Gladis and Roose, 1991);
- Potential benefit to individuals who decline medication, cannot tolerate it, or for whom medication is inadvisable; lower dropout rate for CBT than medication in some studies (Agras et al., 1992);
- More effective in ameliorating core bulimic symptoms and more likely to result in abstinence from binge eating than other psychosocial interventions, including supportive-expressive therapy, behavior therapy, nutritional counseling, group

psychoeducation, and self-help (Fairburn,1986; Fairburn et al., 1991; NICE, 2004; Shapiro et al., 2007);

- Wide availability of treatment manuals based on prototypes used with documented effect in clinical trials (Fairburn, 1985; Fairburn, 2008; Fairburn, et al., 1995).

Only interpersonal therapy (IPT) rivaled CBT-BN in outcome at long-term follow-up (Agras et al., 2000; Fairburn et al., 1995). IPT is an empirically supported focal psychotherapy that was originally designed to treat major depression (Klerman, Weissman, Rounsaville and Chevron, 1984). IPT addresses four major areas of interpersonal difficulty: grief, interpersonal role disputes, role transitions and interpersonal deficits. IPT therapists take an active, but non-directive role in teaching patients general and problem- specific strategies for improving interpersonal functioning.

Patients improved more rapidly with CBT-BN than with IPT in two important comparison studies (Agras et al., 2000; Fairburn et al., 1991). The CBT-BN group showed greater improvement in bulimic symptoms than the IPT group after the first few weeks of treatment. The IPT group continued to lag behind the CBT group throughout the formal treatment period. However, when reassessed after longer-term follow-up of eight months to five years, the IPT group had continued to improve, and there was no longer any significant difference in treatment outcome between groups. At the conclusion of successful IPT, patients often feel fully responsible for their improvement and have a sense of interpersonal competence and empowerment, which perhaps accounts for their continued improvement after formal treatment ends.

That IPT can be effective without explicitly focusing on food and weight underscores the importance of interpersonal conflict in triggering the negative affective states that are common precipitants for bulimic behaviors. During the past decade, the cognitive-behavioral model has expanded to more explicitly acknowledge non-weight related factors such as problems with relationship skills or affect regulation that can lead to a cascade of negative thoughts, feelings, and actions that may end in a final common bulimic pathway (Figure 2). The therapist is encouraged to adopt a broad cognitive-behavioral focus that allows for examination of dysfunctional interpersonal and emotional processes that may contribute to the bulimic cycle.

Limitations of Standard CBT-BN

- Only 30-50% of intent to treat samples typically achieves abstinence from binge eating and purging, with substantial variation across studies (Agras et al., 2000; Fairburn et al., 1995; Wilson et al., 2007).
- Reported measures of statistically significant improvement may not translate into clinically significant change; for example, statistically significant change in bulimic attitudes does not necessarily equate with improvement in bulimic behaviors (Openshaw, Waller and Sperlinger, 2004).
- Dramatic reductions in average binge and purge frequencies following CBT-BN may convey a deceptively rosy picture as patients who are bingeing and purging multiple

times daily at the outset of a study still remain quite symptomatic even if treatment reduces binge and purge frequencies by 50%.

DIETING:	A perfectionist who has low self-esteem and overvalued beliefs about the importance of weight and shape begins rigid, restrictive dieting. Social reinforcement temporarily boosts self-esteem and sense of control.	Self Esteem ⬆
BINGEING:	Negative moods as well as physiological and psychological responses to food restriction lead to preoccupation with food, and overwhelming urges to binge. Inevitable violation of the diet's restrictive rules leads the all-or- nothing thinker to conclude that she has "blown everything" so she "might as well" binge.	⬇
PURGING:	Purging can follow, commonly triggered by: Sensations of physical fullness paired with cognitions equating feeling full with "feeling fat" or having overeaten; Negative affect, including feelings of guilt and shame; Distorted belief that purging erases the caloric effects of binge eating can remove Such cognitions can disinhibit binge eating and encourage larger binges, which facilitate self-induced vomiting.	⬇

Figure 2. Typical Cognitive-Behavioral Cycle Leading to Development and Maintenance of BN.

Incorporating CBT-BN into Eclectic Treatments

In practice, clinicians commonly combine elements of CBT with other psychological treatments or with medications. There is inconclusive evidence as to whether combining or sequencing CBT-BN and medications confers an advantage over using CBT-BN alone (Shapiro et al., 2007), and combined treatments may have higher dropout rates than CBT-BN alone (Goldbloom et al., 1997).

There is no empirical support for the common practice of combining elements of CBT with elements of psychodynamic therapy, IPT or addiction-based approaches. Combining conceptually or procedurally incompatible approaches (Fairburn, 2008; Wilson et al., 2007) might confuse the patient, dilute the focus of CBT, and undermine its effectiveness (Wilson et al., 2007). Despite these caveats it is common practice for clinicians to combine approaches, especially CBT and IPT (Fairburn, 2008; Hendricks and Thompson, 2005).

A preset timeframe for brief treatment may have its advantages; it has been argued that the brief treatment structure serves to optimally concentrate the minds of patient and therapist, conveys concrete expectations for rapid improvement, and enables the patient to take ownership of the improvements that often continue in the weeks and months following cessation of treatment (Wilson et al., 2007).

What is Cognitive *Behavioral* Therapy?

CBT draws from the cognitive formulations of Aaron Beck, Albert Ellis, and others (Beck, 1976; Beck, Rush, Shaw and Emery, 1979) and from the theories of Watson, Skinner, and other behaviorists (Skinner, 1950). Behaviorist explanations of psychopathology are based primarily on principles of learning and conditioning. For example a basic tenet of behaviorism is the prediction that the probability that a behavior will recur in the future generally increases if it has positive consequences and decreases if it is ignored or penalized . Behaviorists look for direct or indirect "rewarding" or stress-reducing effects that may be perpetuating dysfunctional behaviors; they also search for possible adaptive "functions" that a behavior—even a behavior that is, on the whole, maladaptive or dysfunctional —may have in a patient's life. Such "functional analyses" of behavioral logs inform suggestions for environmental change. The behaviorist model is based on the tenet that environmental change can shape behavioral changes and that behavioral changes will lead to changed thoughts and feelings.

If the behaviorist model aims to use behavioral change to foster cognitive and affective change, then the cognitive model is in some ways the behaviorist model turned on its head. The cognitive model focuses on cognitive determinants of moods and behavior and the ways in which cognitive change can foster behavioral and mood change.

The cognitive approach to the treatment of BN is modeled on Aaron Beck's cognitive therapy for depression (Beck et al., 1976). Particularly helpful are the examples of ten common cognitive distortions and interpretive errors synthesized by David Burns (1989). These include all-or-nothing thinking, overgeneralization, jumping to conclusions, magnifying negatives, and catastrophization. Cognitive therapy teaches patients to identify interpretive errors in general and distorted thoughts and attitudes about shape, weight and eating, in particular. Self-monitoring exercises teach patients to notice the circumstances and cognitions that precede episodes of restrictive dieting, binge eating or purging. Therapists and patients then examine the self-monitoring logs together, noting problematic thoughts that may have preceded episodes of disordered eating.

Clinical Vignette

Directly before an episode of binge eating, Linda, a 19-year-old college student with BN, wrote the following in her log: "I'm such a loser, I have no self control. I stayed on my 800-calorie diet perfectly for two days ... and then what? I had three Oreos. Here I go again...Either I am doing great on my diet or I blow it all. I already feel fat."

To help Linda to recognize her distorted cognitive processes, which include all or nothing thinking, emotional reasoning ("I feel fat, so I must be fat"), catastrophization, overgeneralization and labeling, the clinician working with Linda asks her to objectively evaluate the statement that three cookies constitutes "blowing it all" as if she were providing evidence in a court of law. She is asked to list arguments or evidence that supports or casts doubt on the statement's conclusion and then to arrive at a different reasoned conclusion or alternative statement. Such restatements are sometimes called "reframes," a metaphorical reference to the way in which the same painting may look different in a different frame. A template for the technique of cognitive challenge is provided in Table 1, below.

Table 1. [Template for a] Cognitive Challenge of a Problematic Thought

Record the problematic thought:	
List arguments or evidence that support the statement: • _____ • _____ • _____	List arguments or evidence that cast doubt on the conclusion: • _____ • _____ • _____
REFRAME: Arrive at a reasoned conclusion or alternative statement	

While "negative self-talk," and distorted interpretations of reality such as Linda's (above) certainly may contribute to anxiety or negative mood states, few clinicians today would endorse the simplistic perspective that distorted cognitions in themselves actually cause depression and anxiety.

Our current understanding of brain circuitry, supported by neuroimaging evidence, has made it apparent that emotional states and behavioral responses are strongly influenced by forces beneath the level of our conscious awareness (Viamontes and Beitman, 2006).

Among the unconscious determinants of behavior and mood are sensory stimuli that are registered and responded to by the brain without ever reaching the level of our conscious awareness, and knowledge and associations held in unconscious pathways such as our implicit memory system.

Since behaviors and emotional responses may be inaccessible to cognitive notice or modulation, there are inherent limitations to cognitive therapy. Likewise, general principles of operant conditioning and behaviorism have limitations in their ability to explain complex behaviors such as binge eating and purging, which are likely to have genetic and evolutionary determinants. General laboratory principles of behaviorism do not account for the fact that humans can develop certain behavior patterns more readily than others. Evolutionary priming or preparedness makes particular behavioral habits relatively easy to learn and hard to extinguish (for example, overeating or bingeing on foods high in fat and sugar). Finally, our individual genetic makeup as it is expressed as a result of our interaction with our particular environment determines many characteristics that may contribute to the development of BN - for example, a tendency toward weight gain or particular personality dimensions.

Integrated cognitive-behavioral models provide a framework for attempting to assess and modulate psychopathological behaviors that result from the dynamic interaction of genes, environment, and stress-inducing maladaptive patterns of thought and behavior.

CBT Tailored for the Treatment of BN

CBT-BN targets the specific maladaptive cognitive-behavioral patterns that characteristically contribute to the development and maintenance of BN. CBT-BN also uses general CBT techniques to defuse nonspecific "negative self-talk" and other dysfunctional cognitive-behavioral habits that can trigger negative moods and bulimic behaviors.

The BN-specific cognitive behavioral vicious cycle is set in motion in the context of intersecting environmental stress and genetic vulnerability. Among the most vulnerable to developing BN are individuals with low self-esteem who are subject to sociocultural pressures to be thin. Such individuals may develop a belief in the importance of shape and weight as a principal determinant of their self-worth. As a result, they may come to equate dieting and weight loss with control and enhanced self-worth. Under certain circumstances, especially if they have a tendency toward dichotomous thinking and perfectionism, and are subject to other stressors, some of these vulnerable individuals may make radical attempts to bolster their self-esteem by implementing severely restrictive, inflexible diets in an attempt to rapidly lose weight. *(Figure 2)*

Restrictive diets and rigid dietary rules can cause strong feelings of physical and emotional deprivation, which may trigger binge eating. Purging may begin as an attempt to take charge of the out-of-control situation. The myth that purging can effectively prevent the absorption of calories may have the result of disinhibiting binge eating by uncoupling it from the deterrent fear of weight gain. Purging may in fact lead to larger binges, because it is easier to self-induce vomiting after a large binge than a small overindulgence.

In the years since the development of the cognitive-behavioral model for BN, emerging data have both supported the basic tenets of the model and suggested the need for expansion and modification. Recent studies in neuroscience and neuroimaging have provided support for the observation that cognitions are distorted and biased toward the negative in patients with BN (Legenbauer, Vocks and Ruddel, 2008) as well as in patients with depression and other psychiatric diagnoses. Neuroimaging studies are beginning to demonstrate that successful treatment with CBT results in observable changes and even apparent normalization of pre-treatment abnormalities in neural circuitry that have been observed in patients with depression and anxiety disorders (Baxter et al., 1992; Goldapple et al., 2004; Linden, 2006).

The CBT-BN assumption that dieting is a key precipitant for the onset of BN in susceptible individuals has been generally supported by empirical data (Brewerton, Dansky, Kilpatrick, and O'Neil, 2000). However, it has become apparent that subsets of individuals develop BN by purging and then beginning to binge eat, without having previously engaged in strict dieting (Byrne and McLean, 2002). This is one example of a variant or alternate pathway to the development and maintenance of BN that was not part of the original model.

Several researchers have experimented with broadening and individualizing basic CBT-BN, guided by functional analyses and other methods of identifying thoughts, feelings or behaviors that may play a role in the perpetuation of the eating disorder (Fairburn, Cooper and Shafran, 2003; Fairburn, 2008; Ghaderi, 2005). The Oxford group and others have suggested that CBT should be individualized transdiagnostically -- not on the basis of categorical diagnostic categories, but on the basis of symptom clusters and pathological cognitive-behavioral patterns that might be addressed in a modular fashion in conjunction with standard CBT. Examples of individualized areas which might be targeted as potentially contributing to the maintenance of the disorder include "clinical" perfectionism and dichotomous thinking, interpersonal difficulties, core low self-esteem, problems with affect regulation and mood intolerance, and obsessional focus on the control of shape and weight. Whether the enhanced, more individualized CBT-BN will have greater efficacy than standardized CBT-BN remains unclear (Ghaderi, 2006).

CBT-BN: 20 Sessions, "from Soup to Nuts"

The following section outlines the structure and content of Fairburn's CBT-BN (Fairburn et al, 1993), describes some of the features of the broader approach, or "Enhanced" CBT (Fairburn, 2008), and includes clinical vignettes. (As the majority of individuals with BN are female, they are referred to in the female gender for the sake of stylistic simplicity).

Initial Evaluation

Standardized CBT-BN is generally conducted in 16 - 20 sessions over the course of 4 or 5 months. A detailed initial assessment should precede the sessions. The most important purpose of this assessment is to begin establishing a working alliance with the patient and to engage her in treatment.

It is recommended that approximately 90 minutes be allotted for the initial evaluation.

A. Topics Should Include:

- Hopes, expectations and fears about treatment;
- Detailed information about current eating patterns;
- Bulimic behaviors, including binge eating, restricting, purging exercising or other compensatory behaviors;
- Attitude about weight and shape
-

- Feelings about the bulimic behaviors and their ramifications: What aspect most distresses the patient, her friends and her family? What positive and negative role or "function" does the bulimia serve in her life? What might motivate her to change or to resist change?
- Development and evolution of the disorder, and weight history
- Current life circumstances

B. Additional Information to be Obtained
(Screening questionnaires may be used to gain supplemental information if desired):

1) Current and past psychiatric, medical and substance abuse problems;
2) History of psychological or pharmacological treatment
3) Brief social and developmental summary;
4) Family history.

A workbook or text dedicated to CBT for eating disorders (such as those listed at the end of this chapter before the references) can prove helpful for both clinician and patient. It can help the clinician structure the assessment and treatment. Such books usually provide templates for patient self-monitoring records and psychoeducation handouts that can be distributed to patients in order to reinforce the topics that are covered in session.

The Three Phases Of CBT-BN: Objectives

Phase I: Objectives At A Glance

CBT–BN can be divided into three phases. During Phase I of treatment, the main emphases are on establishing a treatment alliance, orienting the patient to treatment, and educating the patient about the cognitive-behavioral mechanisms that maintain eating disorder behaviors. An additional important objective is to normalize and structure eating patterns. The first four to eight sessions may be held at a frequency of once or twice weekly.

Principal Objectivesfor the First Few Sessions:

Introduction to Treatment

- Establish a working alliance with the patient
- Establish treatment framework and expectations
- Outline timeframe, structure and goals of the different phases of treatment
- Describe structure and content of individual sessions
- Introduce weekly weighing
- Explain importance and rationale of self-monitoring of food-related behavior and associated thoughts, feelings and environmental circumstances

Initial Behavior Modification

- Implement self-monitoring
- Implement weekly weighing
- Institute a regular but flexible daily pattern of three discrete meals and one or two planned snacks

Presenting the Basic Cognitive Behavioral Model For BN

Using Figure 1 and Figure 2, formulate an individualized cognitive behavioral model of the forces maintaining the individual patient's eating disorder pathology.

- Review general principles such as the bi-directional influence between behaviors and thoughts, feelings and beliefs.
- Explain the rationale for targeting both cognitive and behavioral change.
- Review the bi-directional relationship between binge eating and dieting: Binge eating motivates patients to diet; dieting also leads to binge eating.
- eview the bi-directional relationship between binge eating and purging: Binge eatingleads to purging, but purging promotes bingeing and sets the stage for larger binges.

Additional Objectives of Phase I

- Assess eating disorder patterns
- Discuss treatment expectations and past treatment experiences
- Document specific details about the patient's binge eating and purging and the perceived function that they serve (e.g. weight management, self-soothing)
- Harness the expectation effect: Provide information about the effectiveness of treatment
- Assess patient's motivation to change and enhance motivation using psychoeducation;
- Educate patient about health consequences of bulimic behaviors:
- Short and long-term physical and psychological consequences of restrictive dieting, binge eating, self-induced vomiting, laxative abuse, and compulsive exercise
- Negative psychological and metabolic consequences of starvation, including anxiety, preoccupation with food, risk of bingeing
  Ineffectiveness of purging for weight control
- Assess patient's resistance to change

Identify, validate and address potential obstacles to treatment, including fear of failure, fear of change, and fear of giving up the behaviors

Phase 2 Objectives:

In the weekly meetings during the second phase of treatment, further emphasis is placed on identifying binge triggers, learning cognitive restructuring techniques and establishing healthy eating patterns. Self-monitoring tasks and cognitive strategies are used to analyze the thoughts, beliefs and values that trigger and maintain the bulimic behaviors. Patients work on cognitive restructuring and modifying the environmental factors that contribute to the perpetuation of the disorder.

Phase 3 Objectives:

During phase three, the focus is on maintenance of change and planning for relapse prevention. The last few sessions are often conducted at bi-weekly intervals.

Self-Monitoring: A Keystone of Treatment

A keystone of CBT treatment is the self-monitoring of eating behavior. Patients are asked to record the time and setting of all food intake and associated thoughts and feelings. Since self-monitoring can be tedious and time-consuming, the therapist must set up conditions during the first session and reinforce them in later sessions so that the patient will be likely to follow through with this treatment requirement. Some suggestions for how to do this follow:

1) Explain the importance of self-monitoring to allow the detailed focus on thoughts and behaviors outside of the session.
2) Educate the patient about the widespread endorsement of self-monitoring as central to the treatment of BN and the fact that self-monitoring alone may help to reduce symptoms (Agras, Schneider, Arnow, Raeburn and Telch, 1989).
3) Outline the requirements for self-monitoring, and focus early in each session on the logs, praising the patient for completing them. If the logs are incomplete, devote some effort to understanding why they have not been completed, but praise the patient for any acts approximating working on the logs (e.g. thinking about filling them out, etc.).

If any episode is perceived as a binge, the patient is asked to record the emotional, physiological and environmental circumstances that preceded it. After recording these incidents for a week or so, patterns usually emerge quite clearly. For example, some people typically binge when they are bored, others when they feel lonely; still others binge on vacations, or after they drink or use drugs.

In many instances, the patient's self-monitoring records allow the clinician to present hypotheses about the factors that may trigger bulimic behaviors. For example, it may become apparent that a patient not only typically binges at night, but that she binges on nights when more than six hours have elapsed since her last meal and she is exposed to a sensory temptation such as a buffet or a nearby bowl of candy.

In CBT-BN, each session has an agenda, and the clinician manages the pace of the session to adhere to the agenda. To preempt the possibility that the patient might feel that she is being "pushed around" or might become passive and allow the therapist to take over, the therapist must establish a therapeutic stance that has been referred to as "collaborative empiricism." The therapist and patient must collaborate as an investigative team intent on taking note of the cognitive and behavioral patterns associated with the bulimic behaviors, and developing and testing hypotheses about these patterns with the aim of instituting alternative ways of thinking and behaving.

Clinical Vignettes Modeling the Essential Elements of CBT-BN

In the following section, essential elements of CBT-BN are modeled in several clinical vignettes. Table 2 on pages 221-226 describes Pamela, a 33-year old accountant.

Clinical Vignette: Mark, a 25-Year Old Professional Ballet Dancer

Another example of how to fit a patient's story into the cognitive behavioral model follows: Mark, a 25-year-old dancer, has a genetic predisposition for weight gain. In a typical Western social environment, there would not be great social pressure for Mark, as a male, to attain a weight that was more ideal than average. However, in certain male microenvironments such as ballet, wrestling, acting, modeling or gymnastics, there is an extreme emphasis on thinness and ideal shape. In keeping with a stress-diathesis model for the pathogenesis of psychiatric disorders, the cognitive behavioral model reflects the importance of the interaction between genes and environment in the pathogenesis of eating disorders.

Mark is at risk for developing an eating disorder because of his genetic predisposition to deviate from the exacting weight expectations of his social group, combined with his low self-esteem and dependence upon the praise of others to sustain a sense of self-worth (which also may be genetically primed) (Fairburn et al., 1997).

Mark is lonely after breaking up with his girlfriend and has gained a few pounds. After a ballet rehearsal that did not go well he has been ruminating obsessively about how fat he looks compared with the other dancers. He goes on a strict 900-calorie diet that drastically restricts carbohydrates.

He sticks to the diet scrupulously, loses five pounds, and is praised by his instructor. After the next performance, he has a few drinks at the troupe party, and can't resist a piece of chocolate cake. Feeling depressed and angry with himself, he thinks about how he is a real "loser" who is unable to stick to a diet when everyone else can. He goes back on the low carbohydrates diet. Over time, the effects of physiological and psychological deprivation build up. After dancing, he feels irritable and exhausted due to the lack of carbohydrates and frequently violates the strict diet, leading him to have the repeated experience of feeling like a failure.

Episodes of simply overeating or violating the diet's rules alternate with episodes of binge eating, eroding his already low self-esteem and sense of control. He adopts even more rigid and restrictive rules, believing that without them he would be completely out of control and would be binge eating all of the time. As this cycle progresses and he feels more and more out of control and fearful of weight gain, he begins "compensatory" vomiting and excessive exercising. The erroneous belief that vomiting removes most calories ingested during a binge erodes his constraints against both binge eating and purging. His binges become larger, as that makes it easier for him to self-induce vomiting. His body and brain's system of appetite regulation and satiety, which relies on predictable absorption of nutrients after food ingestion, becomes increasingly dysregulated.

Mark's therapist explains to him the way in which purging and restricting fuel the fires of binge eating. The therapist helps Mark to challenge the assumption that a very low carbohydrate diet is realistic for a dancer and that other people could adhere to it. He encourages Mark to consider the possibility that his repeated experiences of failure may be a result of having set such unrealistic standards.

Standard supportive psychotherapy might explore the origins of his low self-esteem and perfectionism at this point. The CBT-BN therapist however, stays focused on the current dysfunctional eating. In doing so, the therapist is able to address the way in which bulimic behaviors are triggered by the negative affective states that indirectly result from rigid perfectionism, dichotomous thinking, and self-deprecating cognitions.

Mark agrees to institute a regimen of three meals and two planned snacks, each one containing a balance of carbohydrates (with an emphasis on complex carbohydrates), protein, and fats. After two weeks of self-monitoring and the balanced food regimen, Mark is relieved to find that he has ceased binge eating and feels less irritable and more energetic.

CBT-BN helps patients such as the ones described above appreciate that their problem is not solely binge eating, but a cycle in which dieting, purging and dysfunctional attitudes about weight and shape all interact to perpetuate the binge eating and the entire eating disorder. Once patients understand and accept this concept, they may be willing to experiment with behavioral changes such as instituting a structured pattern of meals and snacks.

In addition, with the modified and broader model of more individualized CBT-BN, clinicians can use the powerful tools of CBT to address distorted non-food-related cognitions that may underlie the negative affective states that commonly trigger dysfunctional eating. The tools and exercises learned in CBT can help patients to recognize the positive results of behavioral changes in interpersonal domains as well as in eating behavior, which can further motivate them to experiment with alternative patterns of thought and behavior.

Table 2. Presenting Essential Elements of CBT-BN

Session 1: Therapist Objectives	Vignette and commentary
Establish rapport and a therapeutic alliance	The strength of the therapeutic alliance has consistently been correlated with treatment outcome in various types of psychotherapy, including CBT-BN (Loeb et al., 2005). The strength of the alliance has been related to expectation effects, attunement, and the therapist's communication of a coherent treatment framework to the patient.
Establish a stance of collaborative investigation	To establish a positive working relationship, it is helpful for the therapist to convey a sense of confidence and positive expectation but to avoid any stance that might be interpreted as controlling or patronizing. Individuals with eating disorders are often particularly sensitive to control issues. Parents and competitive peers may have scrutinized them and used coercive force to try to get them to eat differently, to gain weight, or to stop purging. Patients may be in the habit of lying and hiding bulimic behaviors in order to avoid scrutiny. Therefore, it is vital that the therapist establish a collaborative stance and a tone of investigative curiosity as opposed to one of accusation or argument. The therapist must convey to the patient the sense that, for example, a question such as, "Why did you delay dinner until 8 pm?" is meant to communicate neutral curiosity and interest in the reasoning that led to the delay, not an accusation about, "Why did you do something so stupid as to delay dinner?"
Validate the patient's concerns, using language that is as neutral as possible	During the first session, the therapist explores the patient's motivation to engage in treatment as well as her concerns about treatment. The therapist validates the patient by acknowledging that the patient has these trepidations and concerns, without trying to "talk her out of" them at this point.

Table 2. Presenting Essential Elements of CBT-BN

Session 1: Therapist Objectives	Vignette and commentary
	Pamela (P): "I came here because I am fed up with this disgusting out-of-control eating. But I'm worried that if I stop purging I will gain weight."
	Therapist (T): "I appreciate your letting me know that you are concerned about what might happen to your weight when you stop bingeing and purging. When I explain our treatment model today, I will specifically address those concerns."
Avoid reinforcing the patient's negative cognitions	T is already applying cognitive-behavioral principles in addressing P's concern. Behavior modification is based upon the premise that behaviors that are rewarded or reinforced will occur more often, and behaviors that are punished or ignored will occur less frequently. Rewards come in many forms -- including positive thoughts and feelings and positive environmental or social consequences—such as getting attention from others. Similarly, punishment can involve internal or external consequences, including negative emotions and being ignored by others.
Communicate positive expectations about treatment outcome Communicate the importance of fact-finding in developing a joint formulation	A premise of cognitive therapy is that negative cognitions play an important role in the chain of events precipitating dysfunctional behaviors. In the dialog above, T provides immediate and selective reinforcement of P's adaptive cognitions and avoids giving attention (even negative attention) to maladaptive cognitions. T does not ignore or trivialize P's fear of weight gain; however, T avoids reinforcing her "worry thoughts" by reiterating them verbatim. Instead, T reframes P's worries that "I will gain weight" in more neutral language as concern about "what may happen to your weight." In addition, T communicates positive expectations about the outcome of the treatment by rephrasing P's speculation about "if I stop purging" to a projection about "when you stop bingeing and purging."

Table 2. Continued

Session 1: Therapist Objectives	Vignette and commentary
Find out which bulimic behaviors most concern the patient and apply the cognitive behavioral model to formulate (together with the patient) an explanation of the maintenance of those behaviors.	T: "Since your main concern is 'out-of-control binge eating', why don't we start with your telling me about your last out-of-control binge. I would like you to describe, as if you were an unbiased observer or news reporter, what was going on internally and what was going on around you before, during, and after the binge. Then we can use a cognitive behavioral model to figure out what forces are driving you to keep binge eating even though you have been trying so hard to stop."

P: "I was actually really good all day Monday… I had lost weight two years ago on this lemon cleansing diet, and I have been trying to get back on it again. On Sunday night, I binged and was disgusted with myself. I swore that first thing Monday morning I would go back to the lemon cleansing diet."

"On Monday morning, I wasn't even hungry. I had the lemon drink for lunch and resisted everything else all day, even though I could see my favorite kind of chocolate in my office-mate's candy jar."

"At the last minute, though, my boss asked me to stay late. I did not have more of the special lemon drink with me, so I decided that I should not eat anything at all until I got home. I was perfect until around 8 pm. I don't know what came over me then. I grabbed a handful of chocolate and then was really angry with myself for blowing the diet. I had a few more handfuls of chocolate and then was embarrassed that my co-worker would know what a pig I am." |
| Explain to the patient the cognitive behavioral model for purging and dieting as driving forces that perpetuate binge eating | "I made up my mind that I would go back on a strict lemon cleanse regime the first thing in the morning. I decided that I had to buy another package of chocolates to put in my co-worker's jar before she got to work, but I was angry at having to buy them. I was also angry that I'd blown the diet when I had been so perfect up until then. I had the thought that it might be a long time before I could eat chocolate again once I got back on board with the diet. So I decided that I might as well finish the chocolate in front of me. I ate everything left in the jar, even though I was stuffed. When I got home I felt so fat and my stomach was so huge that I used a whole package of laxatives." |

Table 2. Continued

Session 1: Therapist Objectives	Vignette and commentary
Relate patient's dieting, bingeing and purging patterns to the conceptual framework of the treatment model	T now has an opportunity to review with the patient the cognitive behavioral model of the maintenance of bulimia nervosa (Figure 1) in terms of the patient's particular issues. While patients commonly consider binge eating to be the problem and vomiting and strict dieting ("being good" or "perfect", in P's words) to be the solution or attempted solution (even though it may be a dysfunctional one), T explains that laxatives have very little effect on the absorption of the calories taken in during a binge; they mainly affect fluid balance, and that dieting not only does not counteract binge eating but actually perpetuates it.
Discuss the physiological, cognitive, emotional and environmental triggers that may be involved in perpetuating P's BN	T gives P a factual handout about the psychological and physiological effects of severe food restriction. It includes a description of the famous Minnesota study of semi-starvation, conducted during World War II (Keys et al., 1950). During this study, male volunteers were put on a very low calorie diet for six months; by the end of this period, they had lost approximately 25% of their original body weights. Although the men had no previous history of eating disorders, while on the diet they became preoccupied with thoughts about food and eating, and many became irritable, apathetic and depressed. During the refeeding phase of the experiment, many of these normal volunteers were overwhelmed by urges to binge eat. For months after the restriction ended, many had difficulty stopping themselves once they started eating, even after they felt very full.

T explains to P that an extremely low calorie diet such as the lemon cleanse is interpreted by the body as starvation. The body's response can include a lowering of metabolism and urges to binge eat as well as irritability, obsession with food, and other psychological responses noted in the Minnesota experiment. |

Table 2. Continued

Session 1: Therapist Objectives	Vignette and commentary
	T points out to P that her episode of binge eating on Monday was preceded by a period of many hours during which P had eaten very little. T notes that since P has stated during the intake assessment that she always skips breakfast, she is habitually going for 14-hour periods between nighttime eating and lunch. T discusses how P's dieting behavior and long periods without eating are indistinguishable to her body from a famine or starvation. The long periods without food can be reframed to be viewed as likely precipitants or "set-ups" for a binge eating episode. In addition, she would have been less vulnerable to having a binge had she eaten more flexibly with her dietary rules, and gotten a healthy meal or snack instead of attempting to fast.
Formulate an individualized cognitive behavioral model for the maintenance of the patient's bulimic behaviors.	T then returns to P's concern that she will gain weight during treatment. T explains that the initial focus of treatment is on gaining control of the chaotic eating behaviors, not on weight change. T will explain that most patients do not gain weight, and in fact may lose weight because they are reducing binge eating. However, T will also educate P about the fact that habitual laxative abuse can cause dehydration and can cause temporary constipation and water retention after the laxative abuse is discontinued. T can explain that while P may experience fluctuations in water weight and sensations of being bloated, these are usually temporary. P is reminded that by not weighing herself until her weigh-in next week she can avoid unnecessary distress about temporary water weight fluctuations and focus on the important task of gaining control of her binge eating and dangerous laxative abuse.
	In addition, T explores the emotional and environmental circumstances surrounding the binge, noting that sometimes negative cognitions and mood states trigger binge eating and purging:
	T: "Now that we understand some of the physiological factors that might have made you vulnerable to binge eating on Monday, it would also be helpful to examine what you were feeling and thinking, as negative moods and thought processes also commonly trigger binge eating."

Table 2. Continued

Session 1: Therapist Objectives	Vignette and commentary
	P: "Well, Mondays are never great days; I was tired and looking forward to getting home when my boss asked me-- at the last minute-- to work late. I was angry that he was asking again, but I felt trapped; I felt that I couldn't refuse. He asks me to work late more than my co-workers because he knows that I don't have anything better to do at night. I remember thinking how pathetic it is that I don't have a husband or family, and that I only had myself to blame for having to work overtime." T comments that P was feeling tired, angry at her boss and at herself, ashamed about eating her co-worker's chocolates, and angry at having to buy more. T asks if she ever binged on other occasions when tired or angry. P recalls that she has binged on previous occasions when she has felt angry with someone but has felt powerless to change the situation. Now T can review Figure 1 with P and draw up an individualized model illustrating some of the factors that may be maintaining P's BN. T can also discuss the negative role of perfectionism, all-or-nothing thinking and other distorted cognitions. Examples include the notion that a few chocolates constitute the difference between being "good" or "perfect" and being "a pig" who has "blown it all," and the idea that since she has gone off the diet, she "might as well" finish the rest of the chocolate.

Conclusion

CBT-BN remains the first line treatment of choice for BN. Controlled outcome studies have demonstrated that it is more effective than pharmacotherapy and alternative psychotherapies, it is brief and cost effective, and it is widely available to clinicians in manualized form. It is hoped that individualizing this treatment and focusing more on interpersonal skills and affect regulation may further augment the effects of treatment and possibly result in higher rates of long-term abstinence.

CBT-Oriented Workbooks

(Cited in *The American Psychiatric Association Practice Guideline for the Treatment of Patients with Eating Disorders*, 2006).

Agras WS, Apple RF. (2007).* *Overcoming Eating Disorders: A Cognitive-Behavioral Therapy Approach for Bulimia Nervosa and Binge-Eating Disorder.* Patient Manual, 2nd edition. Oxford University Press*)*.

Agras WS, Apple RF. (2007). *Overcoming Eating Disorders: A Cognitive-Behavioral Therapy Approach for Bulimia Nervosa and Binge-Eating Disorder.* Therapist Guide, 2nd edition. Oxford University Press,

Cash TF. (1997). *The Body Image Workbook: An 8-Step Program for Learning to Like Your Looks.* Oakland, CA, New Harbinger.

Fairburn C. (1995). *Overcoming Binge Eating.* New York, Guilford.

Goodman LJ, Villapiano M. (2001). *Eating Disorders: The Journey to Recovery Workbook.* New York, Brunner-Routledge (client workbook).

Goodman LJ, Villapiano M. (2001). *Eating Disorders: Time for Change. Plans, Strategies, and Worksheets.* New York, Brunner-Routledge (therapist workbook).

Schmidt U, Treasure J. (1993). *Getting Better Bit(e) by Bit(e): A survival kit for Sufferers of Bulimia Nervosa and Binge eating Disorder.* London, Routledge.

*(A.P.A Practice Guidelines cited earlier editions of some of the above books).

References

Agras WS, Schneider JA, Arnow B, Raeburn SD, Telch CF. (1989). Cognitive-behavioral and response-prevention treatments for bulimia nervosa. *Journal of Consulting and Clinical Psychology*, 57, 215–21.

Agras WS, Walsh BT, Fairburn CG, Wilson GT, Kraemer HC. (2000). A multicenter comparison of cognitive-behavioral therapy and interpersonal psychotherapy for bulimia nervosa. *Archives of General Psychiatry*, 57, 459–466.

American Psychiatric Association. (2006). Practice guideline for the treatment of patients with eating disorders, third edition. *American Journal of Psychiatry*, 163:suppl. pp. 1-26.

Anderson CB, Joyce PR, Carter FA, McIntosh VV, Bulik CM. (2002). The effect of cognitive-behavioral therapy for bulimia nervosa on temperament and character as measured by the temperament and character inventory. *Comprehensive Psychiatry*, 43(3), 182-188.

Baxter L, Schwartz JM, Bergman K, Szuba MP, Guze BH, Mazziotta JC, Alazraki A, Selin CE, Ferng HK, Munford P, Phelps ME. (1992). Caudate glucose metabolic rate changes with both drug and behavior therapy for obsessive-compulsive disorder. *Archives of General Psychiatry*, 49(6) 181-89.

Beck AT. (1976). *Cognitive therapy and the emotional disorders*. NY: International Universities Press.

Beck AT, Rush AJ, Shaw BF, Emery G. (1979). *Cognitive therapy of depression*. NY: Guilford Press.

Brewerton TD, Dansky BS, Kilpatrick DG, O'Neil PM. (2000). Which comes first in the pathogenesis of bulimia nervosa, dieting or bingeing? *International Journal of Eating Disorders*, 28, 259-264.

Bulik CM. (2005). Exploring the gene–environment nexus in eating disorders. *Journal of Psychiatry and Neuroscience*, 30(5), 335-9.

Burns DD. (1989). *The Feeling Good Handbook.* New York: William Morrow and Co.

Byrne SM, McLean NJ. (2002). The cognitive-behavioral model of bulimia nervosa: a direct evaluation. *International Journal of Eating Disorders*, 31, 17-31.

Cooper PJ, Steere J. (1995). -A comparison of two psychological treatments for bulimia nervosa: implications for models of maintenance. *Behaviour Research and Therapy*, 33, 875-885.

Fairburn CG. (1981). A cognitive behavioral approach to the management of bulimia. *Psychological Medicine*, 11, 707-711.

Fairburn CG. (1985). Cognitive-Behavioral Treatment for Bulimia. In *Handbook of Psychotherapy for Anorexia Nervosa and Bulimia.* Edited by Garner DM, Garfinkel PE. New York: The Guilford Press, pp. 160-192.

Fairburn CG, Jones R, Peveler RC, Carr SJ, Solomon RA, O'Connor ME, Burton J, Hope RA. (1991). Three psychological treatments for bulimia nervosa: A comparative trial. *Archives of General Psychiatry*, 48, 463–9.

Fairburn CG, Kirk J, O'Connor M, Cooper PJ. (1986). A comparison of two psychological treatments for bulimia nervosa. *Behaviour Research and Therapy*, 24, 629–43.

Fairburn CG, Marcus MD, Wilson GT. (1993). Cognitive-behavioral therapy for binge eating and bulimia nervosa: a comprehensive treatment manual. In *Binge Eating: Nature, assessment and treatment.* Edited by Fairburn CG, Wilson GT. New York: Guilford Press, pp. 361-404.

Fairburn CG, Norman PA, Welch SL, O'Connor ME, Doll HA, Peveler RC. (1995). A prospective study of outcome in bulimia nervosa and the long-term effects of three psychological treatments. *Archives of General Psychiatry*, 52, 304-312.

Fairburn CG, Welch SL, Doll HA, Davies BA, O'Connor, ME. (1997). Risk factors for bulimia nervosa. *Archives of General Psychiatry*, 54, 509-517.

Garner DM, Rockert W, Davis R, Garner MV, Olmsted M, Eagle M. (1993). Comparison of cognitive-behavioral and supportive-expressive therapy for bulimia nervosa. *American Journal of Psychiatry*, 150, 37-46.

Ghaderi A. (2006). Does individualization matter? A randomized trial of standardized (focused) versus individualized (broad) cognitive behavior therapy for bulimia nervosa. *Behaviour Research and Therapy*, 44, 273-288.

Goldapple K, Segal Z, Garson C, Lau M., Bieling P, Kennedy S. et al. (2004). Modulation of cortical-limbic pathways in major depression: Treatment-specific effects of cognitive behavior therapy. *Archives of General Psychiatry*, 61, 34–41.

Goldbloom DS, Olmsted M, Davis R, Clewes J, Heinmaa M, Rockert W, Shaw B. (1997). A randomized controlled trial of fluoxetine and cognitive behavioral therapy for bulimia nervosa: short-term outcome. *Behaviour Research and Therapy*, 35, 803-811.

Hay PJ, Bacaltchuk J, Stephano S. (2004). Psychotherapy for bulimia nervosa and binging. *Cochrane Database of Systematic Reviews*, 3:CD000562.

Hendricks PS, Thompson JK. (2005). An integration of cognitive-behavioral therapy and interpersonal psychotherapy for bulimia nervosa: A case study using the case formulation method. *International Journal of Eating Disorders,* 37, 171-174.

Jacobi C, Dahme B, Dittmann R. (2002). Cognitive-behavioral, fluoxetine and combined treatment for bulimia nervosa: short- and long-term results. *European Eating Disorders Review*, 10, 179-198.

Keys A, Brozek J, Henschel A, Mickelsen O, Taylor HL. (1950). *The Biology of Human Starvation*. Minneapolis: The University of Minnesota Press.

Klerman GL, Weissman MM, Rounsaville BJ, Chevron ES. (1984). *Interpersonal Psychotherapy of Depression.* NY: Basic Books.

Legenbauer T, Vocks S, Ruddel H. (2008). Emotion recognition, emotional awareness and cognitive bias in individuals with bulimia nervosa. *Journal of Clinical Psychology*, 64(6), 687-702.

Lewandowski LM, Gebing TA, Anthony JL, O'Brien WH. (1997). Meta-analysis of cognitive-behavioral treatment studies for bulimia. *Clinical Psychology Review*, 17, 703-718.

Linden DEJ. (2006). How psychotherapy changes the brain – the contribution of functional neuroimaging. *Molecular Psychiatry,* 11, 528–538.

Loeb KL, Wilson GT, Labouvie E, Pratt EM, Hayaki J, Walsh BT, Agras WS, Fairburn CG. (2005). Therapeutic alliance and treatment adherence in two interventions for bulimia nervosa: A study of process and outcome. *Journal of Consulting and Clinical Psychology*, 73(6), 1097-1107.

Mitchell JE, Agras WS, Wilson GT, Halmi K, Kraemer H, Crow S. (2004). A trial of a relapse prevention strategy in women with bulimia nervosa who respond to cognitive-behavior therapy. *International Journal of Eating Disorders*, 35, 549–555.

Mitchell JE, Agras S, Wonderlich S. (2007). Treatment of bulimia nervosa: Where are we and where are we going? *International Journal of Eating Disorders*, 40(2), 95-101.

Mitchell JE, Halmi K, Wilson GT, Agras WS, Kraemer H, Crow S. (2002). A randomized secondary treatment study of women with bulimia nervosa who fail to respond to CBT. *International Journal of Eating Disorders,* 32, 271-281.

National Institute for Clinical Excellence (NICE) (2004). Eating disorders: Core interventions in the treatment and management of anorexia nervosa, bulimia nervosa and related eating disorders. NICE Clinical Guideline number 9. The British Psychological Society and the Royal College of Psychiatrists. (www.nice.org.uk).

Openshaw C, Waller G, Sperlinger D. (2004). Group cognitive-behavior therapy for bulimia nervosa: statistical versus clinical significance of changes in symptoms across treatment. *International Journal of Eating Disorders*, 36, 363-75.

Pyle RL, Mitchell JE, Eckert ED, Hatsukami DK, Pomeroy C, Zimmerman R. (1990). Maintenance treatment and 6-month outcome for bulimic patients who respond to initial treatment. *American Journal of Psychiatry*, 147, 871-75.

Russell GFM. (1979). Bulimia nervosa: An ominous variant of anorexia nervosa. *Psychological Medicine*, 9, 429-448.

Shafran R, de Silva P. (2003). Cognitive-Behavioural Models. In *Handbook of Eating Disorders*. Edited by Treasure J, Schmidt U, van Furth E. John Wiley and Sons, pp. 121-138.

Shapiro JR, Berkman ND, Brownley KA, Sedway JA, Lohr KN, Bulik CM. (2007). Bulimia nervosa treatment: A systematic review of randomized controlled trials. *International Journal of Eating Disorders*, 40(4), 321-336.

Skinner BF. (1950). Are theories of learning necessary? *Psychological Review*, 57, 193-216.

Viamontes GI, Beitman, B. (2006). Neural Substrates of Psychotherapeutic Change: Part I: The Default Brain. *Psychiatric Annals*, 36(4), 225-236.

Viamontes GI, Beitman B. (2006). Neural Substrates of Psychotherapeutic Change: Part II: Beyond the Default Brain. *Psychiatric Annals* 36(4) 238-246.

Walsh BT, Hadigan CM, Devlin MJ, Gladis M, Roose SP. (1991). Long-term outcome of antidepressant treatment for bulimia nervosa. *American Journal of Psychiatry*, 148, 1206–12.

Wilfley DE, Cohen LR. (1997). Psychological treatment of bulimia nervosa and binge eating disorder. *Psychopharmacology Bulletin*, 33, 437-454.

Wilson GT. (1997). Cognitive behavioral treatment of bulimia nervosa. *The Clinical Psychologist* 50(2), 10-12.

Wilson GT, Fairburn CC, Agras WS, Walsh BT, Kraemer H. (2002). Cognitive-behavioral therapy for bulimia nervosa: time course and mechanisms of change. *Journal of Consulting and Clinical Psychology*, 70(2), 267-74.

Wilson GT, Grilo CM, Vitousek KM. (2007). Psychological treatment of eating disorders. *American Psychologist*, 62(3), 199-216.

Wilson GT, Pike KM. (2001). Eating Disorders. In: *Clinical Handbook of Psychological Disorders, 3rd edition: A Step-by-step treatment manual*. Edited by Barlow DH. New York and London. The Guilford Press, pp. 332-375.

Wilson GT, Vitousek K, Loeb KL. (2000). Stepped-care treatment for eating disorders. *Journal of Consulting and Clinical Psychology*, 68, 564-572.

In: Evidence-Based Treatments for Eating Disorders
Author: Ida F. Dancyger and Victor M. Fornari

ISBN 978-1-60692-310-8
© 2009 Nova Science Publishers, Inc.

Chapter XIII

Evidence-Informed Strategies for Binge Eating Disorder and Obesity

Kimberly A. Brownley, Jennifer R. Shapiro and Cynthia M. Bulik
University of North Carolina at Chapel Hill
North Carolina, USA

Abstract

Obesity is a major public health problem in the United States (US), where approximately two out of every three adults are overweight. Excess food intake is a driving force behind this problem. Binge eating results in excess food intake, and approximately 5% to 8% of obese individuals meet criteria for Binge Eating Disorder (BED). Obesity is associated with increased rates of cardiovascular disease, cancer, and musculoskeletal pain. Independent of obesity, BED is associated with increased rates of depression and other psychiatric problems. This chapter reviews current evidence-based treatments for obesity and BED. Also mentioned are novel therapies that have shown promise in limited clinical studies. Among the available pharmacological treatments, sibutramine, orlistat, and buproprion have demonstrated efficacy in short-term (three months to two years) treatment trials for obesity. Similarly, sibutramine, orlistat, and various antidepressants have shown promise in the short-term treatment of BED. Effective behavioral therapies include cognitive behavioral therapy, dialectical behavioral therapy, and combination diet and exercise therapy. Self-monitoring is an important component of most behavioral strategies. Surgical techniques are generally reserved for treating severe obesity and include gastric banding and bypass. The chapter concludes with a discussion of key challenges and future directions for research and clinical application in the treatment of obesity and BED. The emergence of technology (internet, text messaging, etc.) as an important anti-obesity tool along with the clinically relevant concept of "number needed to treat/harm" (NNT/NNH) are highlighted.

Introduction

The prevalence of overweight [body mass index (BMI) of 25-29.9 kg/m^2] and obesity (BMI ≥30) have increased dramatically in the US population in recent years and have now reached epidemic proportions, with over 65% of adults currently classified as overweight or obese (Manson and Bassuk, 2003). Obesity is associated with high costs and considerable health complications including diabetes, hypertension, cardiovascular disease, sleep apnea, pain, and certain types of cancer (Daniels et al., 2005; de Sousa, Cercato, Mancini, Halpern, 2008; Eckel et al., 2004; Hjartåker, Langseth, and Weiderpass, 2008; Janke, Collins, and Kozak, 2006; McMillan, Sattar, and McArdle, 2006; Thompson and Wolf, 2001). Approximately 5% to 8% of obese individuals meet criteria for binge eating disorder (BED) (Bruce and Agras, 1992; Bruce and Wilfley, 1996). The prevalence of BED is as high as 30% to 70% in obese individuals seeking weight-loss treatment (de Zwaan, 2001). BED becomes more prevalent with increasing severity of obesity and is associated with early onset of obesity (Yanovski, 1993; Yanovski, 2003). Obese individuals with BED report higher lifetime prevalence of affective, anxiety, and personality disorders (Mussell et al., 1996; Specker, de Zwaan, Raymond, and Mitchell, 1994; Yanovski, Nelson, Dubbert, and Spitzer, 1993); greater health dissatisfaction; and higher cumulative rates of major medical disorders (Bulik, Sullivan, and Kendler, 2002) than obese individuals without binge eating. Also, binge eating, independent of BMI, is associated with several psychiatric and medical symptoms in both men and women (Reichborn-Kjennerud, Bulik, Sullivan, Tambs, and Harris, 2004). In short, BED can have debilitating consequences that affect an individual's physical, emotional, and social well-being [see Janice's Story below]. The purpose of this chapter is to address evidence-based approaches for the treatment of obesity and BED. Specifically, we will discuss pharmacological and behavioral approaches for both conditions as well as surgical approaches for obesity.

Vignette – Janice's Story

Janice, a 35 year old woman, lives with her golden retriever, Max, and her best friend, Sarah, in a two bedroom apartment on the east side of town. She has a few close friends but mainly keeps to herself. Janice has been overweight since she was five years old and she remembers as a child sneaking food into her room at night, hiding food from her parents, and always wanting to snack. When she began school, Janice did not like to eat lunch because the other children would tease her about her weight. As a result, she would come home from school and eat large amounts of food until she became uncomfortably full. This persisted throughout high school. Last year, Janice started a new job and began to gain weight. She is 5'3" and weighs about 340 pounds. Her friends never understood why she was very overweight because Janice barely picked at her food when they all went out to eat. Still, the weight gain persisted. Then one day while cleaning, Sarah came across an unfamiliar notebook. Curious, she opened it to find Janice's handwriting and a page that read "I don't know what to do. I feel so out of control. I can go the entire day without having the slightest urge to binge and then something happens—my boss yells at me, the dog chews another hole in the carpet, I lock my keys in my car—anything! It doesn't even have to be negative. The other day my sister told me she was getting married. I was so happy for her that I sat down and ate an entire gallon of chocolate ice cream and two large pizzas, all within two hours. I can't explain it. It is as if something triggers this feeling deep within me. I start eating and lose control. I eat until I can't possibly swallow another bite. I feel disgusted with myself. I feel guilty. I am so embarrassed by how much I eat that I hide my binges from my friends and family. My weight keeps skyrocketing while my health is plummeting. I need help. Every time I've tried to diet, I just fail. I do great all day but then at the end of the night, I blow it. I have never gone a single week without binge eating. About 5 years ago, I lost 25 pounds but gained 40 back after I got a blister on my foot and had trouble walking. I have considered having surgery to take off the excess pounds, but I know that it will only solve half the problem. Sure, I would no longer be physically able to eat the amounts of food that I do now, but what about the cravings? My life revolves around food. I'm always thinking of the next meal. I love eating and once I start, I really can't stop. Food is always there for me—when I am happy, sad, angry, stressed—you name it. Without food, I'd be all alone."

As illustrated by this vignette, Janice's binge eating was deeply troubling to her—a life-long battle, her overeating left her feeling out of control, ashamed, and a failure. She relied on food to cope with strong emotions, perpetuating a vicious cycle of binge eating and self disgust. Janice's weight skyrocketed, increasing her risk of other medical problems and warranting drastic intervention. Janice recognizes that surgery will help with the weight problem but not necessarily with the craving and lack of control around food. She understands the importance of addressing the cognitive and emotional triggers for her binge eating through psychotherapy and possibly medication.

Pharmacological and Surgical Treatment for Obesity

Medications used for weight loss generally fall into three categories based on their mechanism of action: a) drugs that reduce food intake and appetite ("appetite suppressants"), b) drugs that alter metabolism, and c) drugs that increase thermogenesis (heat production or energy expenditure). To date, the Food and Drug Administration (FDA) has not approved any "thermogenic" anti-obesity drugs for use in the US. Here, we summarize what is known regarding the efficacies and limitations of appetite suppressants and lipase inhibitors. Some discussion is also provided of novel, less well-studied anti-obesity agents that have shown promise in small clinical studies. Finally, we address surgical approaches for treating severe obesity. For more in-depth coverage of these topics, the reader is referred to several previously published reviews (Bray, 2000; DeWald, Khaodhiar, Donahue, and Blackburn, 2006; Douketis, Macie, Thabane, and Williamson, 2005; Dunican, Desilets, and Montalbano, 2007; Leung, Thomas, Chan, and Tomlinson, 2003; Norris et al., 2005; Orzano and Scott, 2004; Padwal, Li, and Lau, 2004; Thompson, Cook, Clark, Bardia, and Levine, 2007) and meta-analyses (Li et al., 2005; Padwal, Li, and Lau, 2003).

Appetite Suppressants

There are several FDA-approved appetite suppressants; examples include benzphetamine, diethylpropion, phendimetrazine, and phentermine. These drugs are centrally-acting stimulants that promote the release of brain chemicals known as catecholamines (i.e., dopamine, epinephrine, norepinephrine) (Bray, 2000; Li et al., 2005; Thompson et al., 2007). Early studies suggested that phentermine was superior to placebo in reducing weight over a period of nine months (Munro, MacCuish, Wilson, and Duncan, 1968). However, in part because drugs in this class have some abuse potential and because some are associated with significant cardiovascular and central nervous system side effects, they are approved for short-term (up to 12 weeks) use only. Thus, these medications are not widely prescribed or used for prolonged weight loss.

In contrast to these short-term options, sibutramine is approved for long-term treatment and has been widely studied in longer-term trials (Bray, 2000; Bray et al., 1996; DeWald et al., 2006; Leung et al., 2003; Li et al., 2005; Padwal et al., 2004; Thompson et al., 2007). Sibutramine is thought to inhibit food intake by blocking synaptic reuptake of both norepinephrine and serotonin in the brain. Across studies, sibutramine was superior to placebo in promoting weight loss, with weight loss generally occurring in the initial six months of treatment and being maintained with continued sibutramine administration for up to two years (Bray, 1996; Dujovne, Macie, Thabane, Williamson and the Sibutramine Study Group 2001; James et al., 2000). Sibutramine was also associated with beneficial changes in blood lipids and other biomarkers of cardiovascular disease risk (Dujovne et al., 2001; James et al., 2000). A recent study also suggests that sibutramine safely reduces weight and improves cardiovascular risk profile in adolescents, as well (Daniels et al., 2007).

Overall, this general class of drugs has shown some efficacy in suppressing appetite and promoting satiety; however, because these drugs produce untoward side effects (such as nervousness, insomnia, headache, and elevated blood pressure), their clinical utility as agents of long-term weight loss is quite limited.

Drugs that Alter Metabolism

Limiting dietary intake of fat can be an effective way to reduce caloric consumption and lose weight. However, compliance with low-fat diets is often poor, limiting the success of this approach for long-term weight loss. In the past decade, a relatively new approach to regulating dietary fat has emerged with the development of agents that interfere with fat metabolism and thereby reduce the amount of ingested fat that is available for absorption. The most widely used agent in this class is orlistat (Xenical). Orlistat inhibits gastric and pancreatic lipases, which are enzymes necessary for converting dietary fat (triglycerides) into forms that can be absorbed by the body and used for energy. In clinical studies, orlistat was superior to placebo in promoting initial weight loss and in maintaining weight loss after two years (Drent et al., 1995; Rossner, Sjostrom, Noack, Meinders, and Noseda, 2000; Van Gaal, Broom, Enzi, and Toplak, 1998). Orlistat also reduced blood cholesterol and other cardiovascular disease risk factors (Davidson et al., 1999; Tonstad et al., 1994). Orlistat primarily acts in the stomach and small intestine, with very limited effects elsewhere in the body. Thus, when side effects occur they generally are gastrointestinal in nature, including fecal urgency and incontinence. In most cases, these side effects are mild to moderate, and they often dissipate with continued use (Drent et al., 1995; James, Avenell, Broom, and Whitehead, 1997; Van Gaal et al., 1998).

"Novel" Anti-Obesity Agents

The atypical antidepressant, buproprion, is approved to treat depression and as adjunct therapy for smoking cessation. In clinical studies focusing on these outcomes, buproprion was associated with modest weight loss in a small percentage of participants (Croft et al., 1999; Weisler et al., 1994). In a more recent study focusing on weight loss as the primary outcome in obese women, buproprion was superior to placebo in promoting weight loss after eight weeks of treatment (Gadde et al., 2001). Women who responded well to buproprion were given the opportunity to continue treatment for up to two years. Average weight loss after two years was approximately 14% of initial body weight. Buproprion is associated with mild side effects including dry mouth, nausea, and insomnia but is generally well-tolerated (Settle, Stahl, Batey, Johnston, and Ascher, 1999). Taken together, these studies suggest that buproprion warrants further study to understand its potential long-term efficacy as an anti-obesity agent.

Metformin is an "insulin sensitizing" agent used in the treatment of type 2 diabetes. Metformin also reduces glucose production in the liver. Together, these effects help normalize and stabilize blood glucose levels. In several small clinical studies, metformin consistently was associated with reduced appetite and food intake (Lee and Morley, 1998; Paolisso et al., 1998; Stumvoll, Nurjhan, Perriello, Dailey, and Gerich, 1995). Nonetheless, in these studies, the weight loss attributed to metformin was modest, suggesting that metformin alone is not a good candidate for the treatment of obesity.

Surgical Treatments for Severe Obesity ("Bariatric Therapy")

Surgical approaches are very effective in the treatment of severe ("morbid") obesity (DeWald et al., 2006, for review). Compared to other modalities, surgical treatments usually result in longer-lasting weight loss and they tend to improve comorbid conditions of obesity, such as hypertension, respiratory problems, and diabetes (Foley, Benotti, Borlase, Hollingshead, and Blackburn, 1992; MacDonald et al., 1997; Sugerman et al., 1992). Surgical therapies fall into two broad categories: a) procedures designed to restrict gastric volume and b) procedures designed to decrease the functional length of the small intestine. Thus, certain approaches lead to weight loss by limiting food intake and others lead to weight loss by limiting nutrient absorption. Some "mixed" approaches apply both techniques simultaneously. Gastric bypass is generally superior to banding procedures for weight loss and long-term weight loss maintenance (DeWald et al., 2006), and it now can be performed using minimally invasive laparoscopy (Wittgrove and Clark, 2000). Thus, bypass is currently viewed as the gold standard procedure.

Examples of restrictive procedures include gastroplasty, gastric banding, gastric bypass, and sleeve gastrectomy. In gastroplasty, surgical staples are used to partition the stomach into two compartments. In gastric banding, an adjustable prosthetic band is placed around the stomach to reduce its food-holding capacity. Gastric bypass divides the stomach into a small upper pouch and larger lower pouch, both of which are connected to the small intestine; this leads to a marked reduction in the functional volume of the stomach, accompanied by an altered physiological response to food (referred to as "dumping"). Dumping involves the rapid emptying of hypo-osmolar gut contents from the stomach into the small bowel and results in nausea, pain, diarrhea, and other symptoms. Dumping signals the patient very quickly if he/she has overeaten – particularly sweet or high-carbohydrate foods or liquids – and this signal can serve as a deterrent to further overconsumption. Sleeve gastrectomy reduces the stomach to about one-third its original size by removing a large portion of the stomach, itself. Examples of procedures designed to disrupt absorption include jejunoileal bypass and biliopancreatic diversion. Jejunoileal bypass was the first surgical procedure used to treat obesity (Payne and DeWind, 1969) but is no longer performed due to a high rate of serious liver and metabolic complications. As its name suggests, biliopancreatic diversion shifts biliary and pancreatic secretions to the distal end of the ileum.

Bariatric surgery is the most effective treatment for morbid obesity (Anderson and Wadden, 1999); however, complications do occur and have increased paralleling the increasing numbers of procedures performed (Abell and Minocha, 2006). According to a recent review (Abell and Minocha, 2006), up to 70% of individuals who lose weight quickly may experience gallstones. In addition, "dumping" occurs in about 14.6% of those who undergo "mixed" surgery and can be particularly problematic for patients who struggle with strong food cravings and binge eating. Eleven percent of those who undergo "mixed" surgery experience vitamin and mineral deficiency (e.g. calcium, iron, vitamins B12 and D) (Abell and Minocha, 2006). Other complications include vomiting, staple line failure, infection, bowel obstruction, ulceration, bleeding, and splenic injury. In addition to these complications, a 0.4% mortality rate of patients who undergo combined surgery has been reported (Monteforte and Turkelson, 2000). A recent retrospective cohort study (Adams et al., 2007) compared long-term mortality rate (all-cause and specific cause) in 7925 surgical patients with 7925 control patients from the general population, matched on sex, BMI, and age. Results showed that although the all-cause mortality was 40% lower in the surgery group and mortality from specific diseases (e.g., diabetes, CAD, cancer) was on average 52% lower in the surgery group, non-disease related deaths (e.g., suicide, accidents, other) were 1.58 times as great in the surgery group than in the control group. This suggests that although surgery may indeed decrease all-cause and specific-disease mortality, it cannot address psychological issues and other variables that impact well-being and post-surgical mortality. For this reason, psychological evaluations are an important adjunct to any surgical treatment for obesity. In addition, a prospective study (Sjostrom et al., 2007) that compared 2010 patients who underwent bariatric surgery with 2037 patients who received conventional treatment (lifestyle change, behavior modification, or no treatment) found that after 10.9 year followup the surgery group had a hazard ratio of 0.76 compared with the control group, with death occurring in a significantly higher percentage of the control group (6.3%) compared to the surgery group (5.0%). Although these studies are important, they lack the scientific rigor of a randomized controlled trial; however, conduct of a randomized controlled trial for obesity is difficult given potential ethical concerns about assigning patients to either surgical or behavioral treatment rather than allowing them to select the treatment of their choice.

Pharmacological Treatments for BED

The majority of published randomized clinical trials (RCTs) of pharmacotherapy for BED have been limited in scope. They have generally been small in size (fewer than 500 total participants in eight medication RCTs), and the vast majority of participants have been Caucasian women over age 18 (see Berkman et al., 2006; Brownley, Berkman, Sedway, Lohr, and Bulik, 2007). Thus far, the medications that have received the most attention in the treatment of BED are second-generation antidepressants (Arnold et al., 2002; Hudson et al., 1998; McElroy et al., 2000; McElroy, Hudson et al., 2003; Pearlstein et al., 2003), tricyclic antidepressants (Laederach-Hofmann et al., 1999), anticonvulsants (McElroy, Arnold et al., 2003), and sibutramine (Appolinario et al., 2003). Table 1 summarizes the results of these studies.

Antidepressants (Selective Serotonin Reuptake Inhibitors and Tricyclic Antidepressants

Fluoxetine, fluvoxamine, sertraline, and citalopram are the selective serotonin reuptake inhibitors (SSRIs) most widely studied to date. In short-term studies (12 weeks), both fluoxetine (Arnold et al., 2002) and fluvoxamine (Pearlstein et al., 2003) were effective in reducing binge frequency and depressed mood. Fluvoxamine was superior to placebo in reducing binge frequency and improving illness severity after nine weeks (Hudson et al., 1998). However, remission rates and depression scores did not differ between groups, and BMI at the end of the study was not reported. Thus, the group receiving fluvoxamine experienced more rapid reductions in binge eating and weight than the placebo group, but by the end of the study these changes did not result in clinically meaningful changes (i.e., binge abstinence and weight loss). After 6 weeks, compared with placebo, both sertraline (McElroy et al., 2000) and citalopram (McElroy, Hudson et al., 2003) were associated with reduced binge eating, weight loss, and illness severity ratings in individuals with BED. Citalopram, but not sertraline, was also associated with reduced depression ratings compared to placebo. However, neither sertraline nor citalopram was clearly superior to placebo in terms of remission rate, and the initial rapid response in binge eating observed with citalopram was not sustained over time.

Table 1. Summary of Pharmacological Treatment Studies for Binge Eating Disorder

Medication	Dose	Sample	Results (Significant Group Differences)	Source
Fluoxetine	20 – 80 mg/day	93% female Age (range): 18-60 yrs Age [mean (SD)]: Fluoxetine: 41.9 (9.7) Placebo: 40.8 (9.0) Enrolled: 60 Dropout: 40%	Over six weeks, fluoxetine was superior to placebo in reducing binge frequency, illness severity, and depressed mood, and in controlling weight and BMI gain. At study endpoint, fluoxetine was associated with lower illness severity and depressed mood, and less weight gain, and generally was well-tolerated for subjects.	Arnold et al., 2002
Fluvoxamine	50 – 300 mg/day	93% female Age (range):18-60 yrs Age [mean (SD)]: Fluvoxamine: 41.2 (9.9) Placebo: 43.0 (9.5) Enrolled: 85 Dropout: 12%	Over nine weeks, fluvoxamine was superior to placebo in reducing binge frequency, BMI, and clinical severity. At study endpoint: remission rates and depression scores were not different and there was no clinically meaningful change for binge abstinence and weight loss.	Hudson et al., 1998
Fluvoxamine	150 mg/b.i.d	85% Female Age (range): 41.0 yrs Age [mean (SD)]: NR Enrolled: 25 Dropout: 20%	No significant improvement for binge frequency, depressed mood, or eating psychopathology (eating, shape, or weight concerns). At study endpoint: NR.	Pearlstein et al., 2003

Medication	Dose	Sample	Results (Significant Group Differences)	Source
Topiramate	50-600 mg/day	87% Female Age (range): 18-60 yrs Age [mean (SD)]: Topiramate: 40.9 (8.2) Placebo: 40.7 (9.1) Enrolled: 61 Dropout: 15%	Over 14 weeks, topiramate was superior to placebo in reducing binge frequency, illness severity, eating-related obsessions, compulsions, BMI, and weight, which decreased in the topiramate group but increased in the placebo group. At study endpoint: NR.	McElroy, Arnold et al., 2003
Citalopram	20-60 mg/day	95% Female Age (range): 18-60 yrs Age [mean (SD)]: Citalopram: 42.0 (9.0) Placebo: 39.2 (12.0) Enrolled: 38 Dropout: 18%	Over six weeks, compared to placebo, citalopram was associated with a faster rate of reduction in binge frequency, illness severity, binge eating-related obsessions and compulsions, and weight. At study endpoint: citalopram was associated with greater reduction in frequency of binge days, BMI, and weight.	McElroy, Hudson et al., 2003
Imipramine (added to dietary and psychological counseling)	25 mg / t.i.d	87% Female Age (range): 20-60 yrs Age [mean (SD)]: Imipramine: 40.7 (10.9) Placebo: 35.7 (10.3) Enrolled: 31 Dropout: 7%	Over eight weeks of active treatment and at week 32 followup, imipramine was superior to placebo in decreasing binge frequency, depressed mood, and body weight. At study endpoint: NR.	Laederach-Hofmann et al., 1999
Sertraline	50-200 mg/day	94% Female Age (range0: 18-60 yrs Age [mean (SD)]: Sertraline: 43.1 (9.9) Placebo: 41.0 (12.2) Enrolled: 34 Dropout: 24%	Over six weeks, sertraline was superior to placebo in reducing binge frequency, illness severity, and BMI, and in increasing global improvement. At study endpoint: NR.	McElroy et al., 2000

Table 1. (Continued)

Medication	Dose	Sample	Results (Significant Group Differences)	Source

Sibutramine hydrochloride	15 mg/day	95% Female
		Age (range): 18-60 yrs
		Age [mean (SD)]:
		  Sibutramine: 35.2 (9.0)
		  Placebo: 36.6 (10.2)
		Enrolled: 60
		Dropout: 20%
			Over 12 weeks, sibutramine was superior to placebo in reducing binge frequency and severity.
			At study endpoint: sibutramine was associated with less depressed mood. Groups differed in weight: weight decreased over the treatment period in the sibutramine group but increased in the placebo group.
				Appolinario et al., 2003

Orlistat	120 mg / t.i.d	88% Female
		Age (range): 35-58 yrs
		Age [mean (SD)]:
		  Orlistat: 45.2 (7.4)
		  Placebo: 47.0 (7.0)
		Enrolled: 50
		Dropout: 22%
			Over 12 weeks, CBT plus orlistat was associated with greater total weight loss and % weight loss than CBT plus placebo.
			At study endpoint: greater percentage of CBT+orlistat group remitted and achieved at least 5% weight loss.
			The group difference in weight loss was maintained at 2-month followup.
				Grilo et al., 2005

Abbreviations: BMI (Body Mass Index); CBT (Cognitive Behavioral Therapy); NR (Not reported).

Tricyclic antidepressants have shown some promise in the treatment of BED. When given as adjunct therapy to standard diet counseling and psychological support, imipramine significantly reduced binge eating episodes, depressed mood, and body weight after eight and 32 weeks in 31 individuals with BED (Laederach-Hofmann et al., 1999). Unfortunately, abstinence rates from binge eating were not reported, thus the clinical utility of imipramine in the treatment of BED remains unknown.

Other Agents

The appetite suppressant, sibutramine (which is marketed for the treatment of obesity), and the anticonvulsant agent, topiramate, have demonstrated limited efficacy in the treatment of BED. In a 14-week study of obese individuals with BED, topiramate was superior to placebo in reducing binge frequency (episodes and binge days per week) and scores on the Yale-Brown Obsessive Compulsive Scale for Binge Eating (McElroy, Arnold et al., 2003); however, weight loss, illness severity, and depression scores did not differ between groups after treatment. In contrast, sibutramine given for 12 weeks significantly reduced binge days per week, Binge Eating Scale scores, and self-reported depression scores compared to placebo in individuals with BED (Appolinario et al., 2003). Notably, the sibutramine group lost on average 7.4 kg whereas the placebo group gained weight.

Orlistat has been studied as augmentation therapy for BED patients undergoing cognitive behavioral therapy (CBT) (Grilo, Masheb, and Salant, 2005). Compared to CBT plus placebo, CBT plus orlistat was associated with greater initial weight loss (-1.6 kg vs. -3.5 kg) and remission rates. However, neither effect was maintained at 2-month followup, and other eating-related measures and depression did not differ between groups.

Treatment Limitations and Concerns

Virtually all of the medications reviewed here have side effects commonly associated with second-generation and tricyclic antidepressants (such as sedation, dry mouth, headache, sexual dysfunction/decreased libido, insomnia, constipation, and gastrointestinal upset). Inability to tolerate side effects is clearly a major reason for treatment drop (up to 24% in studies reviewed here). Placebo response rates have also been quite high in medication trials for BED (6% to 39%). These factors, in addition to a general failure to report abstinence rates and long-term follow-up data, limit our understanding of treatment options for BED. Furthermore, there is very little information available about specific factors that contribute to treatment efficacy in BED. For example, early abstinence from binge eating may be associated with greater weight loss (Agras et al., 1994). These findings warrant further study, as do questions regarding treatment efficacy in ethnic, gender, and age subgroups. Initial findings require replication, and larger more culturally diverse samples need to be studied before an accurate picture of individual difference factors in BED outcome can emerge.

Overall Summary of Pharmacological Treatments for BED

Taken together, these studies suggest that there are several viable options for pharmacotherapy in the treatment of BED. Short-term, placebo-controlled trials provide limited evidence that SSRIs reduce target eating, psychiatric, and weight symptoms in individuals with BED. However, this evidence must be viewed cautiously because of high dropout and placebo response rates across studies. Sibutramine, topiramate, and low-dose imipramine may also benefit individuals with BED by reducing weight, but their impact on binge abstinence and remission remain uncertain. Additional studies are needed to confirm the therapeutic potential of these agents in the treatment of BED.

Behavioral Interventions for Weight Control

Prior to the 1960s, psychologists used psychoanalytic theory to treat overweight individuals by focusing on oral fixations and developmental disturbances, which were believed to have caused obesity. In the 1960s, learning theory was applied to weight management. According to learning theory, certain learned behaviors contributed to weight gain and if these behaviors were unlearned and replaced with healthier alternatives, weight loss would follow. This idea launched considerable research into the behavioral approach to weight management.

The behavioral approach for weight control or obesity consists of core techniques including dietary recommendations, exercise, cognitive techniques, stimulus control, relapse prevention, and social support. Although weight loss is certainly the goal of treatment, weight is de-emphasized as it is not a behavior, per se, but a result of the behavior changes. The treatment requires an active participation of the patient; it is goal oriented, problem focused, structured, and it uses many techniques to change distorted thinking, mood, and thus problematic behavior.

Nutrition Education

It is important for patients to understand healthy versus unhealthy eating. Emotional eating (i.e., eating for any other reason than physiological necessity: including boredom, anger, frustration, excitement, etc.), eating in response to cravings or urges (which is also often linked to emotional reasons), and unhealthy dieting (purging, restricting or viewing a "diet" as a "limited time" rather than a healthy permanent lifestyle change) are examples of unhealthy eating behaviors that may result in both physical problems (e.g., intense hunger, low energy, fatigue, headaches, visual problems, weight gain, electrolyte disturbance, dental problems, gastrointestinal problems), cognitive problems (e.g., focus on food, loss of interest, poor concentration, memory problems, difficulty with comprehension and decision making), and emotional problems (e.g., stress, irritability, and anxiety, depression) (Bulik and Taylor, 2005). Incorporating a dietitian into the treatment team is essential so that patients learn healthy, balanced nutrition and the importanceof remaining within a certain calorie range or exchange program necessary for weight control/maintenance. A dietitian will help create a meal plan to consume several small meals per day so that patients do not set themselves up for overeating due to excessive hunger later in the day. Such healthy eating includes designating meal times, not allowing greater than 3 to 4 hours between eating times, not skipping meals, and avoiding eating in between planned meal/snack times.

Self-Monitoring

Self-monitoring of energy intake is a hallmark of weight control interventions and is a critical element in short and long-term weight management (Wing and Hill, 2001). Monitoring helps individuals understand their current eating patterns and identify patterns that need to be changed. For example, some individuals may learn that they go straight to the refrigerator after a long, stressful day at work (even if they are not physiologically hungry yet); others may find they are more likely to eat large portions in the evening if they go seven hours without eating during the day. In addition, monitoring helps individuals learn about the nutritional value of various foods, and it assists in meal planning/preparation and supports healthy choices. Monitoring provides a means for holding oneself accountable which, in turn, aids in helping individuals to avoid overeating or unhealthy eating. Monitoring also helps individuals notice their behavior changes and new patterns.

Physical Activity

It is recommended that patients gradually increase both lifestyle physical activity (e.g., gardening or yard work, climbing stairs, bicycling for transportation) and structured exercise. Exercise is a key component of any weight loss program and is highly correlated with long-term weight management. Accumulation of several short bouts of exercise per day (10 to 15 minute bouts for a total of 30 to 45 minutes per day) is as effective in promoting short-term (3 to 6 months) weight loss as exercising once per day for an equivalent length of time (Haskell et al., 2007; Jakicic, Winters, Lang, and Wing, 1999; Schmidt, Biwer, and Kalscheuer, 2001). In addition, exercising in short bouts may be superior to exercising once per day in maintaining weight loss over longer periods of time (12 to 18 months) but only when coupled with access to and use of home-based exercise equipment, possibly because home-based exercise is more convenient and associated with better adherence (Jakicic et al., 1999).

Cognitive Restructuring

According to cognitive behavioral theory, thoughts and feelings precede actions, and inaccurate thoughts drive unhealthy behaviors. CBT uses cognitive techniques to challenge inaccurate/unhealthy thoughts, and it focuses on current thinking, problematic behavior, precipitating factors, and developmental events. For weight control, patients are asked to maintain daily monitoring logs in which they record foods eaten, eating disordered behaviors (e.g., eating in the absence of physical hunger, purging, avoiding food in social settings, food restriction), thoughts, feelings, and details about the situation in which these behaviors occurred. In addition to revealing information about food consumed and eating patterns, such self-monitoring reveals patterns of automatic thoughts (e.g., "I am fat", "If I eat this, I am weak", "I did good today, I deserve this", "I blew it, now I might as well eat more") that reflect broader core beliefs. Over time, individuals become aware of their automatic thoughts; challenge them; question and evaluate the evidence that supports/opposes the thoughts; consider alternative views; determine the effect of the automatic thoughts on other thoughts, feelings, and behaviors; and identify typical thinking errors. Finally, given that negative mood and stress can result in overeating, cognitive techniques are used to reduce emotional distress, so that individuals refrain from eating during stressful situations.

Behavioral Chaining

Consistent with learning theory, CBT helps individuals identify the antecedents, behaviors, and consequences of their diet, exercise, and other behaviors associated with weight control. Individuals become skilled at understanding both cues/triggers for and consequences of eating behavior. Cues consist of specific thoughts, feelings, or behaviors and can be internal or external. Examples of internal cues include thoughts about the past or future that can generate emotions of sadness or anxiety, and physiological or bodily sensations such as a growling stomach or fatigue. Examples of external cues include social situations or events, interpersonal conflict, walking past a favorite restaurant, and food advertisements. A consequence is the result of behavior and can be either positive or negative. For example, physiological consequences of eating can include: 1) reduced hunger (positive) and 2) high cholesterol (negative). Emotional consequences of eating can include: 1) temporary relief of the negative feeling (positive) and 2) depression, guilt, shame after overeating (negative). Often, when individuals who are attempting weight loss overeat they do not think of the consequences in advance. Thus, behavioral chaining is a tool that helps individuals identify connections between cues, thoughts, behaviors, and consequences, and is used in the therapeutic process to help them resist cues to eating and think about the consequences in advance.

Behavioral Strategies

Specific behavioral strategies are essential to help individuals avoid unhealthy eating behavior and reinforce healthier alternatives. Patients are taught to set realistic, specific goals that are challenging but achievable, and then to gradually modify them to shape their desired behavior. Patients are often encouraged to identify small material rewards for achieving their goals. It is important that rewards are: a) not food-based (e.g., a trip to one's favorite ice cream parlor or pizza restaurant), b) delivered close in time to the desired behavior, and c) something the individual would otherwise not obtain. Individuals learn to control stimuli in their environment by following an eating schedule, food shopping from a list, removing serving dishes from the table, storing food in cabinets (not on the counter top), and buying foods that are healthy and require preparation. Individuals also practice avoiding high risk cues (keeping specific foods out of the house, taking an alternative route so that convenient stores are avoided), doing one thing at a time (e.g., do not eat and watch TV), and strengthening cues for desired behavior (plan an afternoon activity instead of going home alone and eating). Another strategy is to change the response to cues by building in a pause between having thought about eating and the actual act of eating. During this time, individuals may practice thought restructuring, focus on the consequences, or find an alternative behavior. Initially, pause intervals may be short in duration, but with practice they can gradually increase giving the patient greater opportunity to choose a different course of action rather than overeating when the urge arises. For example, patients may choose an alternative behavior to unhealthy eating (e.g., going for a walk, talking on the phone, taking a bath, knitting) or they may elect to "surf the urge" (i.e., allowing the urge or craving to peak, experiencing the peak, and then noticing that the urge decreases over time). Individuals also practice focusing on consequences, including positive consequences from healthy eating and negative short and long term consequences from unhealthy eating. These strategies can help patients learn that their cravings do not always lead to a "point of no return" and can build and reinforce a sense of control in dealing with urges once they arise.

Relapse Prevention

Relapse prevention is essential to long-term weight management. The objective of relapse prevention is to help patients identify ways in which they will continue to practice the skills learned during treatment. They also learn to distinguish between an occasional "slip" or "lapse" versus a "relapse". A "slip/lapse" happens when a patient engages in unhealthy eating behavior but regains control; a "relapse" happens when a patient loses control and then ultimately reverts to his/her original unhealthy eating patterns. Relapse prevention strategies help individuals identify high risk situations in advance, plan for them (e.g., identify alternative behaviors), and cope (practice positive thought restructuring: "Just because I slipped, does not mean that I have fallen off the wagon."). Patients can develop a personal "panic card" on which they list positive self-statements, alternative behaviors, and phone numbers of persons they can call for support. This card can be very useful when patients find themselves in high risk situations and are having difficulty identifying their newly learned healthy behaviors.

CBT-based weight control treatments typically consist of 20- to 30-week programs and are usually offered in group formats. Over the past 30 years, programs have increased from eight weeks to 30 weeks in recognition of the fact that weight loss accumulates at a rate of approximately one to two pounds per week and longer programs result in greater total weight loss (Wadden, Crerand, and Brock, 2005). While some individuals are successful at losing significant amounts of weight on 30 weeks, the majority of patients lose a modest 10% of their initial body weight. This amount of weight loss should not be discounted, however, as it has other important health implications including reductions in hypertension, hypercholesterolemia, diabetes, and all-cause mortality (Pi-Sunyer, 2002). Long-term maintenance of weight loss is associated with continued exercise, healthy diet, self-monitoring, and continued patient-provider contact (Jakicic, et al., 1999; Perri, 1998; Wing and Hill, 2001).

Cognitive-Behavioral Therapy for BED

Since many individuals with BED are overweight and eat in response to certain cues, CBT targeting both decreasing binge eating and managing weight may be useful in the treatment of BED. The primary goal for BED treatment is to achieve abstinence from binge eating; for overweight individuals with BED, a second treatment goal is sustainable weight loss. In addition, treatment often focuses on reducing symptoms of anxiety and depression that are commonly associated with BED and may trigger binge eating episodes (Grilo, Shiffman, and Carter-Campbell, 1994). Specifically, in therapy, patients learn to identify depressive or anxious automatic thoughts that lead to binge eating (e.g., "I'm a loser, nobody wants to be in a relationship with me, I might as well eat and be fat"; "I have to ace this job interview but I'm so nervous, I'll just calm myself down with this piece of chocolate cake"). CBT helps individuals identify and challenge their automatic thoughts, break the connection between such thoughts and eating, and identify alternative behaviors.

Several clinical studies have shown that CBT can be effective in the treatment of BED (Gorin, le Grange, and Stone, 2003; Hilbert and Tuschen-Caffier, 2004; Wilfley et al., 2002). When applied in a group format, patients learn CBT tools while also receiving social support from other group members. Patients can also benefit from individual therapy designed to address specific, personally relevant issues in greater depth. Group CBT for BED has been shown to be effective in reducing the number of binge days and hunger as well as in improving key psychological features of BED including disinhibition, depression, and self-esteem (Gorin et al., 2003; Hilbert and Tuschen-Caffier, 2004; Wilfley et al., 2002). CBT may also increase the likelihood of abstinence from binge eating (Gorin et al., 2003). However, CBT, as currently delivered, does not appear to lead to significant changes in body weight. Augmenting CBT with increased spousal involvement in therapy (Gorin et al., 2003) or body exposure treatment (Hilbert and Tuschen-Caffier, 2004) does not increase the impact of CBT in patients with BED. In sum, CBT may be effective in helping patients improve their sense of control over binge eating behavior but may require enhancements to adequately address weight concerns.

DBT employs both cognitive and behavioral strategies to help patients obtain skills pertaining to mindfulness, emotion regulation, interpersonal effectiveness, and distress tolerance. Telch et al. (Telch, Agras, and Linehan, 2001) studied 20 weeks of DBT versus waiting list control in 44 women with BED and found that DBT resulted in greater reduction in binge days, binge episodes, and in weight, shape, and eating concerns. However, the two groups did not differ in weight loss or in change in depression or anxiety. A recent pilot study found similar benefits of DBT including reductions in binge behavior and eating concerns without consistent reductions in BMI (Chen et al., 2008).

Our understanding of the potential benefits of CBT for BED is limited for several reasons. Controversies exist regarding diagnosis, in part, because the diagnostic criteria continue to undergo revision and there is no universally recognized operational definition of a "binge episode." In addition, validated age-appropriate instruments are only now becoming available for assessing BED in children and adolescents (Bryant-Waugh, Cooper, Tayler, and Lask, 1996; Johnson, Grieve, Adams, and Sandy, 1999; Shapiro, Woolson et al., 2007). Finally, most behavioral treatment studies for BED have been plagued by high drop-out rates, making it difficult to evaluate the true therapeutic impact of CBT in this patient population. Future research should address questions such as whether calories previously consumed as binges become distributed over non-binge meals after treatment (thus explaining lack of weight loss) and whether treatment alters the way in which patients label binges and non-binge meals (T. Walsh, personal communication, September 8, 2007). A recent evidence-based review emphasized that research studies should be more standardized and focus on abstinence from binge eating (not merely reduced binge frequency) as the critical outcome and target relapse prevention (Berkman et al., 2006; Brownley et al., 2007). Future research should control for placebo response, which has been shown to be high (yet possibly transitory) in BED (Carter et al., 2003; Jacobs-Pilipski et al., 2007; Pearlstein et al., 2003). Finally, given the promising preliminary results, additional studies of DBT (e.g., that can articulate which aspects of DBT are most applicable to the complex emotional and behavioral features of BED) are warranted.

Future Directions

In addition to continued research on weight loss and BED, new methods that enhance motivation and retention in intervention trials need to be developed. This endeavor will likely includes new information technologies such as e-mail, the Internet, personal digital assistants, text messaging, and other technological advances. These devices and technologies can be used to enhance treatment, particularly for those patients experiencing shame, denial, and interpersonal deficits or for those facing limited availability of specialty care. Our group (Shapiro, Reba-Harrelson et al., 2007) recently evaluated preliminary feasibility and acceptability of CD-ROM-delivered cognitive behavioral therapy (CD-ROM CBT) and compared it to 10 weekly group CBT sessions and to a waiting list control in 66 overweight individuals with BED. Promising results emerged pertaining to attrition and continued use of the CD post-treatment. Also, the majority of participants who were in the control waiting list group chose to receive CD-ROM CBT over group CBT treatment at the end of the waiting period. Thus, preliminarily, CD-ROM appears to be an acceptable and at least initially preferred method of CBT delivery for overweight individuals with BED. A more rigorous study designed to test these ideas directly is on-going.

Similarly, successful computer based programs have been reported for weight loss in individuals with type 2 diabetes (Tate, Jackvony, and Wing, 2003) and are being piloted for weight loss interventions in the US and United Kingdom for adults (Harvey-Berino, Pintauro, and Gold, 2002; Kirk et al., 2003; Kumanyika and Obarzanek, 2003). Tate and colleagues (Tate et al., 2003) compared an internet-only treatment versus an internet + weekly e-mail check-ins with a counselor treatment and reported significant weight loss in both groups with greater loss in the internet +e-mail group. Both groups showed reductions in caloric intake and increases in energy expenditure indicating that internet-based applications for the treatment of overweight are efficacious. Thus, the use of technology as a means of treatment delivery is emerging (Tate et al., 2003); further studies are needed in order to bridge the gap between clinical research and population-based delivery for the treatment of BED.

When evaluating the overall value of a particular treatment modality, it is useful to understand the "clinical significance" of a "statistically significant" research finding. Such understanding comes in the form of an "effect size" that indicates the size or importance of an observed treatment effect. One approach to determining effect size that is particularly relevant to the practice of evidence-based medicine is NNT (number needed to treat). Simply defined, NNT is the number of patients a clinician would need to treat with a particular modality to prevent one patient from having an adverse outcome over a predefined period of time. When comparing a particular treatment to placebo or another control condition, NNT is the number of patients who would need to receive active treatment in order to achieve one more successful outcome in the treatment group compared to the control group. In a sense, the NNT also represents the likelihood that a patient who receives treatment will benefit from it. For example, if five patients must receive treatment in order to prevent one from having an adverse outcome over the defined treatment period, then the NNT for that treatment is five, and each patient who received the treatment would have a 20% (one in five) chance of benefiting from the treatment. Using more traditional epidemiological terms to describe risk, the NNT is inversely related to absolute risk reduction. Conversely, NNH (number needed to harm) is defined as the number of patients who would need to receive active treatment in order for that group to experience one additional adverse event compared to the control group; NNH is inversely related to the absolute risk increase. The NNT and NNH measures are most useful when applied to the evaluation of binary outcomes (e.g., treatment success vs. treatment failures) and when there are reasonably large differences in the success rates of the treatment vs. the control conditions (Kraemer and Kupfer, 2006). With respect to weight-related and binge eating outcomes, therefore, it would be meaningful to calculate the NNT and NNH for outcomes such as obesity status (achieved BMI below 29.9, yes or no) or binge abstinence (yes/no) that are assessed in treatment trials where the placebo (or control condition) response rate is low. The NNT and NNH measures would be less applicable for outcomes such as % ideal body weight, change in binge frequency, time to remission, etc.

With respect to obesity, the NNT varies somewhat as a function of the treatment modality (medication, surgery, behavioral). In a recent evidence-based review of clinical trials of effective weight loss treatments, Orzano and Scott (Orzano and Scott, 2004) found similar results for surgical procedures such as gastric bypass and gastroplasty (NNT range 2 to 8), medications such as sibutramine and orlistat (NNT range 4 to 8), and combination diet and exercise interventions (NNT = 7). Compared to diet alone, sibutramine was more effective in helping patients achieve 10% or more weight loss, with the NNT being 50% lower for those treated with a higher (15 mg, NNT = 4) versus a lower (10 mg, NNT = 8) dose. While these studies provide some understanding of NNT in the context of obesity, more data are needed to adequately evaluate treatment modality differences in NNT (as well as NNH).

The measures of NNT and NNH have received scant attention in the eating disorders literature thus far. Bacaltchuk and colleagues (Bacaltchuk, Hay, and Trefiglio, 2001) reviewed randomized controlled trials of antidepressants and psychological treatments for bulimia nervosa. In five studies comparing an antidepressant alone to psychotherapy alone over a mean duration of 17.5 weeks, the NNH was four. In seven studies comparing medication/psychotherapy combinations to psychotherapy alone over a mean duration of 15 weeks, the NNH was seven and the NNT was eight. To date, there have been no published studies of NNT or NNH in the context of BED. This may, in part, reflect the relatively weak evidence base for treatment efficacy as it pertains to the benchmark binary outcome of abstinence. As we move forward in our understanding (and management) of placebo response and dropout in treatment trials for BED, and we elevate the scientific rigor of future studies to focus on key outcomes of abstinence and achievement of normal body weight, physicians and clinicians may be well served by presenting our findings in the clinically-relevant terms of NNT and NNH.

Conclusion

Treatments for obesity and BED include medications, behavioral interventions, surgery, and combinations of these approaches. Evidence for long-term success is much stronger for obesity treatment strategies than for BED strategies, in part, because of a lack of long-term BED studies overall. Side effects of certain medications and risks associated with surgery limit the broad application of these interventions; and surgical interventions for obesity are likely to be more successful when paired with psychological evaluations and therapies. Assessing for and treating binge eating behavior is an important aspect of supportive therapy that accompanies surgical interventions. Additional strategies for maintaining initial weight loss and improvements in eating psychopathology are needed, and observations that certain anti-depressants and novel techno-therapies may be beneficial for curbing binge eating and promoting weight loss warrant further investigation. The successful battle against these two serious public health concerns will depend on our ability to tailor treatments to individual patients, incorporating evidence-based strategies that are disseminated easily to both the treating clinician and the patient.

Acknowledgement

The authors wish to thank Xiaofei Mo, M.D. for her valuable editorial contributions.

References

Abell, T. L., and Monocha A. (2006). Gastrointestinal complications of bariatric surgery: Diagnosis and therapy. *American Journal of the Medical Sciences, 331*, 214-218.

Adams, T. D., Gress, R., Smith, S. C., Halverson, C., Simper, S. C., Rosamond, W. D., LaMonte, M. J., Stroup, A. M., Hunt, S. C. (2007). Long-term mortality after gastric bypass surgery. *New England Journal of Medicine, 357*, 753-761.

Agras, W., Telch, C., Arnow, B., Eldredge, K., Wilfley, D., Raeburn, S., Bruce B., Koran, L. M. (1994). Weight loss, cognitive-behavioral, and desipramine treatments in binge eating disorder: An additive design. *Behavior Therapy, 25*, 225-238.

Anderson, D. A., and Wadden, T. A. (1999). Treating the obese patient. Suggestions for primary care practice. *Archives of Family Medicine, 8*(2), 156-167.

Appolinario, J. C., Bacaltchuk, J., Sichieri, R., Claudino, A. M., Godoy-Matos, A., Morgan, C., Zanella, M. T., and Coutinho W. (2003). A randomized, double-blind, placebo-controlled study of sibutramine in the treatment of binge-eating disorder. *Archives of General Psychiatry, 60*(11), 1109-1116.

Arnold, L. M., McElroy, S. L., Hudson, J. I., Welge, J. A., Bennett, A. J., and Keck, P. E. (2002). A placebo-controlled, randomized trial of fluoxetine in the treatment of binge-eating disorder. *Journal of Clinical Psychiatry, 63*(11), 1028-1033.

Bacaltchuk, J., Hay, P., and Trefiglio, R. (2001). Antidepressants versus psychological treatments and their combination for bulimia nervosa. *Cochrane Database of Systematic Reviews, (4)*, CD003385.

Berkman, N., Bulik, C., Brownley, K., Lohr, K., Sedway, J., Rooks, A., Gartlehner, G. (2006). *Management of Eating Disorders. Evidence Report/Technology Assessment No. 135.* Rockville, MD: AHRQ Publication No. 06-E010. (Prepared by the RTI International-University of North Carolina Evidence-Based Practice Center under Contract No. 290-02-0016.).

Bray, G. A. (2000). A concise review on the therapeutics of obesity. *Nutrition, 16*(10), 953-960.

Bray, G. A., Ryan, D. H., Gordon, D., Heidingsfelder, S., Cerise, F., and Wilson, K. (1996). A double-blind randomized placebo-controlled trial of sibutramine. *Obesity Research, 4*(3), 263-270.

Brownley, K. A., Berkman, N. D., Sedway, J. A., Lohr, K. N., Bulik, C. M. (2007). Binge eating disorder treatment: A systematic review of randomized controlled trials. *International Journal of Eating Disorders, 40*(4), 337-348.

Bruce, B., and Agras, W. S. (1992). Binge eating in females: A population-based investigation. *International Journal of Eating Disorders, 12*(4), 365-373.

Bruce, B., and Wilfley, D. (1996). Binge eating among the overweight population: a serious and prevalent problem. *Journal of the American Dietetic Association, 96*(1), 58-61.

Bryant-Waugh, R., Cooper, P., Taylor, C., and Lask, B. D. (1996). The use of the eating disorder examination with children: a pilot study. *International Journal of Eating Disorders, 19*(4), 391-397.

Bulik, C., Sullivan, P., and Kendler, K. (2002). Medical and psychiatric morbidity in obese women with and without binge eating. *International Journal of Eating Disorders, 32*(1), 72-78.

Bulik, C. M., and Taylor, N. (2005). *Runaway Eating: The 8-point plan to conquer adult food and weight obsessions.* USA: Rodale, Inc.

Carter, W. P., Hudson, J. I., Lalonde, J. K., Pindyck, L., McElroy, S. L., and Pope, H. G. Jr. (2003). Pharmacologic treatment of binge eating disorder. *International Journal of Eating Disorders, 34*(Suppl 1), S74-S88.

Chen, E. Y., Matthews, L., Allen, C., Kuo, J. R., Linehan, M. M. (2008). Dialectical behavior therapy for clients with binge-eating disorder or bulimia nervosa and borderline personality disorder. *International Journal of Eating Disorders, 41*(6), 505-512.

Croft, H., Settle, E., Jr., Houser, T., Batey, S. R., Donahue, R. M., and Ascher, J. A. (1999). A placebo-controlled comparison of the antidepressant efficacy and effects on sexual functioning of sustained-release bupropion and sertraline. *Clinical Therapeutics, 21*(4), 643-658.

Daniels, S. R., Arnett, D. K., Eckel, R. H., Gidding, S. S., Hayman, L. L., Kumanyika, S., Robinson, T. N., Scott, B. J., St Jeor, S., and Williams, C. L. (2005). Overweight in children and adolescents: pathophysiology, consequences, prevention, and treatment. *Circulation, 111*(15), 1999-2012.

Daniels, S. R., Long, B., Crow, S., Styne, D., Sothern, M., Vargas-Rodriguez, I., Harris, L., Walch, J., Jasinsky, O., Cwik, K., Hewkin, A., and Blakesley, V. for the Sibutramine Adolescent Study Group. (2007). Cardiovascular effects of sibutramine in the treatment of obese adolescents: Results of a randomized, double-blind, placebo-controlled study. *Pediatrics, 120*(1), 147-157.

Davidson, M. H., Hauptman, J., DiGirolamo, M., Foreyt, J. P., Halsted, C. H., Heber, D., Heimburger, D. C., Lucas, C. P., Robbins, D. C., Chung, J., and Heymsfield, S. B. (1999). Weight control and risk factor reduction in obese subjects treated for 2 years with orlistat: a randomized controlled trial. *Journal of the American Medical Association, 281*(3), 235-242.

DeWald, T., Khaodhiar, L., Donahue, M., and Blackburn, G. (2006). Pharmacological and surgical treatments for obesity. *American Heart Journal, 151*(3), 604-624.

de Sousa, A. G., Cercato, C., Mancini, M. C., and Halpern, A. (2006). Obesity and obstructive sleep apnea-hypopnea syndrome. *Obesity Reviews, 9*(4):340-354.

de Zwaan M. (2001). Binge eating disorder and obesity. *International Journal of Obesity, 25,* S51-S55.

Douketis, J. D., Macie, C., Thabane, L., and Williamson, D. F. (2005). Systematic review of long-term weight loss studies in obese adults: clinical significance and applicability to clinical practice. *International Journal of Obesity, 29*(10), 1153-1167.

Drent, M. L., Larsson, I., William-Olsson, T., Quaade, F., Czubayko, F., von Bergmann, K., Strobel, W., Sjöström, L., and van der Veen, E. A. (1995). Orlistat (Ro 18-0647), a lipase inhibitor, in the treatment of human obesity: a multiple dose study. *International Journal of Obesity and Related Metabolic Disorders, 19*(4), 221-226.

Dujovne CA, Z. J., Rowe E, Mendel CM; Silbutramine Study Group. (2001). Effects of sibutramine on body weight and serum lipids: A double-blind, randomized, placebo-controlled study in 322 overweight and obese patients with dyslipidemia. *American Heart Journal, 142*(3), 489-497.

Dunican, K. C., Desilets, A. R., and Montalbano, J. K. (2007). Pharmacotherapeutic options for overweight adolescents. *Annals of Pharmacotherapy, 41*(9), 1445-1455.

Eckel, R. H., York, D. A., Rossner, S., Hubbard, V., Caterson, I., St. Joer, S. T., Hayman, L. L., Mullis, R. M., and Blair, S. N. (2004). Prevention Conerence VII: Obesity, a worldwide epidemic related to heart disease and stroke executive summary. *Circulation, 110,* 2968-2975.

Foley, E. F., Benotti, P. N., Borlase, B. C., Hollingshead, J., and Blackburn, G. L. (1992). Impact of gastric restrictive surgery on hypertension in the morbidly obese. *American Journal of Surgery, 163*(3), 294-297.

Gadde, K. M., Parker, C. B., Maner, L. G., Wagner, H. R., 2nd., Logue, E. J., Drezner, M. K., and Krishnan, K. R. (2001). Bupropion for weight loss: an investigation of efficacy and tolerability in overweight and obese women. *Obesity Research, 9*(9), 544-551.

Gorin, A., le Grange, D., and Stone, A. A. (2003). Effectiveness of spouse involvement in cognitive behavioral therapy for binge eating disorder. *International Journal of Eating Disorders, 33*(4), 421-433.

Grilo, C. M., Masheb R. M., and Salant S. L. (2005). Cognitive behavioral therapy guided self-help and orlistat for the treatment of binge eating disorder: a randomized, double-blind, placebo-controlled trial. *Biological Psychiatry*, 57(10), 1193-1201.

Grilo, C. M., Shiffman, S., and Carter-Campbell, J. T. (1994). Binge eating antecedents in normal-weight non-purging females: Is there consistency? *International Journal of Eating Disorders, 26*, 239-249.

Harvey-Berino, J., Pintauro, S. J., and Gold, E. C. (2002). The feasibility of using Internet support for the maintenance of weight loss. *Behavior Modification, 26*, 103-116.

Haskell, W. L., Lee, I.-M., Pate, R. R., Powell, K. E., Blair, S. N., Franklin, B. A., Macera, C. A., Heath, G. W., Thompson, P. D., and Bauman, A. (2007). Physical Activity and Public Health: Updated Recommendation for Adults from the American College of Sports Medicine and the American Heart Association. *Medicine and Science in Sports and Exercise, 39*(8), 1423–1434.

Hilbert A, and Tuschen-Caffier, B. (2004). Body image interventions in cognitive-behavioural therapy of binge-eating disorder: a component analysis. *Behaviour Research and Therapy, 42*, 1325-1339.

Hjartåker, A., Langseth, H., and Weiderpass, E. (2008). Obesity and diabetes epidemics: cancer repercussions. *Advances in Experimental Medicine and Biology, 630*, 72-93.

Hudson, J. I., McElroy, S. L., Raymond, N. C., Crow, S., Keck, P. E., Jr., Carter, W. P., Mitchell, J. E., Strakowski, S. M., Pope, H. G., Jr., Coleman, B. S., and Jonas, J. M. (1998). Fluvoxamine in the treatment of binge-eating disorder: a multicenter placebo-controlled, double-blind trial. *American Journal of Psychiatry, 155*(12), 1756-1762.

Jacobs-Pilipski, M. J., Wilfley, D. E., Crow, S. J., Walsh, B. T., Lilenfeld, L. R., West, D. S., Berkowitz, R. I., Hudson, J. I., and Fairburn, C. G. (2007). Placebo response in binge eating disorder. *International Journal of Eating Disorders, 40*(3), 204-211.

Jakicic, J. M., Winters, C., Lang, W., and Wing, R. R. (1999). Effects of intermittent exercise and use of home exercise equipment on adherence, weight loss, and fitness in overweight women: A randomzied trial. *Journal of the American Medical Association, 282*, 1554-1560.

James, W. P., Astrup, A., Finer, N., Hilsted, J., Kopelman, P., Rössner, S., Saris, W. H., and Van Gaal, L. F. (2000). Effect of sibutramine on weight maintenance after weight loss: a randomised trial. *Lancet, 356*(9248), 2119-2125.

James, W. P., Avenell, A., Broom, J., and Whitehead, J. (1997). A one-year trial to assess the value of orlistat in the management of obesity. *International Journal of Obesity and Related Metabolic Disorders, 21*(Suppl 3), S24-S30.

Janke, E. A., Collins, A., and Kozak, A. T. (2007). Overview of the relationship between pain and obesity: What do we know? Where do we go next? *Journal of Rehabilitation Research and Development, 44*(2), 245-262.

Johnson, W., Grieve, F., Adams,C. , and Sandy, J. (1999). Measuring binge eating in adolescents: Adolescent and parent version of the questionnaire of eating and weight patterns. *International Journal of Eating Disorders, 26*(3), 301-314.

Kirk, S. F., Harvey, E. L., McConnon, A., Pollard, J. E., Greenwood, D. C., Thomas, J. D., and Ransley, J. K. (2003). A randomised trial of an internet weight control resource: The UK Weight Control Trial [ISRCTN58621669]. *BMC Health Services Research, 3*(1), 19.

Kraemer, H. C., and Kupfer, D. J. (2006). Size of treatment effects and their importance to clinical research and practice. *Biological Psychiatry, 59*(11), 990-996.

Kumanyika, S. K., and Obarzanek, E. (2003). Pathways to obesity prevention: report of a National Institutes of Health workshop. *Obesity Research, 11*, 1263-1274.

Laederach-Hofmann, K., Graf, C., Horber, F., Lippuner, K., Lederer, S., Michel, R., and Schneider, M. (1999). Imipramine and diet counseling with psychological support in the treatment of obese binge eaters: a randomized, placebo-controlled double-blind study. *International Journal of Eating Disorders, 26*(3), 231-244.

Lee, A., and Morley, J. E. (1998). Metformin decreases food consumption and induces weight loss in subjects with obesity with type II non-insulin-dependent diabetes. *Obesity Research, 6*(1), 47-53.

Leung, W. Y., Thomas, G. N., Chan, J. C., and Tomlinson, B. (2003). Weight management and current options in pharmacotherapy: Orlistat and sibutramine. *Clinical Therapeutics, 25*(1), 58-80.

Li, Z., Maglione, M., Tu, W., Mojica, W., Arterburn, D., Shugarman, L. R., Hilton, L., Suttorp, M., Solomon, V., Shekelle, P. G., and Morton, S. C. (2005). Meta-analysis: pharmacologic treatment of obesity. *Annals of Internal Medicine, 142*(7), 532-546.

MacDonald, K. G., Jr, Long, S. D., Swanson, M. S., Brown, B. M., Morris, P., Dohm, G. L., and Pories, W. J. (1997). The gastric bypass operation reduces the progression and mortality of non-insulin-dependent diabetes mellitus. *Journal of Gastrointestinal Surgery, 1*(3), 213-220.

Manson, J. E., and Bassuk, S. S. (2003). Obesity in the United States: a fresh look at its high toll. *Journal of the American Medical Association, 289*(2), 229-230.

McElroy, S. L., Arnold, L. M., Shapira, N. A., Keck, P. E. Jr., Rosenthal, N. R., Karim, M. R., Capece, J. A., Fazzio, L., and Hudson, J. I. (2003). Topiramate in the treatment of binge eating disorder associated with obesity: a randomized, placebo-controlled trial. *American Journal of Psychiatry, 160*(2), 255-261.

McElroy, S. L., Casuto, L. S., Nelson, E. B., Lake, K. A., Soutullo, C. A., Keck, P. E., Jr., and Hudson J. I. (2000). Placebo-controlled trial of sertraline in the treatment of binge eating disorder. *American Journal of Psychiatry, 157*(6), 1004-1006.

McElroy, S. L., Hudson, J. I., Malhotra, S., Welge, J. A., Nelson, E. B., and Keck, P. E., Jr. (2003). Citalopram in the treatment of binge-eating disorder: a placebo-controlled trial. *Journal of Clinical Psychiatry, 64*(7), 807-813.

McMillan, D. C., Sattar, N., and McArdle, C. S. (2006). ABC of obesity. Obesity and cancer. *British Medical Journal, 333*(7578), 1109-1111.

Monteforte, M. J., and Turkelson, C. M. (2000). Bariatric surgery for morbid obesity. *Obesity Surgery, 10*, 391-401.

Munro, J. F., MacCuish, A. C., Wilson, E. M., and Duncan, L. J. (1968). Comparison of continuous and intermittent anorectic therapy in obesity. *British Medical Journal, 1*(5588), 352-354.

Mussell, M., Mitchell, J., de Zwaan, M., Crosby, R., Seim, H., and Crow, S. (1996). Clinical characteristics associated with binge eating in obese females: a descriptive study. *International Journal of Obesity and Related Metabolic Disorders, 20*, 324-331.

Norris, S. L., Zhang, X., Avenell, A., Gregg, E., Schmid, C. H., and Lau, J. (2005). Pharmacotherapy for weight loss in adults with type 2 diabetes mellitus. *Cochrane Database of Systematic Reviews, 25*(1), CD004096.

Orzano, A. J., and Scott, J. G. (2004). Diagnosis and treatment of obesity in adults: An applied evidence-based review. *Journal of the American Board of Family Practice, 17*(5), 359-369.

Padwal, R., Li, S. K., and Lau, D. C. W. (2003). Long-term pharmacotherapy for overweight and obesity: a systematic review and meta-analysis of randomized controlled trials. *International Journal of Obesity, 27*(12), 1437-1446.

Padwal, R., Li, S. K., and Lau, D. C. W. (2004). Long-term pharmacotherapy for obesity and overweight. *Cochrane Database of Systematic Reviews, 3*(4), CD004094.

Paolisso, G., Amato, L., Eccellente, R., Gambardella, A., Tagliamonte, M. R., Varricchio, G., Carella, C., Giugliano, D., and D'Onofrio F. (1998). Effect of metformin on food intake in obese subjects. *European Journal of Clinical Investigation, 28*(6), 441-446.

Payne, J. H., and DeWind, L. T. (1969). Surgical treatment of obesity. *American Journal of Surgery, 118*(2), 141-147.

Pearlstein, T., Spurell, E., Hohlstein, L. A., Gurney, V., Read, J., Fuchs, C., and Keller, M. B. (2003). A double-blind, placebo-controlled trial of fluvoxamine in binge eating disorder: a high placebo response. *Archives of Women's Mental Health, 6*(2), 147-151.

Perri, M. (1998). The maintenance of treatment effects in the long-term management of obesity. *Clinical Psychology: Science and Practice, 5*(4), 526-543.

Pi-Sunyer, F. X. (2002). Medical complications of obesity in adults. In C. G. Fairburn and K. D. Brownell (Eds.), *Eating disorders and obesity: A comprehensive handbook* (pp. 467-472). New York: Guilford.

Reichborn-Kjennerud, T., Bulik, C. M., Sullivan, P. F., Tabmbs, K., and Harris, J. R. (2004). Psychiatric and medical symptoms in binge eating in the absence of compensatory behaviors. *Obesity Research, 12*(9), 1445-1454.

Rossner, S., Sjostrom, L., Noack, R., Meinders, A. E., and Noseda, G. (2000). Weight loss, weight maintenance, and improved cardiovascular risk factors after 2 years treatment with orlistat for obesity. European Orlistat Obesity Study Group. *Obesity Research, 8*(1), 49-61.

Schmidt, W. D., Biwer, C. J., and Kalscheuer, L. K. (2001). Effects of Long *versus* Short Bout Exercise on Fitness and Weight Loss in Overweight Females. *Journal of the American College of Nutrition, 20*(5), 494-501.

Settle, E. C., Stahl, S. M., Batey, S. R., Johnston, J. A., and Ascher, J. A. (1999). Safety profile of sustained-release bupropion in depression: results of three clinical trials. *Clinical Therapeutics, 21*(3), 454-463.

Shapiro, J. R., Reba-Harrelson, L., Dymek-Valentine, M., Woolson, S. L., Hamer, R. M., and Bulik, C. M. (2007). Feasibility and acceptability of CD-ROM-based cognitive-behavioural treatment for binge-eating disorder. *European Eating Disorders Review, 15*, 175-184.

Shapiro, J. R., Woolson, W., Hamer, R. M., Kalarchian, M. A., and Bulik, C. M. (2007). Evaluating binge eating in children: development of the Children's Binge Eating Scale (C-BEDS). *International Journal of Eating Disorders, 40*(1), 82-89.

Sjostrom, L., Narbro, K., Sjostrom, D., Karson, K., Larsson, B., Wedel, H., Lystig, T., Sullivan, M., Bouchard, C., Carlsson, B., Bengtsson, C., Dahlgren, S., Gummesson, A., Jacobson, P., Karlsson, J., Lindroos, A., Lonroth, H., Naslund, I., Oblers, T., Stenlof, K., Torgerson, J., Agren, G., and Carlsson, L. M. S. (2007). Effects of bariatric surgery on mortality in Swedish obese subjects. *New England Journal of Medicine, 357*(8), 741-752.

Specker, S., de Zwaan, D., Raymond, N., and Mitchell, J. (1994). Psychopathology in subgroups of obese women with and without binge eating disorder. *Comprehensive Psychiatry, 35*(3), 185-190.

Stumvoll, M., Nurjhan, N., Perriello, G., Dailey, G., and Gerich, J. E. (1995). Metabolic effects of metformin in non-insulin-dependent diabetes mellitus. *New England Journal of Medicine, 333*(9), 550-554.

Sugerman, H. J., Fairman, R. P., Sood, R. K., Engle, K., Wolfe, L., and Kellum, J. M. (1992). Long-term effects of gastric surgery for treating respiratory insufficiency of obesity. *American Journal of Clinical Nutrition, 55*(2 Suppl), 597S-601S.

Tate, D. F., Jackvony, E. H., and Wing, R. R. (2003). Effects of Internet behavioral counseling on weight loss in adults at risk for type 2 diabetes: a randomized trial. *Journal of the American Medical Association, 289*(9), 1833-1836.

Telch, C. G., Agras, W. S., and Linehan, M. M. (2001). Dialectical behavior therapy for binge eating disorder. *Journal of Consulting and Clinical Psychology, 69*(6), 1061-1065.

Thompson, D., and Wolf, A. M. (2001). The medical-care cost burden of obesity. *Obesity Reviews, 2*, 189-197.

Thompson, W. G., Cook, D. A., Clark, M. M., Bardia, A., and Levine, J. A. (2007). Treatment of Obesity. *Mayo Clinic Proceedings, 82*(1), 93-102.

Tonstad, S., Pometta, D., Erkelens, D. W., Ose, L., Moccett, T., Schouten, J. A., Golay, A., Reitsma, J., Del Bufalo, A., Pasotti, E. et al. (1994). The effect of the gastrointestinal lipase inhibitor, orlistat, on serum lipids and lipoproteins in patients with primary hyperlipidaemia. *European Journal of Clinical Pharmacology, 46*(5), 405-410.

Van Gaal, L. F., Broom, J. I., Enzi, G., and Toplak, H. (1998). Efficacy and tolerability of orlistat in the treatment of obesity: a 6-month dose-ranging study. Orlistat Dose-Ranging Study Group. *European Journal of Clinical Pharmacology, 54*(2), 125-132.

Wadden, T. A., Crerand, C. E., and Brock, J. (2005). Behavioral treatment of obesity. *Psychiatric Clinics of North America, 28*(1), 151-170.

Weisler, R. H., Johnston, J. A., Lineberry, C. G., Samara, B., Branconnier, R. J., and Billow, A. A. (1994). Comparison of bupropion and trazodone for the treatment of major depression. *Journal of Clinical Psychopharmacology, 14*(3), 170-179.

Wilfley, D. E., Welch, R. R., Stein, R. I., Spurell E. B., Cohen, L. R., Saelens B. E., Dounchis, J. Z., Frank, M. A., Wiseman, C. V., and Matt, G. E. (2002). A randomized comparison of group cognitive-behavioral therapy and group interpersonal psychotherapy for the treatment of overweight individuals with binge-eating disorder. *Archives of General Psychiatry, 59*, 713-721.

Wing, R. R., and Hill, J. O. (2001). Successful weight loss maintenance. *Annual Review of Nutrition, 21*, 323-341.

Wittgrove, A. C., and Clark, G. W. (2000). Laparoscopic gastric bypass, Roux-en-Y- 500 patients: technique and results, with 3-60 month follow-up. *Obesity Surgery, 10*(3), 233-239.

Yanovski, S. Z. (1993). Binge eating disorder: Current knowledge and future directions. *Obesity Research*, 1(4), 306-324.

Yanovski, S. Z. (2003). Binge eating disorder and obesity in 2003: Could treating an eating disorder have a positive effect on the obesity epidemic? *International Journal of Eating Disorders, 34*, S117-S120.

Yanovski, S. Z., Nelson, J. E., Dubbert, B. K., and Spitzer, R. L. (1993). Association of binge eating disorder and psychiatric comorbidity in obese subjects. *American Journal of Psychiatry, 150*(10), 1472-1479.

In: Evidence-Based Treatments for Eating Disorders   ISBN 978-1-60692-310-8
Author: Ida F. Dancyger and Victor M. Fornari   © 2009 Nova Science Publishers, Inc.

Chapter XIV

Interpersonal Psychotherapy (IPT) for Eating Disorders

Rebecca Murphy, Suzanne Straebler, Zafra Cooper,
and Christopher G. Fairburn
University of Oxford, United Kingdom

Abstract

This chapter is concerned with the use of interpersonal psychotherapy (IPT) to treat patients with eating disorders. IPT is a short-term focal psychotherapy which was initially developed as a treatment for clinical depression but has been applied to many other clinical problems. Its leading indications are as a treatment for depression and bulimia nervosa. The goal of treatment is to help patients identify and resolve current interpersonal difficulties, the rationale being that doing so will result in recovery from the target disorder.

The chapter opens with a detailed consideration of the rationale for using IPT to treat patients with eating disorders. Then the evidence supporting this use of IPT is presented. There follows a description of the treatment and a comparison of IPT with cognitive behavior therapy (CBT). The chapter closes with a discussion of the ways in which IPT might operate.

Introduction

This chapter focuses on the use of interpersonal psychotherapy (IPT) in the treatment of eating disorders (IPT-ED). IPT is a short-term focal psychotherapy which was initially developed as a treatment for clinical depression. The goal of treatment is to help patients identify and resolve current interpersonal difficulties. The rationale for such a treatment is that interpersonal problems are known to contribute to the onset and maintenance of clinical depressions and as such their modification is likely to facilitate recovery. The efficacy of IPT in the treatment of depression has led to it being applied to other clinical problems, including recurrent depressive disorder, bipolar disorder, dysthymia, substance abuse, marital problems, anxiety disorders and eating disorders (Weissman, Markowitz, and Klerman, 2007). It has also been adapted for use with adolescents (Mufson, Moreau, Weissman, and Klerman, 1993), older adults (Frank, Frank, Cornes, Imber, Miller, and Morris, 1993), and pregnant women (Weissman, Markowitz, and Klerman, 2007).

First we consider the rationale for using IPT to treat patients with eating disorders. Then we review the evidence supporting this use of IPT. This is followed by a concise description of the treatment and a comparison of IPT with cognitive behavior therapy (CBT). Finally, we consider how IPT might achieve its effects and suggest avenues for future research.

The Rationale for Using IPT to Treat Patients with Eating Disorders

There are good reasons for using IPT to treat patients with eating disorders. Most patients with eating disorders have interpersonal difficulties. These may have been evident before the eating disorder developed or they may be more recent and possibly a consequence of it. The majority of adult cases are in their twenties or early thirties and have had an unremitting eating disorder for on average eight years (Fairburn et al, 2007). Not uncommonly, the eating disorder has had a profound effect on interpersonal development as late adolescence and early adulthood are crucial periods for growth in this regard. For example, many patients have had little experience developing and maintaining intimate relationships, in part because of the social withdrawal that is a feature of eating disorders and in part because of accompanying low self-esteem. Some have also had to abandon career plans and are essentially "at sea" in terms of their life aspirations and goals. As a result, the interpersonal impact of the eating disorder may be profound. These interpersonal difficulties tend to contribute to the maintenance of the eating disorder through a variety of mechanisms. First, patients' psychopathology tends to persist unchallenged as a result of their isolation from the normalizing influence of their peers. Second, some eating disorder features are maintained by interpersonal difficulties. For example, both binge eating and dietary restraint tend to occur, or be intensified, by the occurrence of adverse interpersonal events. Third, interpersonal difficulties often serve to worsen self-esteem which in turn tends to magnify patients' attempts to control their eating, shape and weight (Fairburn et al, 2008). IPT is designed to help patients overcome their interpersonal difficulties, thereby removing a major factor maintaining their eating disorder.

The Empirical Standing of IPT for Eating Disorders

Bulimia Nervosa

There have been two main randomized controlled trials of IPT for bulimia nervosa. The first of these was conducted by Fairburn and colleagues in Oxford (Fairburn et al, 1991,

1993). Seventy-five patients were randomized to cognitive behavior therapy for bulimia nervosa (CBT-BN; Fairburn, Marcus and Wilson, 1993), a behavioral version of CBT-BN (BT) or IPT, and at the end of treatment were entered into a closed (i.e., treatment-free) 12-month follow-up period. The treatments were carefully monitored for adherence. Patients in all three treatment conditions gave equivalent ratings of treatment suitability and expectancy. CBT was found to be significantly more effective at reducing the key behavioral features of bulimia nervosa than IPT at post-treatment, but this difference disappeared over the following eight months due to continuing improvement in the IPT group (see Figure 1). The behavioral version of CBT was least effective overall due to substantial post-treatment relapse. Thus IPT was as effective as CBT in the long term, but comparatively slower-acting. In a longer term follow up of these patients Fairburn et al. (1995) found that on average six years after treatment the majority of patients who had received IPT and CBT had maintained the changes seen at 12 months. Indeed, 72% of those who had received IPT no longer met DSM-IV criteria for an eating disorder (Fairburn, Norman, Welch, O'Connor, Doll and Peveler, 1995). IPT and CBT also resulted in an equivalent and lasting decrease in general psychiatric features and an improvement in self-esteem and social functioning. The fact that both CBT and IPT were superior to BT indicates that the improvements were not simply the result of non-specific psychotherapeutic processes.

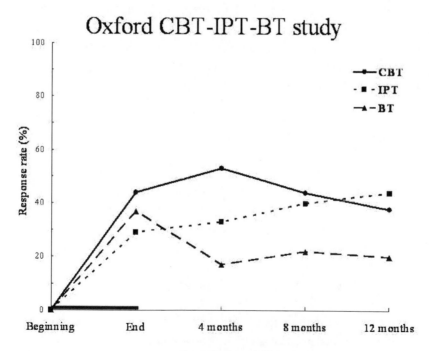

Fairburn et al. *Archives of General Psychiatry* 1993; 50: 419-428

A second, much larger (N=220), two-centre study conducted at Stanford and Columbia replicated the main Oxford findings (Agras, Walsh, Fairburn, Wilson and Kraemer, 2000). Again, CBT was found to be superior to IPT at the end of treatment but the two treatments were equivalent by eight-to-12-month open follow-up. An additional goal of this second CBT-IPT study was to identify differential predictors of response to IPT and CBT, the hope being that this would allow the matching of patients to the two treatments. However, no differential predictors were found (Fairburn, Agras, Walsh, and Wilson, 2004).

Mitchell, Halmi, Wilson, Agras, Kraemer, and Crow (2002) carried out a study to explore whether women with bulimia nervosa who did not respond to CBT would respond to IPT or antidepressant medication. Unfortunately, the findings of this study are difficult to interpret because of a high rate of non-acceptance of the second-line treatment. Overall, there was no evidence to suggest that IPT was a good treatment for patients who do not make a full response to CBT.

Anorexia Nervosa

There has been one study of the use of IPT in the treatment of anorexia nervosa (McIntosh, Jordan, Carter, Luty, McKenzie, Bulik, Frampton and Joyce, 2005). Fifty-six patients were randomized to IPT, CBT or non-specific supportive clinical management. At the end of treatment, IPT was found to be the least effective of the three treatments. No data on follow-up have been presented so it is not yet known whether IPT has the same delayed effect in anorexia nervosa as seen in bulimia nervosa. It should also be noted that the sample was an unusual one in that many of the patients were subthreshold cases of anorexia nervosa with a weight above the widely used diagnostic cut-off point.

Eating Disorder NOS

There has also been one major study of the use of IPT in the treatment of patients with eating disorder NOS. This focused on a subgroup of these patients, namely those with binge eating disorder accompanied by obesity (Wilfley, Welch, Stein, Borman Spurrell, Cohen, Saelens, Zoler Dounchis, Frank, Wiseman and Matt, 2002). In this study, 162 patients were randomized to group CBT or group IPT and then followed up for 12 months. The patients in the two treatment conditions showed an almost identical, and substantial, response over treatment and open follow-up. Overall, the findings are suggestive of a non-specific psychotherapeutic response.

No studies have addressed the use of IPT with patients with other forms of eating disorder NOS. This is a serious omission since it is now recognized that eating disorder NOS is the most common eating disorder diagnosis made in routine clinical practice, and that these patients have as severe and longstanding an eating disorder as patients with bulimia nervosa (Fairburn et al, 2007).

Conclusion

Four conclusions may be drawn from this body of research:

1) IPT is an alternative to CBT in the treatment for bulimia nervosa but it takes longer to achieve its effects. Indeed, systematic review conducted by the UK National Institute for Health and Clinical Excellence (NICE) concluded that IPT was the leading empirically supported alternative to CBT (NICE, 2004). There are no empirical grounds for matching patients to CBT or IPT.
2) IPT cannot be recommended as a treatment for anorexia nervosa, at least not as a sole form of treatment (as provided in the McIntosh et al, 2005 study).
3) IPT is one of many treatments for binge eating disorder, the other leading treatments being an adaptation of the CBT for bulimia nervosa (Fairburn et al, 1993) and guided cognitive-behavioral self-help (Grilo, 2006).
4) There is a pressing need for research on the use of IPT with patients with eating disorder NOS.

The Practice of IPT for Eating Disorders

IPT for eating disorders (IPT-ED) is based on IPT for depression and closely resembles it. In essence, it is a slight modification of the empirically-supported adaptation of IPT for patients with bulimia nervosa (Fairburn, 1997). IPT for bulimia nervosa (IPT-BN) has been extended for use with patients with any form of form of eating disorder (IPT-ED) so long as the patient is not significantly underweight (defined in this context as a BMI ≤ 17.5) and IPT-ED addresses a new type of interpersonal problem that we have termed "life goals". This is described later.

As IPT-ED is an outpatient-based treatment, it is essential that it is safe for patients to be managed this way. Patients with eating disorders are at risk of suicidal behavior and various physical complications. Establishing that it is appropriate to provide outpatient treatment is therefore an essential preliminary to embarking upon IPT. Guidelines for doing so are provided by Fairburn, Cooper and Waller (2008).

IPT-ED generally involves 16 to 20 50-minute treatment sessions over about four to five months. Like IPT for depression, the treatment has three phases.

Phase One - This generally occupies three-to-four sessions. The first aim of this phase is to describe the rationale and nature of IPT-ED. This is part of the process of engaging patients in treatment. The second aim is to agree jointly upon the current interpersonal problem, or problems, which will be the focus of the rest of treatment.

Phase Two - This is the main part of treatment and occupies up to ten weekly sessions. The goal is that the patient first characterizes the identified interpersonal problem(s), and then addresses it (them). IPT for depression categorizes interpersonal problems into one of four overarching "problem areas"; grief, interpersonal role disputes, role transitions and interpersonal deficits. Both problem area-specific and generic IPT strategies and procedures are used to address these problems.

Phase Three - This generally occupies the final three sessions. There are two goals; the first being to ensure that the changes made in treatment are maintained, and the second being to minimize the risk of relapse in the longer-term. .

For details about the practice of IPT, readers should consult the original IPT "manual" (Klerman, Weissman, Rounsaville and Chevron, 1984) or the more recent version of it (Weissman, Markowitz and Klerman, 2000).

Phase One

Phase One usually occupies three-to-four sessions. As noted above, there are three goals.

1. *Engaging patients in treatment and describing the rationale and nature of IPT-ED* - It is explained that to help people break out of a self-perpetuating problem such as an eating disorder it is necessary to find out what is keeping it going and then to address the maintaining processes in treatment. The therapist informs the patient that interpersonal difficulties are common in patients with eating disorders, although many people have limited awareness of them due to the distracting influence of their preoccupation with thoughts about eating, shape and weight. Interpersonal difficulties maintain the eating disorder through a number of mechanisms. These were summarized earlier. It is often useful to give patient's specific examples (related to their individual circumstances) of how interpersonal issues may maintain their type of eating disorder. It is then explained that treatment will focus on the patient's current interpersonal difficulties, rather than on the eating problem, because the goal is to help patients overcome their eating problem by resolving difficulties in their life and relationships. Focusing too much on the eating problem would tend to distract the patient and therapist from this task.

Patients are also forewarned that the treatment will change in style over time. Initially, during the first three or four sessions, the goal is to identify those interpersonal difficulties on which the rest of treatment will focus. The therapist may say something along these lines:

> "This initial phase of treatment will involve a review of your past and present relationships, and during this stage I will take the lead in asking you questions. This phase of treatment will end with us agreeing upon the problem or problems that should be the focus of the remainder of treatment. Thereafter our sessions will change in style. You will become largely responsible for the content of the sessions and I will take more of a back seat role. Gradually we will learn more about your interpersonal difficulties and ways of changing them. Your role will be not only to explore these difficulties in our treatment sessions but also to think about what we have discussed between the sessions. Furthermore, whilst you are having treatment it is important to experiment with making changes in your life. Doing so will help us better understand the nature of your problems and may suggest further ways of changing."

It is important that the patient understands that the treatment is time-limited. The fact that the treatment has a fixed number of sessions helps the therapist stress the importance of working hard at treatment.

"This is an opportunity to change - an opportunity to break out of what has been a longstanding problem. It is essential that you make the most of this opportunity by giving the treatment priority in your life. Not doing so is likely to limit the progress that we can make."

2. Identifying current interpersonal problems - Three sources of information are used to identify current interpersonal problems:

i)   *A history is taken of the interpersonal context in which the eating problem developed and has evolved* – As part of this history-taking the therapist asks about how the eating problem has evolved (e.g. the ages at which the patient first began to diet, binge and purge, and any significant changes in weight). The therapist also asks about the patient's interpersonal functioning prior to and since the development of the eating problem, including relationships with family and peers. The therapist will also take a history of co-existing psychiatric disorders if these are present. The review highlights links between changes in the eating problem and interpersonal events and circumstances, thereby stressing the importance of interpersonal processes. This helps the patient see the relevance of IPT and gives clues as to current interpersonal problems. For most patients the review of the past should be relatively brief and take only two sessions. It should be noted that the earlier description of IPT for BN encouraged the construction of a detailed 'life chart' (Fairburn, 1997). This has been abandoned as it can become too time-consuming and adds little to the identification of current interpersonal difficulties.

ii) *An assessment is made of the quality of the patient's current interpersonal functioning and life circumstances* - This involves conducting an "interpersonal inventory" in which the therapist asks about the patient's social network and current circumstances. Enquiry is made about family members, the patient's partner (if any), confidants, friends, work contacts and other acquaintances. The topics addressed include frequency of contact, positive and negative aspects of each relationship, mutual expectations, intimacy and reciprocity. In addition, the therapist asks about significant interpersonal changes over the last few years. In particular this encompasses interpersonal "exits" (i.e. where the patient has lost a relationship, including bereavements). Patients are also asked about recent significant changes in their life circumstances (for example, in terms of their home-life, family, social life, health, and so on) and about their future life goals.

iii) *The precipitants of changes to eating are identified* - In each of the assessment sessions, the therapist also asks whether there have been any changes in the patient's eating since the last session (i.e., intensification of dieting, binge eating, purging, etc) and, if so, enquires about the interpersonal circumstances preceding them. Since it is common for changes in eating to be precipitated by interpersonal events, they may serve as "markers" of current interpersonal problems. In this way the relationship between the eating problem and interpersonal events can be carefully explored. Some secondary accounts of the treatment have implied that this is not done in IPT for eating disorders (e.g., Weissman, Markowitz and Klerman, 2007). This is incorrect.

3. Choosing which problems should become the focus of treatment - By the third or fourth session, the nature of the patient's interpersonal difficulties should be clear. The next step is to decide which should become the focus of the remainder of treatment. This decision should be a collective one.

The Problem Areas

Five types of interpersonal problem tend to be present in patients with eating disorders. These differ somewhat from those identified by Weissman and colleagues in patients with depression. This is not surprising given the age of these patients and the nature of their psychiatric difficulties. These patients are quite different from those with depression who tend to be older and suffering from an episodic disorder rather than an unremitting one.

1. *Lack of intimacy and interpersonal deficits* - The most common interpersonal problem encountered is lack of close or satisfactory intimate relationships, romantic or otherwise. We use a slightly broader definition of 'deficit' than Weissman, Markowitz and Klerman (2000), one which is exclusively present-focused and therefore does not require patients to have long-standing unfulfilling relationships. Although some patients describe a scarcity in general of interpersonal relationships and feelings of isolation, many more specifically lack intimate relationships. Treatment aims to encourage these patients to consider what they want from a relationship and to take steps to achieve this. It may be helpful to review past significant relationships and consider any recurrent problems in order to make changes in the present.

2. *Interpersonal role disputes* - Interpersonal role disputes are also common. Disputes of this nature may be with any figure of importance in the patients' lives, including partners, family members, friends and employers. Such disputes are often the result of each party having differing expectations of each other. The aim of treatment is to help clarify the nature of the dispute, consider the possibilities for change on both sides (including communicating expectations), and then to actively explore them. The outcome may be a renegotiation of the relationship or its dissolution.

3. *Role transitions* - Problems with role transitions are seen when the patient has difficulty coping with a life change. Life changes are common in this patient group given their age. Frequently encountered examples include: moving away from home and establishing independence from parents, starting a first job or having a partner for the first time. However, difficulties in this area are not confined to the problems of late adolescence and early adulthood. They include problems coping with other life changes such as changing jobs, getting married and becoming a parent. The goal of treatment is to help the patient abandon the old role and adopt a new one. This involves exploring exactly what the new role involves and how it can be mastered as well as examining and re-evaluating the old role, which may have become idealized.

4. *Grief* - Problems associated with the death of a loved one are not common in patients with eating disorders given their age. If such difficulties are apparent it is important to help the patient think in detail about the events surrounding the loss and express their feelings about it. Reconstructing the lost relationship, both its' positive and negative aspects, is also of central importance, as it counters the idealization that commonly occurs. As patients become

less focused on the past, they are helped to think about the future and to create new interests and relationships.

5. *"Life goals"* - Problems concerning future life plans are frequently encountered in this patient group. They are characterized by patients' uncertainty over what course their life should take in terms of career, lifestyle and relationships. It is broader in nature than difficulty coping with role transitions because in this instance patients need to develop new roles in their life and reconsider their goals (rather than to adjust to the current role) and it is for this reason that we view "life goals" as a new problem area. Treatment is an opportunity for patients to reconsider their aspirations, to consider taking steps towards meeting them and to make changes in their life. Typically this is a second problem area and one that is addressed after the patient has made progress in another area and is feeling more hopeful about the future.

If more than one problem is identified a decision needs to be made about which problems will be addressed and in what order. In general it is only possible to tackle one or two problems in treatment. Our strategy is to address those whose resolution is likely to have the greatest impact on the patient's eating disorder. Given our view of how IPT is likely to work (see below) we choose those problems that we think will have the greatest impact on the patient's overall interpersonal functioning and self-esteem. Clearly, they also have to be viewed by the patient as a problem. When there are two problems to be tackled they are generally addressed sequentially, with the simpler and more easily solved being tackled first. Progress on one front often bolsters the patient's morale and sense of interpersonal competence thereby facilitating their tackling of other difficulties.

Phase Two

Once the problem area(s) has (have) been agreed by both patient and therapist, the treatment enters phase two. The second and third phases of the treatment are very similar to IPT for depression, as described in the IPT manual, although in IPT-ED the patient is placed under greater general pressure to change. At the end of Phase One the therapist reminds the patient that the treatment will now alter in character.

"As we discussed at the outset, from this point on the nature of our sessions will change. Instead of my asking you questions, you will take the lead. Your task will be to focus on the problems we have identified and consider them in depth and from all possible angles. In this way we will come to a better understanding of them. A key part of treatment is thinking about what changes you could make and how to bring them about. While you are in treatment it is important that you make changes as we will learn much more about your problems from your attempts to change them"

The sessions from this point on are largely patient-led. The therapist is active but not directive and throughout the focus remains on the present. Sessions begin by reminding patients of the session number and how many remain, followed by a general enquiry such as *'How have things been since we last met?'*

The initial task in Phase Two is for the patient to characterize the identified problem(s). The therapist's role is to ensure that the patient remains focused on this task. The therapist asks questions to facilitate this (although this does not extend to making "interpretations" which depend on a particular theoretical view of the disorder and its treatment). In doing this the therapist aims to help patients gain a better understanding of their problems.

Generally, after several sessions, the patient has moved on to consider ways of changing. Using the IPT technique of "decisional analysis" (Weissman, Markowitz and Klerman, 2000), the therapist helps the patient think through all the options available together with their implications in order to arrive at a course of action. As the therapist is not directive, possible solutions are not offered nor are opinions expressed about what the patient should do. The therapist praises all efforts to identify solutions and change. Patients' attempts to change become the focus of subsequent sessions.

As part of the process of understanding interpersonal difficulties and considering ways of changing, the IPT technique of "communication analysis" may be used to better understand key interpersonal exchanges. This involves reviewing these exchanges in detail to identify exactly what was said by both parties, what the patient had intended to communicate, and how the patient interpreted the communication of the other party. The therapist always encourages the patient to consider the perspective of the other person. In this way, ambiguities and misunderstandings may be identified and clarified. This helps patients consider how effectively they communicate with others. It is often useful to ask patients to report exchanges verbatim, using the same tone of voice and words as in the original. Role playing may also be used to prepare patients for key forthcoming exchanges. It is worth noting that this is in contradiction to some reports which have claimed that IPT-ED does not include role play (Weismann, Markowitz and Klerman, 2007).

The need for the patient to change is stressed at regular intervals. It is important to note that this is general pressure to change rather than pressure to take a specific course of action. Progress in treatment becomes an iterative process. Through making changes patients gain a greater understanding of their problems and as a result are able to make progressively more strategic and influential changes. Furthermore, as patients experience successes resulting from such changes their confidence about making further life changes increases.

At the end of each session the therapist provides a brief summary of what has been covered in the session using the patient's own words. This summary is simply an account of the content of the session and does not involve any additional processing or interpretation from the therapist. The therapist also encourages the patient to think further about the matters discussed between this appointment and the next one. In addition, on one or two occasions during Phase Two, the therapist and patient informally review progress by considering each of the agreed upon problems and assessing what has been achieved and what remains to be done.

The therapist's role in Phase Two is to help patients change, to help them appraise the consequences of these changes and then to make further changes. Reference is rarely made to the therapist-patient relationship since doing so can complicate and undermine IPT. However, one exception is patients who have such severe interpersonal deficits that one of the very few relationships available for examination is that between the therapist and patient. Such patients may benefit from feedback about how they come across to others.

Interestingly, most patients make few, if any, references to their eating disorder. If they do, the therapist shifts the topic on to the interpersonal context of the eating problem perhaps by saying "*It is understandable that you are binge eating a lot just now, given what is going on ....*" Detailed discussion of the eating disorder is not part of IPT-ED as it distracts patients and therapists from the interpersonal focus of the treatment. Furthermore, it can trigger extreme ruminative thinking about shape, weight and eating that can prevent patients from reflecting on their interpersonal difficulties. However, at times it can be helpful to restate the rationale of the treatment as this often helps address concerns patients may have about the absence of a direct focus on the eating disorder.

Phase Three

The third phase of treatment comprises the final three sessions. Ending treatment is an interpersonal event in its own right and an important part of treatment. The final sessions are held at two-week intervals, thus allowing patients increased time to continue to make changes on their own with less input from the therapist. There are two related goals. The first is to ensure that the changes that have been made continue following termination, and the second is to minimize the risk of relapse.

Unlike the transition between Phases One and Two, there is no sharp change in style between Phases Two and Three. Instead, the sessions continue much as before except that there needs to be a review of what has been achieved in treatment and a consideration of the future. When progress on a particular problem is being discussed, the therapist should help the patient project forwards to the future perhaps by saying: "*As you know, we only have three more sessions to go. What do you envisage happening regarding .... over the coming months? How can you make sure that you build upon what you have achieved so far?*" By this point, it will be clear what changes are likely to be made during the period of treatment and what changes may well not take place. The therapist should ensure that the patient has realistic expectations in this regard. For example, the therapist might say: "*Given what has emerged during treatment, it seems that you think it unlikely that .... will start to behave differently in the foreseeable future. If this is the case, what do you think you should do?*"

The therapist should also help the patient predict areas of future interpersonal difficulty. Both problems in the areas addressed in treatment and broader interpersonal issues should be discussed. Therapists should ask patients what they plan to do to overcome such difficulties should they arise.

In Phase Three, as well as at appropriate points earlier in treatment, the interpersonal competence of the patient should be highlighted so that patients attribute any changes made to themselves rather than to the therapist. The therapist should explain that, although he or she acted as a guide during treatment, the patient has actually made the changes that have taken place.

An assessment of the state of the patient's eating problem should also be made in Phase Three. Patients are reminded that it often takes a further four to eight months for the full effects of IPT-ED to be realized. We advise patients not to seek further treatment in the meantime. However, patients are also told that their eating problem is likely to remain an Achilles heel in the sense that they may experience a lapse in the future at times of interpersonal difficulty. We encourage patients to view any deterioration in their eating problem (e.g., a return of binge eating or loss of weight) as a potential "early warning sign" of a developing interpersonal problem and as a cue to review what is happening in their personal life and, perhaps, to take corrective action.

It is unusual for patients receiving IPT-ED to have difficulty accepting the ending of treatment. This is because it is made clear at the outset that treatment is time-limited and at the beginning of each session they are reminded of the number of sessions remaining. Nevertheless, therapists should always ask patients how they feel about the ending of treatment, not least because this provides an opportunity to emphasize what has been achieved and to stress their competence at dealing with future areas of difficulty.

An Illustrative Case History

The patient was a 21-year-old college student, referred by her primary care physician, for the treatment of bulimia nervosa. This was a longstanding problem, which had begun in adolescence.

Phase One

Treatment began by taking a history of the interpersonal context in which the eating problem had developed. The patient began dieting at school and started to binge eat and vomit about a year later. During this time, she described feeling that she did not have friends who she could turn to for support. Although she felt unsure as to whether she wanted to continue her education, she went to college because of pressure from her parents. When she started college the eating problem became more severe. She reported that her shame and secrecy over binge eating and vomiting prevented her from making friends. Eventually she decided to drop-out of school. At the time she requested treatment she was working as a waitress.

During the first few treatment sessions, the therapist asked her about each occurrence of binge eating and vomiting and the interpersonal context in which they occurred. This revealed that they usually occurred in the evenings, when feeling lonely or when bored at work.

At the end of the third session, the patient and therapist agreed that the patient's lack of close relationships should be the problem area on which treatment should focus. The patient explained that she preferred to keep others at 'arm's length' as she was afraid of becoming too dependent on them and eventually being let down. She also described being reluctant to reveal her feelings to her friends especially when she was experiencing any problems in case they thought that she wasn't a "fun person" and that she was a burden to them. The patient found these initial sessions particularly difficult since she had previously been trying to avoid thinking about problems in her life and relationships. The therapist was able to keep the patient engaged in treatment by praising her efforts to think about these matters and by explaining that understanding more about her problems was a necessary first step if she was to overcome them. At the end of this initial phase of treatment the therapist reminded the patient of the change in session style that was about to take place.

Phase Two

In the first few sessions of Phase Two, the patient's past friendships were reviewed. This revealed that the patient had never felt that they were reciprocal. Although she was able to listen to her friends' worries she did not allow herself to talk about her own insecurities. She also felt uncertain about whether her friends really liked her and so would avoid taking the initiative in agreeing to meet. The therapist encouraged the patient to consider her options for developing closer friendships. This involved helping her think about the sorts of friendships she wished to develop and the expectations she had of them. At this time, the patient was particularly concerned with a problem at work and decided that she would mention this to a friend. The therapist helped the patient to role play how she could elicit her friend's support without risking the friend feeling burdened. The patient was subsequently pleased that her friend was supportive so she decided to invite the friend to a family party. The friend did not come to the party with the result that the patient came to the next session saying that treatment was not working and she was tired of making efforts to change. The therapist and patient decided to review what had taken place. It emerged that when she had invited her friend she had said that she was going to a family party which would most likely be boring but she was welcome to come. On reflection, the patient realized that from her friend's perspective it was not obvious that the patient wanted her to attend the party. It was clear that the patient needed to learn how to communicate clearly and unambiguously.

During the following weeks the patient continued to make interpersonal changes and developed new friendships through joining a book group. In one session, the patient asked what she should do about her eating since she was still struggling in this regard. The therapist reminded the patient about the rationale underpinning the treatment. The therapist explained that the patient should be focusing on overcoming difficulties in her life and relationships, and that over time this would lead to improvements in her eating.

About two-thirds of the way through treatment the therapist asked the patient to review the progress that she had made. The patient described realizing that she was a likeable person with whom people wanted to be friends and that her friends accepted that sometimes she needed support from them. The patient also mentioned that she had recently been feeling more dissatisfied and bored with her work. Previously, she had welcomed the fact that she found working as a waitress less demanding than being a student. However, even though she had been given greater responsibilities at work, she did not find the job challenging enough. As the addressing of the initial problem area was progressing so well, the therapist and patient agreed to spend time during the remaining sessions reflecting on the patient's goals in life.

The patient was encouraged to think about what she wanted to do in the future. She came to the conclusion that she wanted to be a teacher. She realized that going back to finish her college degree would be the best way of working towards this goal and so she negotiated a return to her studies. She subsequently described looking forward to returning to college because she felt that she had made the decision to be there rather than being there because of pressure from her parents.

Phase Three

In the last phase of treatment, the therapist and patient considered what had been achieved in treatment. The patient felt pleased about the changes that she had made in her life both regarding her friendships and her plan to return to college. As a result she described feeling more confident about herself. The patient was encouraged to consider any potential problems that might occur and how she might use what she had learned in treatment to address them. She reported that she was more aware of difficulties in her life and that, instead of avoiding thinking about them; she was able to think about options for resolving them.

In the penultimate session the therapist asked the patient about her eating. The patient explained that in the initial weeks of treatment she had been concerned that the eating problem was getting worse but that in the last month or so she had been binge eating and vomiting much less frequently. She said that she had realized that overcoming the eating problem did not require her to be more disciplined about eating but rather it involved her addressing what was happening in her life. The therapist told her that continued improvement was likely and advised her to regard problems in eating as a marker of other difficulties in her life and relationships.

Follow-up

The therapist saw the patient for two follow-up sessions, one approximately six months after treatment and one six months after that. During this time the patient had resumed her studies and was living with other college students. She described being much happier in her life and having several close friends. She also reported that she had not been thinking much about food, eating, shape or weight. More detailed assessment revealed that she had few residual eating disorder features.

How IPT-ED Differs from CBT

The distinctive feature of IPT is its interpersonal focus and its interpersonal strategies, rather than its use of particular specific techniques (Weissman, Markowitz and Klerman, 2007). Although IPT employs techniques used in many other therapies, there are certain procedures that are not utilized. As CBT is considered the leading empirically-supported treatment for eating disorders (Wilson and Fairburn, 2007), an examination of the differences and similarities between these two forms of treatment is warranted. It is important to note that it is a very specific form of CBT that is empirically supported (Fairburn, 2008). It is therefore this version that is compared with IPT-ED.

IPT-ED and CBT share a range of common features. Both are time limited, short-term focused psychological treatments which explore current problems; the aim being to change maintaining mechanisms, rather than to uncover past causes. However, the theory underpinning each treatment differs. CBT focuses on cognitive and behavioural maintaining processes and the goal is their direct modification. In contrast, IPT-ED aims to treat the eating disorder indirectly through the addressing of current interpersonal problems.

Consistent with these differing rationales, the content of CBT and IPT-ED sessions differs markedly. IPT-ED makes little reference to the eating disorder but focuses on the identified interpersonal problems, while CBT focuses on the modification of the cognitive and behavioural processes thought to be maintaining the individual patient's eating disorder. Interpersonal difficulties are only addressed in CBT if they appear to be directly maintaining the disturbances of eating. [A variant of CBT has been developed that also addresses interpersonal problems – see Fairburn et al, 2002; Fairburn et al, 2008)].

The role of the therapist is similar in the two treatments with respect to being both active and an advocate for the patient although the sessions differ in form. In IPT, the sessions are patient-led (except during Phase One) and unstructured, whereas in CBT the sessions are agenda-led and structured. The IPT therapist is non-directive, whereas the CBT therapist is more so. The IPT therapist does not encourage patients to change their behaviour in specific ways: instead IPT relies upon in-session verbal dialogue to produce change, together with encouragement to continue thinking about the matters discussed between sessions. In CBT, behaviour change is a major focus of treatment. Indeed, as discussed by Fairburn, Cooper and Shafran (2008), in CBT the goal is to help patients make personalised and highly strategic changes to the way that they behave, and then help them analyze their effects and implications. In IPT, there is only general pressure to make interpersonal change and no homework. In both treatments, the patient is seen as largely responsible for change with the therapist guiding them through this process. Both treatments regard much of the therapeutic progress made during treatment as being the result of work done between the therapy sessions

How IPT Works

There has been little research on how psychological treatments work and IPT is no exception. This is true of IPT in general and IPT-ED. There has been no research on the precise relationship between the therapeutic interventions and changes in interpersonal functioning and eating disorder features. The research findings indicate IPT-BN has a distinctive course of action with it taking longer than CBT to achieve its full effects (see Figure 1). This supports the view that it is likely to work through mechanisms that are specific to it, although another possibility is that it operates through the same mechanisms as CBT but less efficiently.

Clinical observations can provide insight into the mechanisms of action of treatments. In conducting IPT-ED we have observed repeated instances of patients making major positive changes in the identified problem areas and in their life generally. Often these changes set in progress other positive changes, many of which are still evolving at the end of treatment. In the absence of research evidence it is possible to suggest several possible processes which might explain how interpersonal changes might have a beneficial effect on the eating disorder.

- Improved functioning in the identified problem area(s) might result in there being fewer interpersonal triggers of dysfunctional eating.
- Patients' realization that they are capable of bringing about changes in what have often been entrenched interpersonal problems might lead them to feel more capable of solving relationship problems in general. Alternatively or additionally, improved

interpersonal functioning might produce an improvement in overall self-esteem. Either of these changes might result in patients believing that they are capable of changing other problems in their life, including their eating disorder, with the result that they start to actively address it.

- Alternatively, an improvement in overall self-esteem might result in a decrease in the extent to which patients attempt to control their eating, shape or weight, thereby resulting in the gradual erosion of the eating disorder.

The operation of processes of this type might explain how IPT-ED works (see Murphy, Cooper, Hollon & Fairburn, in press). It would also explain why the full effects of IPT-ED take longer to be expressed than those of CBT, since CBT focuses directly on changing the disturbed eating habits and attitudes whereas with IPT-ED these changes are secondary to interpersonal change.

Future Directions

There is a clear need for more research on the use of IPT in the treatment of patients with eating disorders. The body of evidence supporting its use in the treatment of bulimia nervosa is more modest than it is for CBT. Furthermore, there is a paucity of research on the effectiveness of IPT for patients with other forms of eating disorder. As well as there being a need for more data to establish the effectiveness of IPT, research is also required on how IPT operates. Identification of mediators of change should enhance understanding of eating disorder psychopathology and its relationship to interpersonal processes, as well as help in the eventual identification of the active components of IPT. This is the research strategy that we are pursuing in Oxford (see Murphy, Cooper, Hollon & Fairburn, in press).

Acknowledgements

CGF is supported by a Principal Research Fellowship from the Wellcome Trust (046386). RM, SS and ZC are supported by a programme grant from the Wellcome Trust (046386).

References

Agras, W. S., Walsh, B. T., Fairburn, C. G., Wilson, G. T., and Kraemer, H. C. (2000). A multicenter comparison of cognitive-behavioral therapy and interpersonal psychotherapy for bulimia nervosa. *Archives of General Psychiatry*, 57, 459-466.

Fairburn, C. G., Jones, R., Peveler, R. C., Carr, S. J., Solomon, R. A., O'Connor, M. E., Burton, J., and Hope, R. A. (1991). Three psychological treatments for bulimia nervosa: A comparative trial. *Archives of General Psychiatry*, 48, 463-469.

Fairburn, C. G., Jones, R., Peveler, R. C., Hope, R. A., and O'Connor, M.E (1993). Psychotherapy and bulimia nervosa: the longer-term effects of interpersonal psychotherapy, behaviour therapy and cognitive behaviour therapy. *Archives of General Psychiatry*, 50, 419-428.

Fairburn, C.G., Marcus, M.D., and Wilson, G.T. (1993). Cognitive behaviour therapy for binge eating and bulimia nervosa: A comprehensive treatment manual. In C.G. Fairburn and G.T. Wilson (Eds.). *Binge Eating: Nature, Assessment, and Treatment* (pp. 361-404). New York: Guilford Press.

Fairburn, C. G., Norman, P. A., Welch, S. L., O'Connor, M. E., Doll, H. A., and Peveler, R. C. (1995). A prospective study of outcome in bulimia nervosa and the long-term effects of three psychological treatments. *Archives of General Psychiatry*, 52, 304-312.

Fairburn, C.G. (1997). Interpersonal psychotherapy for bulimia nervosa. In D.M. Garner and P. E. Garfinkel (Eds.), *Handbook of Treatment for Eating Disorders*. (pp. 278-294). New York: Guilford Press.

Fairburn, C.G., Cooper, Z., and Shafran, R. (2003). Cognitive behaviour therapy for eating disorders: A "transdiagnostic" theory and treatment. *Behaviour Research and Therapy*, 41, 509-528.

Fairburn, C. G., Agras, W. S., Walsh, B. T., Wilson, G. T., and Stice, E. (2004). Prediction of outcome in bulimia nervosa by early change in treatment. *American Journal of Psychiatry*, 161, 2322-2324.

Fairburn, C.G., Cooper, Z.C., Bohn, K., O'Connor, M.E., Doll, H.A., and Palmer, R.L. (2007). The severity and status of eating disorder NOS: Implications for DSM-V. *Behaviour Research and Therapy*, 45, 1705-1715.

Fairburn, C.G., Cooper, Z., and Shafran, R. (in press). Enhanced cognitive behavior therapy for eating disorders ("CBT-E"): An overview. In C.G. Fairburn, *Cognitive Behavior Therapy and Eating Disorders*. New York: Guilford Press.

Fairburn, C. G., Cooper, Z., Shafran, R., Bohn, K., and Hawker, D. (in press). Clinical perfectionism, core low self-esteem and interpersonal problems. In C.G. Fairburn, *Cognitive Behavior Therapy and Eating Disorders*. New York: Guilford Press.

Fairburn, C.G., Cooper, Z., Shafran, R., Bohn, K., Hawker, D., Murphy, R., Straebler, S. (in press). Enhanced cognitive behavior therapy for eating disorders: The core protocol. In C.G. Fairburn, *Cognitive Behavior Therapy and Eating Disorders*. New York: Guilford Press.

Fairburn, C.G., Cooper, Z., and Waller, D. (in press). The patients: Their assessment, preparation for treatment and medical management. In C.G. Fairburn, *Cognitive Behavior Therapy and Eating Disorders.* New York: Guilford Press.

Frank, E., Frank, N., Cornes, C., Imber, S. D., Miller, M. D., and Morris, S. M. (1993). Interpersonal psychotherapy in the treatment of late-life depression. In G. L. Klerman and M. M. Weissman (Eds.), *New Applications of Interpersonal Psychotherapy*. (pp. 167-198). Washington.: American Psychiatric Press.

Grilo, C.M. (2006). *Eating and Weight Disorders*. (pp. 158-160). New York: Psychology Press.

Kraemer, H.C., Wilson, G.T., Fairburn, C.G., and Agras, S. (2002). Mediators and moderators of treatment effects in randomized clinical trials. *Archives of General Psychiatry,* 59, 877–883.

Klerman, G. L., Weissman, M. M., Rounsaville, B. J., and Chevron, E. S. (1984). *Interpersonal Psychotherapy of Depression*. New York: Basic Books

McIntosh, V.V.W., Jordan, J., Carter, F. A., Luty, S. E., McKenzie, J. M., Bulik, C. M., Frampton, C.M.A., and Joyce, P.R. (2005). Three psychotherapies for anorexia nervosa: A randomized, controlled trial. *American Journal of Psychiatry*, 162:4, 741- 747.

Mitchell, J. E., Halmi, K., Wilson, G. T., Agras, W. S., Kraemer, H., and Crow, S. (2002). A randomized secondary treatment study of women with bulimia nervosa who fail to respond to CBT. *International Journal of Eating Disorders*, 32, 271-281.

Murphy, R., Cooper, Z., Hollon, S.D., & Fairburn, C.G. (in press). How do psychological treatments work? Investigating mediators of change. *Behaviour Research and Therapy.*

Mufson, L., Moreau, D., Weissman, M. M., and Klerman, G. L. (1993). *Interpersonal Psychotherapy for Depressed Adolescents*. New York: Guilford Press.

National Institute for Clinical Excellence (NICE, 2004). *Eating disorders: core interventions in the treatment and management of anorexia nervosa, bulimia nervosa, related eating disorders*. NICE Clinical Guideline No. 9. London: National Institute for Clinical Excellence.

Weissman, M. M., Markowitz, J. C., and Klerman, G L. (2000). *Comprehensive Guide to Interpersonal Psychotherapy*. Basic Books: New York.

Weissman, M. M., Markowitz, J. C., and Klerman, G .L. (2007). *Clinicians Quick Guide to Interpersonal Psychotherapy.* Oxford University Press: New York.

Wilfley, D.E., Welch, R.R., Stein, R.I., Borman Spurrell, E., Cohen, L. R., Saelens, B. E., Zoler Dounchis, J., Frank, M., Wiseman, C. V., and Matt, G. E. (2002). A randomized comparison of group cognitive behavioral therapy and group interpersonal psychotherapy for the treatment of overweight individuals with binge-eating disorder. *Archives of General Psychiatry*, 59, 713-721.

Wilson, G.T., and Fairburn, C.G. (2007). Treatment of eating disorders. In P.E. Nathan and J.M. Gorman (Eds.), *A Guide to Treatments that Work* (Third Edition). New York: Oxford University Press.

In: Evidence-Based Treatments for Eating Disorders
Author: Ida F. Dancyger and Victor M. Fornari

ISBN 978-1-60692-310-8
© 2009 Nova Science Publishers, Inc.

Chapter XV

Using Dialectical Behavioral Therapy for the Treatment of Eating Disorders: A Model for DBT Enhanced CBT

Lucene Wisniewski*, Kelly Bhatnagar and Mark Warren
Case Western Reserve University
Cleveland, Ohio, USA

Abstract

Dialectical Behavior Therapy (DBT) is a behavioral treatment that has become of interest to clinicians and researchers in the eating disorder field. There is empirical evidence for the use of DBT with Binge Eating Disorder and Bulimia Nervosa and interest in its use with patients suffering from Anorexia Nervosa. The treatment focuses on the effective regulation of emotions via the teaching of a comprehensive set of change and acceptance-based skills while promoting strategies for treatment compliance and retention. The current chapter describes DBT, reviews relevant literature, and offers a novel approach for fusing principles of the current field standard, Cognitive Behavioral Therapy (CBT), with those of DBT to create a functional model adapted to meet the specific needs of difficult-to-treat ED patients. Although this model has yet to empirically establish itself as an evidence-based treatment, it holds great promise as it attempts to move in this direction.

Manual-based cognitive-behavioral therapy (CBT) is currently considered the treatment of choice for adults suffering from eating disorders (ED) (National Institute for Clinical Excellence, 2004). CBT, along with interpersonal psychotherapy (IPT), has solidly demonstrated its overall effectiveness (Wilfley et al., 1993), however, there continues to be a

---

* Correspondence concerning this manuscript should be sent to Lucene Wisniewski, Clinical Director, Cleveland Center for Eating Disorders, 25550 Chagrin Boulevard, Suite 200, Beachwood, OH 44122. E-mail may be sent via Internet to lwisniewski@edcleveland.com.

substantial number of individuals that do not successfully recover using these approaches (Anderson and Maloney, 2001; Lundgren *et al.*, 2004), especially those suffering from anorexia nervosa (AN) (Ball and Mitchell, 2004; Channon et al., 1989; McIntosh et al., 2005). These data, along with clinical experiences, have prompted clinicians and researchers alike to look to other empirically-validated treatments for guidance managing patients with EDs (e.g. Fairburn et al., 2003; Wonderlich et al., 2001).

DBT as a Potential Alternative Treatment

It is not surprising that Dialectical Behavior Therapy (DBT) was quickly identified as an alternative treatment for ED patients. DBT is a behavioral therapy, modified to include techniques of validation, acceptance and mindfulness, while simultaneously utilizing a manualized approach for skill-building to better manage emotional dysregulation. It was originally developed by Marsha Linehan, Ph.D. to treat patients with chronic suicidality who also suffered from Borderline Personality Disorder. Linehan has noted that a central characteristic of BPD patients was the presence of impaired emotional regulation and the lack of successful strategies to cope with this impairment (Linehan, 1993a). As a result, self destructive behaviors become the "solution" to this dysregulation, often creating life threatening situations. Linehan also discovered that treatment as usual for suicidal individuals, CBT, was often unsuccessful for this patient population (Linehan, 1993a). DBT was then derived as an alternative approach for these individuals. In doing so, she modified not only the content of the therapy, but also its structure, goals, techniques and theory of change.

While drawing from a wide variety of sources, DBT is based on a unique set of principles. DBT assumes that the most effective path to health begins by first changing behaviors. It further assumes that if a patient with emotion regulation problems is faced with an expectation to change without a concomitant focus on acceptance, then emotional dysregulation will ensue, resulting in the impairment of the patient's ability to learn new behaviors. DBT therefore expects that the balance of acceptance and change is more likely to produce lasting effectiveness than a focus on change alone. To accomplish this goal, DBT focuses on problem solving and skill-building while embracing validation of the patient's experience as a primary task of the therapist. DBT stresses the acceptance of one's current reality, regardless of the pain this acceptance may cause, as the first step to lasting life improvement. In DBT terminology, this is referred to as "radical acceptance." Rather than the traditional therapeutic goal of ending misery or finding happiness, DBT is concerned primarily with giving patients the opportunity to experience a "life worth living" (Linehan, 1993a).

A central tenet of DBT is that, "patients do not fail therapy, therapy fails patients" (Linehan, 1993a). This belief, long evident in other aspects of health care, often does not penetrate the psychotherapeutic setting. A significant number of patients have heard that their failure to heal is due to their being a non-compliant patient, or being unmotivated or unwilling to do the difficult work. DBT firmly rejects this conceptualization, instead asserting that it is the job of the therapy to help the patient, not the job of the patient to conform to therapy. At the same time, DBT holds that therapy can fail even when the therapist does not fail. This stance in DBT makes the therapy, not the patient or the therapist, the central concern in effectiveness.

Why Use DBT for the Treatment of Eating Disorders?

The rationale for applying DBT to the treatment of EDs, has been described in the literature by our group and others (McCabe, LaVia and Marcus, 2004; Wiser and Telch, 1999; Wisniewski and Kelly, 2003; Wisniewski, Safer and Chen, 2007). The rationale proposed suggests that alternative approaches are necessary for EDs because, as previously discussed, current empirically founded treatments (e.g. CBT and IPT) may only be partially effective or ineffective for a select number of patients (Anderson and Maloney, 2001; McIntosh et al., 2005). DBT can be considered a logical alternative because unlike the other approaches, it is based on an affect regulation model of treating ED symptoms. Eating pathology (e.g. binge-eating, self-induced vomiting, restriction, etc.) may now be understood as mechanisms to cope with emotional vulnerability (Telch et al., 2000), as opposed to errors in cognition or faulty interpersonal relationships alone (Fairburn, 1981; Fairburn et al., 1993). In its pure form, DBT is specifically designed to teach adaptive regulation skills and to address target behaviors that result from emotional dysregulation (Linehan, 1993b). Taken together, this provides a strong theoretical justification for applying DBT to the treatment of EDs (Telch et al., 2000, 2001; Wisniewski and Kelly, 2003).

In addition to its use of the affect regulation model, other components of DBT may make it a practical alternative for the treatment of EDs. Its unique synthesis of behavioral principles, dialectical philosophy, and Zen influences makes it particularly useful to ED patients, especially in helping those patients who may be struggling with issues of motivation and commitment. For example EDs, especially AN, differ from other mental illnesses (such as depression and anxiety) in the considerable degree of ambivalence patients hold about symptoms and treatment. Treatment of ED symptoms, therefore, requires a sophisticated use of commitment strategies and must focus not only on helping patients change their behaviors, but also on coaching patients to accept their present state and condition. This dialectical tension is a key aspect of DBT and its emphasis on both change-based and acceptance-based therapeutic strategies. For ED patients, who must accept their current progress in treatment, their fluctuating weight and shape, and other difficult-to-change aspects of their current situation, DBT's acceptance strategies are especially valuable. The focus on acceptance is equally important for the therapist and family members in that it provides a useful framework for relinquishing control over the time course for lasting change to occur.

Other crucial elements of DBT, such as the therapist and patient consultation case management strategies, are similarly suited for work with ED patients. For example, given the tendency for ED patients and their symptoms to evoke intense feeling and emotion in their treatment providers, the consultation team for therapists draws upon the expertise of a diverse group of trained professionals (e.g. psychologists, counselors, social workers, medical doctors, nutritionists, nurses, etc.) to ensure that primary therapists remain committed to treating a patient within a DBT framework, even when treatment appears to be slow and frustrating for all. We believe this support is fundamental in the successful treatment of chronic EDs. Also, by aiding patients in the management of an often extensive health provider network, DBT therapists may contribute to the development of their patient's sense of mastery, control, and self-efficacy, which reinforces the collegial nature of the therapeutic alliance. Thus, the DBT strategy of team consultation to the patient promotes respect for the patient's capacity to learn new behaviors and meet developmental and interpersonal goals.

Finally, similarities in clinical presentation between BPD and ED also distinguish DBT as an appropriate treatment for EDs. For example, ED symptoms are often minimized as insignificant problems despite the high mortality rates found with AN (Steinhausen, 2002) and the significant impairment of functioning found with other EDs (Hayaki *et al.*, 2003). Also ED behaviors, similar to symptoms related to BPD, are easily perceived as conniving, dishonest and superficial by therapists, family and friends. Such negative attributions can lead to significant difficulties in patient's treatment, especially if they are held by the therapist. DBT's solution to this problem is to place great emphasis upon the importance of working within a non-judgmental framework. Within this framework, behaviors are viewed non-critically, and thus usefully defined, as reinforced responses that are within a patient's current skill repertoire, but are able to be substituted for more adaptive responses through the therapeutic process.

Existing Data Demonstrating the Effectiveness of DBT for Eating Disorders

Because the use of DBT for ED treatment is still considered to be relatively new, the efficacy literature on the topic is limited. However, preliminary research, spearheaded by a group at Stanford University, shows great promise for the adaptation of DBT theory and techniques to the ED population. A case report published by Safer, Telch and Agras (2001a) applied a DBT approach for the treatment of a previously unresponsive adult female with a long history of BN symptoms. This approach consisted of an abridged DBT skills training program to address ED symptoms, as well as consultation team meetings used for the support of the clinician. This treatment did not include individual therapy per se (sessions were seen as a proxy for group skills training), the Interpersonal Effectiveness Skill module (see below), or telephone skills coaching—all of which are typically included in traditional DBT. Nonetheless, this patient experienced a rapid decline in both binge-eating and purging behaviors, showing drastic change at both post-treatment and at six-month follow-up (Safer et al., 2001a).

Other studies have examined the effects of a similar DBT adaptation for the treatment of binge/purge behaviors (Safer et al., 2001b) or BED (Telch et al., 2001). In both studies, significant improvements on measures of binge-eating and related eating pathology were demonstrated. Additionally, a DBT program consisting of weekly consultation team, all four traditional DBT skills modules, plus the addition of one novel skills-training module designed specifically to treat individuals with ED and co-morbid BPD appeared to be effective in treating both eating disorder and self-harm behaviors (Palmer et al., 2003).

The significant results from these studies are encouraging and support further research for the use of DBT with individuals who suffer from ED. Preliminary findings suggest that DBT, if adapted correctly, could serve as a powerful treatment for ED patients, especially those who have traditionally been difficult to treat or who have been previously unresponsive to the more standard treatment approaches.

Cleveland Center for Eating Disorders Model

The paucity of research notwithstanding, many ED treatment programs around the country have begun to use DBT with their ED patients. A recent Google search using the key words DBT and Eating Disorder Treatment resulted in over 107,000 hits! DBT's popularity may be moving ahead of the data, however, and guidelines concerning DBT's use with ED patients are therefore needed.

The DBT skills group model tested by the Stanford research group shows promise in the treatment of Binge Eating Disorder (BED) and Bulimia Nervosa (BN) patients but currently does not have a widely available published treatment manual. In addition, the ED patients studied in this research had relatively low symptom severity as they were selected to be those without life threatening behaviors and exhibiting ED symptoms that could be managed in weekly outpatient treatment, as per the American Psychiatric Association practice guidelines for eating disorders (APA, 2000). Furthermore, the authors of this chapter were interested in providing DBT to a more broad patient population, for example, patients who present with *all* ED diagnoses, moderate to severe symptoms, significant medical and psychiatric co-morbidity (that may also include, but does not require self harm/suicidality) and previous failed treatment attempts.

A treatment model was therefore developed to meet the needs of a broader and more difficult to treat ED population. The standard DBT model was chosen as its basis, as it has been the most studied and has a widely available treatment manual (Linehan, 1993a). However, given the potential symptom severity of the targeted population, with many patients dangerously underweight, it did not seem prudent to omit the effective CBT for ED techniques which have been well validated (e.g., meal planning, self-monitoring of intake; psychoeducation regarding ED). Thus the current model of DBT-enhanced CBT or DBT-CBT for EDs was developed (see Wisniewski and Kelly, 2003; Wisniewski, Safer, and Chen, 2007).

The assimilation of DBT into traditional CBT treatments for EDs appeared viable to the authors because first and foremost, the foundation of DBT draws heavily from cognitive-behavioral theory. There are therefore many areas of overlap between the two treatments, the most striking of which is the focus on change via self-monitoring and strategies to promote behavioral self-control. The second rationale for incorporating DBT into standard CBT treatment for EDs was the assumption that DBT could enhance traditional ED treatments by integrating these complementary treatment components of acceptance and change.

Therefore, for clinicians who value empirically-researched models such as CBT yet who also are keenly interested in DBT and its potential application to the treatment of EDs, the following section on DBT-CBT outlines how appropriately trained clinicians can integrate DBT into existing cognitive-behavioral approaches for the treatment of EDs.

The Focus of DBT for Eating Disorders

The treatment described below employs techniques from Standard DBT with two exceptions: the diary card and behavior chain.

Diary Cards. The diary card, which is used in standard DBT treatment (Linehan, 1993a), focuses on targeted behaviors for individuals experiencing suicidality. The authors felt that to be used effectively with ED patients, the diary card needed to be adapted on several levels, the most important of which is to include an opportunity for patients to record food intake, as many patients present in a malnourished state. The diary card, which has been described extensively elsewhere (Wisniewski, Safer, and Chen, 2007), may be considered a blend of the standard DBT diary card and a CBT self monitoring form.

As seen in Figure 1, the DBT for ED diary card includes space to record daily intake, whether or not the patient has engaged in targeted behaviors and a place to report daily skill use. To complete a diary card, patients are first asked to write their name and the date at the top of the page. In the "time" column, the patient is to record the time that each meal or snack was consumed. This information serves as a helpful time indicator for key behaviors or urges. In the column labeled "plan," the patient is to write down the number of dietary exchanges that his or her current meal plan requires as designated by the team dietician. Meal plans tend to change frequently, thus updates are required on a regular basis. In the "act" column, the patient should indicate the actual amount of each exchange that was consumed at that meal or snack. For example, if the patient ate three protein exchanges but the meal plan only required two, the patient would write that they consumed three exchanges. In the column titled "hunger scale," patients are to indicate their subjective sense of hunger immediately before and immediately after a meal or snack. This scale ranges from "empty" to "stuffed," and can be helpful to patients as they are relearning physiological signs of hunger. Beneath this scale, the patient is to describe the approximate quantity and type of foods consumed during the meal or snack. For example, a patient may record for her morning meal "1 slice of turkey bacon, 2 fried eggs prepared with butter, 2 slices of wheat bread with grape jelly, etc." The patient then writes the place the meal or snack was consumed in the "location" column (e.g. restaurant, home). Patients are asked to be as specific as possible when describing location, especially when meals are consumed at home (e.g. " home in the living room while watching television"). In the "fluids" column, the patient records the amount of fluid that was consumed during the meal or snack in either cups or ounces.

The next several columns are for the patient to record any urges to engage in a "targeted behavior" (i.e. urges to binge, purge, use dietary pills, restrict, exercise, etc.) as identified by the patient or treatment team. If the patient actually engages in a targeted behavior, an asterisk should be drawn under the appropriate column. If the patient had an urge but did not actually engage in the behavior, a zero to five scale is used to rate the intensity of the urge (0 = no urge; 5 = strongest urge).

Patients should be reminded that if they do not meet all exchanges at any meal or snack, an asterisk should be placed in the "restriction column." It is important that all columns have a rating or asterisk in them at all times. The column titled "emotion" is used to indicate any emotions that the patient may have experienced during the meal or snack. Emotions should be indicated at every meal. Examples of emotions include calm, anxious, sad, angry, guilty, overwhelmed, etc. Body image issues that may be occurring may be recorded in this space as well. The final column, entitled "skills used," should be used to record any DBT skills (e.g, distraction, act opposite) that the patient used during the meal or snack.

CCED

DIARY CARD

	Name:			Day/Date:			binge	purge	pills	restrict	exercise		Mark (*) if you engaged in behavior. Rate (0-5) if you had an urge but did not engage in behavior.	
Time	PLAN	MEALS	ACT	Food Intake – Include approximate quantity and description of food Hunger Scale – Graph hunger level from start to end of meal	Location	Fluid Intake (cups/ ozs.)							Emotion	Skill Used
		BREAKFAST		empty 2 3 4 neutral 6 7 8 9 stuffed										
		Protein												
		Vegetable												
		Grain												
		Lipid Nutr.												
		Fruit												
		Dairy												
		SNACK												
		LUNCH		empty 2 3 4 neutral 6 7 8 9 stuffed										
		Protein												
		Vegetable												
		Grain												
		Lipid Nutr.												
		Fruit												
		Dairy												
		SNACK												
		DINNER		empty 2 3 4 neutral 6 7 8 9 stuffed										
		Protein												
		Vegetable												
		Grain												
		Lipid Nutr.												
		Fruit												
		Dairy												
		SNACK												
		VITAMINS												

Figure 1. Diary card example.

If the patient is not yet familiar with many of the DBT skills, the patient is to indicate what he or she did to help get herself through the meal (e.g. watch television, call a friend, use paging services, etc.).

When used correctly, diary cards can provide a wealth of information to the clinician and the patient. In order for diary cards to serve as an effective component of treatment, however, they must be completed on a daily basis. It is often helpful to coach patients to keep the diary card in plain view to serve as a reminder to fill it out immediately after each meal, thus providing the greatest amount of accuracy.

Behavior Chain Analysis (BCA). A behavior chain is a detailed analysis of specific behaviors, automatic thoughts, and emotions experienced by a patient preceding, during and after a targeted behavior. The BCA used in the DBT-CBT model is similar in spirit to the BCA used in standard DBT; the authors simply prefer the altered format (see Figure 2).

Patients are asked to complete a BCA for each episode of targeted behavior that occurs between sessions.

For ED patients who are not concurrently suicidal or engaging in self harm, these behaviors include typical ED behaviors (e.g., binge eating, purging, restricting, compulsive exercise, diet pill use). When completing a BCA, the patient is first asked to describe the targeted behavior. In Figure 2, the patient, "Char", "*purged evening snack.*"Detail is encouraged in the description of the target behavior and Char was coached to avoid using vague terms [e.g., purged (vague) versus purged evening snack (more specific)]. The next step in completing a behavior chain is to describe the specific precipitating event(s) that led up to the targeted behavior. In Char's case, she identified the precipitant as having followed her meal plan at lunch and dinner, but having felt as though it was "too much food."

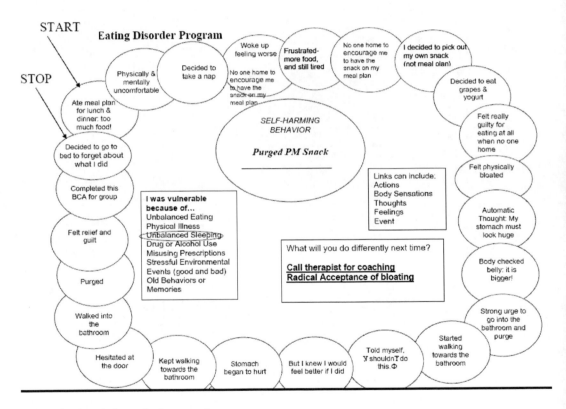

Figure 2. Behavior chain analysis example.

Char was then asked to detail the sequence of events leading up to the targeted behavior (e.g., feeling uncomfortable, no one home at snack time, body checking), factors that may have contributed to feelings of vulnerability (e.g., sleeping and feeling worse after nap), as well as the emotional and behavioral consequences of the targeted behavior (e.g., feeling relief and guilt after purging). The final and arguably most important step in the completion of a BCA is to have the patient brainstorm alternative solutions to the problem behavior. In other words, the patient will determine what they "will do differently next time." In our example, Char was able to identify two DBT skills that she would be willing to try the next time this scenario occurred: 1) calling for Telephone Skills Coaching (described below) and

2) using Radical Acceptance to tolerate the bloating. This in session, non-reinforced, exposure to and focus on the emotions and thoughts related to symptoms has been posited as one of DBT's potential mechanisms of change (Lynch *et al.*, 2006).

DBT-CBT for Eating Disorders: The Model

Individual Therapy. In DBT-CBT for ED, individual therapy includes: a behavioral review of the preceding week, examination of diary cards and behavior chains, exploration of thoughts, feelings and behaviors that led to self-destructive acts, and consideration of alternative strategies going forward. As in standard DBT, the patient meets weekly with an individual therapist, who functions as the primary therapist for that patient on the treatment team. The goals of the individual therapy are to promote skill generalization (using skillful behavior to replace ED behavior outside of treatment) and to aid in the maintenance of motivation and commitment to treatment. The patient and individual therapist typically meet once per week for approximately 60 minutes.

Standard DBT provides a structure for managing and prioritizing behaviors to be addressed in treatment. Standard DBT provides a treatment hierarchy that helps the therapist to identify which behavior(s) to address first in session, thus providing clear path to prioritizing the goals of treatment (Linehan, 1993). DBT assumes that by definition, patients who are difficult to treat have several co-occurring problems making the focus of treatment a challenge. Take, for example, the dangerously low weight patient who comes late to session, reports current passive suicidal ideation, as well having had two episodes of self-harm and multiple purging episodes over the course of the week. However, in the moment she is clearly upset and wants to talk about having broken up with her boyfriend that morning. Without the described targeting framework, deciding how to focus the session could be a challenge. Linehan asserts that the target hierarchy is core to the treatment and goes so far as to assert "a therapist who ignores the targeting strategies is not doing DBT. That is, in DBT what is discussed is as important as how it is discussed" (Linehan, 1993a). DBT's target hierarchy provides a theoretical justification for how to manage these multiple behaviors. As is discussed below, the use of a Target Hierarch in DBT-CBT for ED is only slightly different than in standard DBT as there is a need to accommodate ED behaviors.

Target I: Life threatening behaviors (suicide, parasuicide). As in standard DBT, suicidal ideation and self-injury are the first targets to be addressed in treatment. ED behaviors may be moved to Target I, however, when they present an imminent threat to the patient's life as in a medical emergency (e.g., evidence of bradycardia, orthostatic blood pressure, electrolyte imbalances, EKG abnormalities, syrup of ipecac use).

Target II: Therapy interfering behaviors. The active attention to behaviors that interfere with treatment compliance and progress is one of several reasons that DBT has the potential to contribute to the CBT treatment of EDs. Therapy interfering behaviors that may occur within the context of ED treatment include: not completing diary cards, an inability to focus in session due to malnourished state, refusing to be weighed, engaging in behaviors to surreptitiously alter weight, exercising against medical advice, absence from treatment due to the need for medical intervention, and engaging in purging that interferes with medication efficacy.

Target III: Quality of life interfering behaviors. ED behaviors that are not associated with imminent medical risk are focused on within Target III and are considered behaviors that interfere with one's quality of life. These behaviors include, but are not limited to, restricting, binge eating, vomiting, laxative use, diuretic use, diet pill use, and excessive exercise. The bulk of treatment for ED patients who are not suicidal or at imminent medical risk will occur within Targets II and III.

It is important to note here that the same behavior may be considered a different Target depending on the context. Take, for example, "Cathy," whose primary ED symptom is purging. Her purging was considered Target I after having been diagnosed with hypokalemia, as further purging could result in imminent death. Once the hypokalemia was resolved, purging then moved to Target III. However, when it became clear that Cathy's purging was likely interfering with the effectiveness of her antidepressant (she took the medicine at breakfast, and purged soon afterward), purging moved to Target II. Focus on purging behavior in session, therefore changed with the change in Target status..

Skills Training Group. DBT skills are taught in a group format as is described in the Skills Training Manual (Linehan, 1993b). The focus of skills training is to offer patients alternative ways to manage their problems. Skills fall into four categories: Mindfulness, Distress Tolerance, Interpersonal Effectiveness and Emotion Regulation and are taught as outlined in the Linehan's Skills Training Manual, using examples relevant to patients suffering from EDs.

Mindfulness Skills

As acceptance-based strategies, Core Mindfulness skills help patients to become intentionally aware of thoughts, feelings, and behaviors (Linehan, 1993b) with a strong emphasis on being "present in the moment" and promoting self- awareness without attempts to alter or suppress the experience. Patients are taught mindfulness techniques through the basic methods of observation, description, and participation. Mindfulness can be incorporated into the treatment of ED as it provides a framework for patients to observe and accept previously avoided emotions thoughts, and sensations, including hunger and fullness.

Mindful eating is a skill that has been suggested to be useful for patients with ED. With few exceptions (Kristeller et al., 2006), there is little research and writing, on the use of mindfulness approaches to ED. In the authors' experience, patients with BN or BED can benefit from a mindful-approach to eating with a focus on paying attention to hunger and fullness. This approach is very similar to appetite awareness training (Craighead and Allen, 1995). The authors have also found, however, that for patients with AN, mindful eating can be extremely anxiety-provoking early in treatment. Distraction techniques, with the intent of progressive movement towards mindful eating over time, may be more useful in the beginning stages of treatment with these patients.

Interpersonal Effectiveness Skills

Interpersonal Effectiveness (IE) skills are used to help patients become more assertive and to teach them to use effective problem-solving to handle difficult interpersonal situations (Linehan, 1993b). Specifically, patients are trained to say "no" in undesirable situations, to practice asking for help when necessary, and to resolve interpersonal conflict in a manner that gets their own needs met without damaging the interpersonal relationship or the person's self-respect. ED patients can greatly benefit from such skills as they begin to use these IE skills to manage unsatisfying relationships in their lives as well as to negotiate interpersonal situations around the ED itself (e.g., managing triggering comments made by others, explaining to a dinner partner why she needs to eat at a certain restaurant, etc.).

Distress Tolerance Skills

Distress Tolerance (DT) skills aim to teach patients techniques to manage stressful and upsetting events without engaging in targeted/self-harming behaviors (Linehan, 1993b). Patients are coached to "bear pain skillfully," (Linehan, 1993) and to view distress as something with a purpose. In this module, patients are taught to survive personal crises through the use of distraction, self-soothing, engaging in activities to improve the present moment, and by radically accepting that one may not be able to change the current circumstances. For ED patients, these techniques are also useful in the management and tolerance of urges to engage in disordered eating behaviors.

Emotion Regulation Skills

Similar to patients with BPD, ED patients may frequently experience intense and labile moods. These emotions may become the "problem to be solved" (Linehan, 1993b) from the patient's perspective. Clinically, we often hear "I was upset about what happened at work so I, binged, purged, or restricted." Emotion regulation (ER) skills are taught to help the patient to find more effective ways to experience feelings (Linehan, 1993b). Patients are taught to identify and label emotions aided by Mindfulness Skills, increase pleasant events to promote positive emotion, avoid self-defeating moods by acting in a manner opposite to what they feel (e.g. if while at work, one begins to experience intense anger and has the urge to shout; "acting opposite" would encourage him or her to listen to upbeat music and attempt to laugh in order to produce positive emotion), and identify obstacles to changing one's current mood.

In the DBT-CBT for EDs approach, as in standard DBT, all skills training modules are taught through group discussion and activity. Additionally, patients are asked to complete outside homework assignments in order to promote skill generalizability.

Consultation Team

The consultation team is the component of DBT that primarily functions to monitor and enhance the therapist's motivation and adherence to the treatment model. The weekly consultation team meeting serves as an opportunity for therapists to practice the skills they teach to their patients and to receive clinical feedback and support from other members of the treatment team. This is done in the spirit of providing the most effective care possible while maintaining therapist motivation and commitment to the work. The consulation team treatment approach outlined in DBT differs from many other models; especially in its conceptualization of equality. While some team members may be more experienced or may hold more or higher-level degrees, all members are considered to be equal. There is no one expert who makes the decision for the team; similarly, the consultation team is not to be considered "rounds" as in a medical model, where patients are referred to one-by-one with a to-do list for each person.

The consultation team is crucial for a therapist working with ED patients. The stress of working with patients who may be near death and whose illness often denies them sound judgment and insight into their sickness, are prone to frustration and burnout. The consultation team provides therapists with a validating environment where they can feel understood and simultaneously be shaped non-judgmentally to be more effective.

Telephone Skills Coaching. Telephone Skills Coaching (TSC) is a unique and powerful component of DBT. The goal of TSC coaching in standard DBT is to assist therapists in balancing the dialectic of providing contact to patients during crises, while simultaneously extinguishing passive, dependent behaviors while reinforcing active, effective skill use. It is standard practice for patients enrolled in DBT treatment to be given access to their therapists between sessions and after hours in order to assist in the generalization of skills learned during treatment (Linehan, 1993). In CBT-DBT for EDs, unlike other published models of DBT for EDs (e.g., Stanford), this component is utilized extensively.

The first goal of telephone skills coaching is to decrease suicidal crisis behaviors (Linehan, 1993a) as well as ED behaviors that could cause imminent death (Wisniewski and Ben-Porath, 2005). Patients are instructed to call their therapist prior to engaging in parasuicidal/suicidal behaviors. The hope is that with the therapist's in vivo coaching, a patient could learn to manage the urges to self harm without acting on them.

The second goal of telephone skills coaching is to increase generalization of behavioral skills. This means that telephone coaching may be used to assist patients in generalizing the skills they are learning in treatment to everyday situations (Linehan, 1993a). For example, when patients are learning the skill of distraction to manage urges to purge, they may call the therapist after having tried to use the skill and feel that the attempt has not been wholly effective. The therapist may work with patients to first ensure that they are using the skill appropriately and then to offer other skills patients may use so that they will refrain from purging in that instant. An example of this is "Kerri" who called for coaching because she was feeling the urge to purge after eating breakfast. She tried unsuccessfully to reach several friends by telephone and to watch TV as a distraction, but felt her urges to continue to increase. She called her therapist for help coming up with additional suggestions. After assessing her current attempts to use skills, the therapist and Kerri were able to collaboratively develop a plan that included leaving the house and going to the library (Kerri only purges at home) until her job started two hours later. This plan was effective in having Kerri avoid purging breakfast, thereby reinforcing skill use and the likelihood that Kerri will attempt to use skills the next time she feels urges to purge.

The final goal of telephone skills coaching is to decrease the sense of conflict, alienation, and/or distance from the therapist (Linehan, 1993a). Patients are encouraged to phone their therapist in between sessions to make a repair in the therapeutic relationship. Therefore, ED patients are encouraged to call their therapist if they are feeling alienated or angry rather than waiting for the next session to discuss this. In standard DBT, patients who engage in self harm do not have telephone access to their therapist for 24 hours (Linehan, 1993a). This rule was developed to prevent therapist contact from inadvertently reinforcing ineffective behaviors. It is the authors' experience that the 24-hour rule does not translate well for use with ED patients. Unlike in episodes of self-harm, ED patients who are in treatment likely have a scheduled exposure to a potentially triggering stimulus (i.e., a meal or snack) every four to six hours of the day at a minimum. Therefore each meal or snack will represent a unique opportunity to engage or not engage in targeted behaviors. Given the potential frequency of these events, behavioral principles would likely suggest reinforcement of any attempt to "get back on track" (i.e., engaging in adaptive behavior).

A modification of the 24-hour rule, called the Next Meal/Snack rule (NM/S rule) has therefore been proposed for use with targeted ED behaviors (see Wisniewski and Ben-Porath, 2005). Like the 24-hour rule, the NM/S rule dictates that if an individual has already engaged in a targeted behavior prior to calling for telephone skills-coaching, the call is to be terminated. Take, for example, the patient who calls the therapist after having already purged. In the short phone call, the therapist explains that the patient should call prior to the behavior in the future, that they will talk about the purging episode in the next session, and quickly terminates the call. Unlike the 24-hour rule described above, however, the patient is able to call back for skill-coaching at the next scheduled meal or snack. For a patient in treatment, the next scheduled meal or snack is likely to occur within two to four hours. If the patient does call for coaching later that day however, it is stipulated that the focus of that call be on the present episode only. The prior episode may be discussed only as a contributing factor to the current episode (e.g., restricted lunch resulting in heightened feelings of hunger at dinner). This adaptation reflects a potentially important modification for using the DBT telephone protocol with ED patients.

For those who read the above section with trepidation related to offering patients telephone access, it is relevant to note the following. Our research suggests that ED patients are actually very unlikely to use this service unless required to do so by their therapist (Lindbrunner, Milstein, Ben-Porath and Wisniewski, 2005). It is often the case that the therapist needs to require patients to call for coaching as a way to practice and shape this behavior.

Conclusion

Although still in its introductory stages, DBT is beginning to demonstrate its usefulness for the treatment of non-responsive and difficult-to-treat ED patients. Its unique blend of behaviorist principles with mindfulness techniques and skills that emphasize understanding the delicate balance between change and acceptance make it an appealing intervention for those individuals that struggle with more traditional treatments such as CBT and IPT. DBT employs a non-judgmental team working relationship between the clinician and patient which serves to foster a strong alliance and prevent burnout until therapeutic goals are achieved.

The DBT model presented in this chapter (DBT-CBT for ED) attempts to marry functional aspects of CBT to the beneficial aspects of DBT to create a useful and practical intervention that best meets the needs of individuals suffering from ED. The empirical evidence for using DBT with EDs as described throughout the chapter lends support and promise to the treatment and programming decisions for which this intervention requires. It is important to note, however, that the present model should be test empirically before being widely adopted in order for it to truly establish itself as an evidenced-based treatment.

Author Note

Lucene Wisniewski, Clinical Director, Cleveland Center for Eating Disorders.
Kelly Bhatnagar, Department of Psychology, Case Western Reserve University.
Mark Warren, Medical Director, Cleveland Center for Eating Disorders.

References

Agras, W. S., Walsh, T., Fairburn, C. G., Wilson, G. T., and Kraemer, H. C. (2000). A multicenter comparison of cognitive-behavioral therapy and interpersonal psychotherapy for bulimia nervosa. *Archives of General Psychiatry, 57*(5), 459-466.

Albers, S. (1993). *Eating Mindfully.* New Harbinger Publications.

American Psychiatric Association (2001). *Diagnostic and statistical manual of mental disorders* (4th—Text Revision ed.). Washington, D.C.

Anderson, D. A., and Maloney, K. C. (2001). The efficacy of cognitive-behavioral therapy on the core symptoms of bulimia nervosa. *Clinical Psychology Review, 21*(7), 971-988.

Ball, J., and Mitchell, P. (2004). A randomized controlled study of cognitive behavior therapy and behavioral family therapy for anorexia nervosa patients. Eating Disorders: *The Journal of Treatment and Prevention, 12*(4), 303-314.

Channon, S., de Silva, P., Hemsley, D., and Perkins, R. E. (1989). A controlled trial of cognitive-behavioural and behavioural treatment of anorexia nervosa. *Behaviour Research and Therapy, 27*(5), 529-535.

Craighead, L. W., and Allen, H. N. (1995). Appetite awareness training: A cognitive behavioral intervention for binge eating. *Cognitive and Behavioral Practice, 2*(2), 249-270.

Fairburn, C. G. (1981). A cognitive behavioural approach to the treatment of bulimia. *Psychological Medicine, 11*(4), 707-711.

Fairburn, C. G., Jones, R., Peveler, R. C., Hope, R. A., and et al. (1993a). Psychotherapy and bulimia nervosa: Longer-term effects of interpersonal psychotherapy, behavior therapy, and cognitive behavior therapy. *Archives of General Psychiatry, 50*(6), 419-428.

Fairburn, C. G., Marcus, M. D., and Wilson, G. T. (1993b). Cognitive-behavioral therapy for binge eating and bulimia nervosa: A comprehensive treatment manual. In C. Fairburn and T. Wilson (Eds.) *Binge eating: Nature, assessment, and treatment* (pp. 361-404). New York: Guilford Press.

Fairburn, C. G., Cooper, Z., and Shafran, R. (2003). Cognitive behaviour therapy for eating disorders: A "transdiagnostic" theory and treatment. *Behaviour Research and Therapy, 41*(5), 509-528.

Garner, D. M. (1997). Psychoeducational principles in treatment. In D. Garner and P. Garfinkel (Eds.) *Handbook of treatment for eating disorders (2nd ed.)*. New York: Guilford Press.

Garner, D. M., Vitousek, K. M., and Pike, K. M. (1997). Cognitive-behavioral therapy for anorexia nervosa. In D. Garner and P. Garfinkel (Eds.) *Handbook of treatment for eating disorders—Second edition*. New York: Guilford Press.

Hayaki, J., Friedman, M. A., Whisman, M. A., Delinsky, S. S., and Brownell, K. D. (2003). Sociotropy and bulimic symptoms in clinical and nonclinical samples. *International Journal of Eating Disorders, 34*(1), 172-176.

Kristeller, J. L., Baer, R. A., and Quillian-Wolever, R. (2006). *Mindfulness-based approaches to eating disorders*. In R. Baer (Ed.) *Mindfulness-based treatment approaches: Clinician's guide to evidence base and applications*. San Diego: Elsevier Academic Press.

Limbrunner, H.M., Milstein, S.B., Ben-Porath, D.D., and Wisniewski, L. (2005). An exploratory study of the use of telephone skill-coaching by eating disorders clients. Poster presented at the International Conference on Eating Disorders, Montreal, Canada.

Linehan, M. M. (1993a). *Cognitive-behavioral treatment of borderline personality disorder*. New York: Guilford Press.

Linehan, M. M. (1993b). *Skills training manual for treating borderline personality disorder*. New York, NY: The Guilford Press.

Lundgren, J. D., Danoff-Burg, S., and Anderson, D. A. (2004). Cognitive-behavioral therapy for bulimia nervosa: An empirical analysis of clinical significance. *International Journal of Eating Disorders, 35*(3), 262-274.

Lynch, T. R., Chapman, A. L., Rosenthal, M. Z., Kuo, J. R., and Linehan, M. M. (2006). Mechanisms of change in dialectical behavior therapy: Theoretical and empirical observations. *Journal of Clinical Psychology, 62*(4), 459-480.

McCabe, E., LaVia, M, and Marcus, M. (2004). The use of dialectical behavior therapy in the treatment of eating disorders. In J. Kevin Thompson (Ed.). *Handbook of eating disorders and obesity* (pp. 232-244). New Jersey: John Wiley and Sons.

McIntosh, V. V. W., Jordan, J., Carter, F. A., Luty, S. E., McKenzie, J. M., Bulik, C. M., et al.(2005). Three psychotherapies for anorexia nervosa: A randomized, controlled trial. *American Journal of Psychiatry, 162*(4), 741-747.

National Institute for Clinical Excellence (2004). *Core interventions in the treatment and management of anorexia nervosa, bulimia nervosa, and binge eating disorder.* London: British Psychological Society.

Palmer, R. L., Birchall, H., Damani, S., Gatward, N., McGrain, L., and Parker, L. (2003). A dialectical behavior therapy program for people with an eating disorder and borderline personality disorder-description and outcome. *International Journal of Eating Disorders, 33*(3), 281-286.

Safer, D. L., Telch, C. F., and Agras, W. S. (2001a). Dialectical behavior therapy adapted for bulimia: A case report. *International Journal of Eating Disorders*, 30(1), 101-106.

Safer, D. L., Telch, C. F., and Agras, W. S. (2001b). Dialectical behavior therapy for bulimia nervosa. *American Journal of Psychiatry, 158*(4), 632-634.

Steinhausen, H.C. (2002). The outcome of anorexia nervosa in the 20th century. *American Journal of Psychiatry, 159*(8), 1284-1293.

Telch, C. F., Agras, W. S., and Linehan, M. M. (2000). Group dialectical behavior therapy for binge-eating disorder: A preliminary, uncontrolled trial. *Behavior Therapy, 31*(3), 569-582.

Telch, C. F., Agras, W. S., and Linehan, M. M. (2001). Dialectical behavior therapy for binge eating disorder. *Journal of Consulting and Clinical Psychology, 69*(6), 1061-1065.

Wilfley, D. E., Agras, W. S., Telch, C. F., Rossiter, E. M., Schneider, J. A., Cole, A. G., et al. (1993). Group cognitive-behavioral therapy and group interpersonal psychotherapy for the nonpurging bulimic individual: A controlled comparison. *Journal of Consulting and Clinical Psychology, 61*(2), 296-305.

Wilson, G. T., Fairburn, C. C., Agras, W. S., Walsh, B. T., and Kraemer, H. (2002). Cognitive-behavioral therapy for bulimia nervosa: Time course and mechanisms of change. *Journal of Consulting and Clinical Psychology, 70*(2), 267-274.

Wilson, G. T., and Fairburn, C. G. (2002). Treatments for eating disorders. In P. Nathan and J.Gorman (Eds.) *A guide to treatments that work (2nd ed.)* p. 559-592. New York: Oxford University Press.

Wilson, G. T., Grilo, C. M., and Vitousek, K. M. (2007). Psychological treatment of eating disorders. *American Psychologist Special Issue: Eating disorders*, 62(3), 199-216.

Wiser, S., and Telch, C. F. (1999). Dialectical behavior therapy for binge-eating disorder. *Journal of Clinical Psychology, 55*(6), 755-768.

Wisniewski, L., Kelly, E. (2003). The application of dialectical behavior therapy to the treatment of eating disorders. *Cognitive and Behavioral Practice, 10*, 131-138.

Wisniewski, L, Safer, D, and Chen (2007) Dialectical Behavior Therapy and Eating Disorders. In L. Dimeff and K. Koerner (Eds). *Dialectical Behavior Therapy in Clinical Practice* (pp.174-221). New York: Guilford Press.

Wonderlich, S. A., Mitchell, J. E., Peterson, C. B., and Crow, S. (2001). Integrative cognitive therapy for bulimic behavior. In R. Striegel-Moore and L. Smolak (Eds.) *Eating disorders: Innovative directions in research and practice.* (pp. 173-195). American Psychological Association, Washington, DC, US xii, 305pp.

In: Evidence-Based Treatments for Eating Disorders
Author: Ida F. Dancyger and Victor M. Fornari

ISBN 978-1-60692-310-8
© 2009 Nova Science Publishers, Inc.

Chapter XVI

Evidenced-Based Approaches to Family-Based Treatment for Anorexia Nervosa and Bulimia Nervosa

James Lock and Kathleen Kara Fitzpatrick
Stanford University School of Medicine
Stanford, California, USA

Abstract

Family-based approaches to the treatment of eating disorders represent important, empirically supported options for addressing the needs of adolescents with Anorexia Nervosa and Bulimia Nervosa. Family-based weight restoration treatment for Anorexia Nervosa, in particular, has mounting empirical evidence to support its use with children and adolescents. Family-based treatments encourage participation of a wider familial network to support re-nourishment, establish independence around food and weight management and encourage appropriate developmental gains. The current chapter provides an evaluation of existing research on family-based treatments as well as providing clinicians with information on phases and skills necessary to implement a family-based model in a clinical setting.

Eating disorders are highly prevalent, devastating illnesses that impact both the individual sufferer and those closest to him or her. Anorexia Nervosa (AN), Bulimia Nervosa (BN) and Eating Disorder Not Otherwise Specified (ED NOS) are associated with a great deal of morbidity and mortality and have a peak age of onset in adolescence, often circumventing the critical developmental milestones that lead to independence in adulthood. Given that most adolescents remain imbedded within a family structure and are dependent upon their parents, it is reasonable to expect that family involvement is viewed by many as a critical component of successful treatment of adolescent eating disorders. It may seem somewhat surprising, then, that family-based approaches to the treatment of eating disorders have been controversial since the earliest documentation of these disorders. As early as 1874, Gull characterized families as the "worst attendants" for those suffering from AN (Gull, 1874). This sentiment was echoed in early individual treatment paradigms that suggested families were not a necessary part of treatment, as treatment sought to empower the individual suffering from AN (Bruch, 1973).

Despite early concerns about the role of family in treatment of AN and a veritable absence of information on family-based treatments for BN, the nesting of treatment within a family setting makes ecological sense when one considers that the average age of onset AN and BN is in adolescence. AN has a prevalence estimated at between 0.48% and 0.70% among females aged 15 to 19 years (Hoek and Hoeken, 2003; Lucas et al., 1999; Pawluck and Gorey, 1998). Similarly, BN occurs in approximately 1-2% of the adolescent population while clinically significant bulimic behaviors (BN-EDNOS) occur in an additional 2-3%. As with AN, adolescence is a critical time for the development of BN, with a peak age of onset at eighteen (Mitchell et al., 1987).

The importance of developmental factors coupled with relatively poor treatment outcomes for the treatment of adults with eating disorders made a focus on family-based interventions and treatment paradigms natural extensions for the burgeoning family treatment models beginning in the 1960s. Nearly one hundred years after Gull's admonishment of family members in treatment, psychological theory swung back toward the inclusion of families in eating disorder treatment as we review below.

Theoretical Underpinnings of Family Treatment for Eating Disorders

Structural, strategic and systemic family therapy models were developed, with a particular focus on the treatment of AN. Minuchin's (Minuchin et al., 1978) seminal family work and characterization of the "psychosomatic family" of AN served to focus on family work as a critical treatment modality. Family treatment was designed as a means to address perceived enmeshment and maintenance of these disorders through maladaptive communication patterns and problem-solving. Minuchin and colleagues focused their work on modifying intergenerational boundaries with a focus on enmeshment, conflict management skills and strengthening alliances with the larger social world (Minuchin et al., 1978).

Salvini Palazzoli at the Milan Center drew upon many of the aspects outlined by Minuchin, while highlighting the rigid organization of families with AN and the ways in which this disorder might serve to maintain homeostasis within the family unit(Selvini Palazzoli, 1974). The therapist's power in Milan System's treatment emphasizes the importance of objective observation and family evaluation of their own processes. By placing oneself outside of the family dynamic, therapists can both shed light on patterns as well as expressing empathy for individual family members (Palazzoli, 1974; Palazzoli et al., 1980). This allows the therapist to remain outside of conflict and supportive of family members in the face of conflicting needs or desires.

Christopher Dare and colleagues at the Maudsley Hospital in London developed an eating disorder specific set of treatment protocols that drew upon separate elements of structural, strategic and systemic models with a behavioral re-feeding focus (Russell et al., 1987). The resulting "Maudsley method" or family-based re-feeding (FBT) model of treatment views the family as a fundamental resource in the treatment of eating disorder symptoms, the identified patient as regressed in his/her ability to manage food independently, and encourages a collaborative approach to systematic re-nourishment of the identified patient to an ideal body weight. Although clearly drawing upon previous theories of family therapy, distinguishing it from other approaches is the injunction placing parents in charge of weight restoration of their child while maintaining an agnostic stance toward the cause of the disorder (Dare and Eisler, 1997). FBT has the added benefit of existing in manualized form (Lock et al., 2001).

Interestingly, despite similarities in symptom profiles and age of onset, research paradigms for the treatment for (BN) have focused largely on the development of individual approaches. To date, large-scale treatment studies of BN have focused on the use of cognitive-behavioral therapy and other individual models in adults. Only a handful of studies have examined BN treatment, whether individual or family based in adolescents. Results from these studies suggest that both individual and family based treatments are promising for symptom amelioration (Fairburn, 1988; Fairburn, 1997; Fairburn and Brownell, 2002; Le Grange and Lock, 2007; Le Grange et al., 2003; Le Grange and Schmidt, 2005).

Existing theoretical models for family treatment of adolescent BN draw upon the same theoretical models discussed in relation to adolescent AN. As outlined by Le Grange and Lock (Le Grange and Lock, 2007), parents are urged to assume control over the adolescent's eating and binge/purge behaviors; however, in contrast to FBT for AN, the stance is more collaborative with the adolescent with BN than AN. The primary reason for this is that BN is generally ego-dystonic and shameful, making a joint effort at changing the behaviors more likely than in AN where the ego-syntonic nature of the disorder makes collaboration extremely challenging at the start of FBT. Nonetheless, the core features of FBT remain the same for both conditions.

Empirical Evaluation of Family Treatment of Eating Disorders

Given the history of family models for the treatment of eating disorders, one would assume that a rich empirical literature would exist. Unfortunately, a relative dearth of empirical evidence for eating disorder treatment exists, particularly in adolescents. Among existing studies focusing on adolescents, two recent reviews (Le Grange and Lock, 2005; Tierney and Wyatt, 2005) highlighted the importance and prevalence of family treatments for the treatment of Anorexia Nervosa. Virtually all randomized clinical studies targeting adolescents utilized a family approach, with virtually of these focusing on FBT for AN. Older, general studies included anxiety-based treatments (Goldfarb et al., 1987) and monitored eating with or without feedback (Touyz et al., 1994).

Controlled studies of family- based treatment for AN have found that family-based treatment to be superior to individual therapy for adolescents with AN (Russell et al., 1987) with this maintained at five year follow-up (Eisler et al., 1997). Russell et al. (Russell et al., 1987) found those with duration of illness less than 3 years, and onset prior to age 18, FBT was superior (60% vs. 9% good) while Robin et al.'s (Robin et al., 1999) comparison of FBT to individualized treatment (EOIT) found both groups improved, although weight restoration was faster for those receiving family-based treatment. In these family studies, "family" was generally defined as the family of origin, although the constitution of these families has not been specified. In general, family-based treatments have been utilized with a multitude of family constellations. Single parent families, grandparents with custody, blended families and much older siblings have been represented in these and other studies.

In a recently completed RCT for adolescents with BN (BN and partial BN) 80 adolescents aged 12-19 years (M=16.1, SD=1.6) were allocated to either manualized FBT-BN or manualized Individual Supportive Psychotherapy (SPT). At the end of treatment and 6 month follow-up significantly more patients in FBT-BN were binge/purge abstinent compared to SPT, suggesting that FBT-BN is superior to SPT. The Chicago study was sufficiently powered to demonstrate the potential benefits of an active treatment (i.e., FBT) over a non-specific control treatment (i.e. SPT), and to demonstrate comparable benefits that were not due to time effects. In addition, there were no differences in remission rates at the end of treatment or at follow-up for those subjects with BN or partial BN (Le Grange and Lock, 2007; Le Grange et al., 2003; Le Grange and Schmidt, 2005).

Results from another randomized controlled trial (RCT) for adolescent BN and partial BN comparing family therapy to CBT-GSC (an individual guided self-help form of CBT), has also been recently published (Schmidt et al., 2006).

Family therapy as described by these authors resembles FBT; however, these authors described "family" as any "close other "rather than specifically requiring that a parent be defined as "family." This occurred in about one quarter of cases. This definition was likely utilized, in part, because the mean age of the subjects in this study was 17.6 years (sd = 0.3), much closer to adulthood, especially in the UK where the age of consent is 16 years. While defining family as a close other may fit well with this older age group, this might not be the most effective way to approach FBT with younger adolescents where parental authority is key to the success of FBT. This point in emphasized further by the take up rates for the UK study, wherein 28% of eligible participants refused the study because they did not want their families involved in treatment. In contrast, for the younger adolescents studied at the University of Chicago, where only 11% dropped out of treatment and none of these reported involving the family as the reason for discontinuing treatment. Nonetheless, Schmidt and colleagues found that abstinence rates (41%) achieved by family therapy are comparable to those achieved using FBT in the Chicago study. However, no statistical differences on abstinence rates were found between FBT and the comparison treatment. Schmidt and her colleagues acknowledge that a limitation of their study was the sample size (n = 85), which was likely too small to detect differences between two active treatments for some of their outcomes and that the absence of a waiting-list or attention placebo-control group prevented them from ruling out that improvement was simply due to passage of time or non-specific effects (Schmidt et al., 2006).

Table 1. Outpatient Psychotherapy Trials of Family Treatment for Adolescent Anorexia Nervosa

Study	Type of therapy	N	Age	Treatment Duration (months)	# sessions	Drop-out rate	End of Tx outcome Morgan-Russell good+intermediate
Russell, Szmukler, Dare, and Eisler, 1987*	Whole family vs. individual therapy**	21	16.6	6-12	13	19%	Family therapy = 90%* Individual therapy=18%
Le Grange, Eisler, Dare, and Russell, 1992	Whole family vs. Separated family therapy***	18	15.3	6	9	12%	68% overall; no differences between groups
Robin et al., 1999****	Family therapy vs. individual therapy	37	13.9	12-18	47	11%	Family therapy = 81%* Individual therapy = 66%
Eisler et al., 2000	Whole family vs. separated family therapy	40	15.5	12	16	10%	63% overall; No differences between groups
Lock, Agras, Bryson, and Kraemer, 2005	Family treatment, 6 vs. 12 months	86	15.1	6 or 12	10 or 20 sessions	12%	No differences in outcome between groups 96% overall

* Denotes statistically significant advantage for this approach.
** Whole family indicates that the family was seen with the identified patient ("Conjoint").
*** Separated family therapy indicates the parents were seen without the identified patient.
**** Denotes statistically significant disadvantage for this approach.

One concern for those considering family based treatment models has been the burden of having an entire family present for treatment. A study comparing separated (parents alone) to conjoint (parents and patient) family based treatment found weight restoration efforts were successful in both groups. The role of family criticism and hostility has also been suggested as a reason for focused individual work. Parental criticism is, indeed, a predictor of treatment drop-out in family-based treatment (Lock, Courturier, Bryson and Agras, 2006), but the role of criticism and hostility has not been evaluated in individual treatments and thus no comparison can be drawn between this and other aspects of treatment. Other predictors of drop-out include co-morbid conditions and length of time to weight gain, with greater early weight gains predicting treatment retention. Interestingly, however, FBT may, lead to faster weight gain (Robin et al., 1999) that may retain families in treatment for longer. In general, treatment is implemented over one year, however, Lock et al (2005) compared short (6 month) to long-term (1 year) FBT and found treatment was equally effective for adolescents with short duration AN.

Family-Based Weight Restoration for Eating Disorders

Given the mounting empirical support for FBT, we provide evaluation of the elements of treatment, utilizing the Treatment Manual for Anorexia Nervosa (Lock et al., 2001). Where relevant, modifications specific to the treatment of BN are discussed, drawing upon the manualized version of this treatment protocol (Le Grange and Lock, 2007).

Family-Based Treatment for AN

FBT AN views the adolescent as regressed in terms of her eating disorder, or inability to maintain an optimal weight for age and height. This regression is viewed as limited in scope, however, and the adolescent is presumed to be able to assume developmentally appropriate independence in other domains. As such, treatment addresses the adolescent's developmental concerns and the ways in which parental control over eating represent a significant infringement of typical independence. Expectation that control over eating will be returned to the adolescent once weight and eating behaviors are stabilized is clearly stated, with a concurrent shift in focus to negotiating more typical adolescent conflicts or family needs. Treatment takes place in three phases over six to twelve months, comprised of 10-20 sessions. Sessions in FBT last 1 hour, with the first ten to fifteen minutes being spent with the patient alone during weigh-in and exploration of patient specific concerns about his or her response to parental efforts appropriate to the goals of each phase.

Phase 1 (sessions 1-10). In the first phase, the eating disorder comprises almost the full focus of treatment sessions. The initial session involves history-taking and presentation of the family's dilemma in a "grave but sincere manner" that fully communicates both the significant danger of the patient's current health crisis as well as a call to action for the family to directly intervene. At the end of the first session the parents are encouraged to provide a meal sufficient to "re-nourish their starving (daughter)" to the next session. The family meal is eaten in the second session to provide the therapist with an opportunity for direct observation of the familial interaction patterns around eating. This is an excellent opportunity for observation of dynamics of family meals, to address views about nutrition, to model and coach parents in ways to approach re-feeding. Paradoxical injunctions, including urging the identified patient not to eat unless he/she really wants to, encourages families to directly address the dilemma of their conflicting goals. A primary goal of the family session is to have the patient eat one bite more than he/she had been planning upon eating at the outset of the session.

In the remainder of phase one sessions, the therapist exhorts parents to unite and direct their efforts toward re-feeding, which is the primary focus of treatment. The patient's weight is graphed and shared with the family to guide intervention and serve as feedback on the process of weight restoration. Parents are also urged to take control of binge/purge behaviors in the subset of patients presenting with a binge/purge subtype. Critical to this is management of parental feelings of guilt or anxiety – by engaging and collaborating with parents, the therapist communicates clearly parents have not caused the eating problem and that they can be empowered to change this pattern in a direct fashion. The therapist builds and reinforces a strong parental alliance re-feeding efforts while simultaneously aligning the patient with his or her siblings. The critical goals of this phase are to manage parental guilt and anxiety sufficiently to spur them to action in taking control of eating. The specific actions of re-feeding are not defined by the therapist, but rather families are encouraged to work out for themselves how best to re-feed their anorexic child. The focus is held on food and eating, with parents being encouraged to review each snack and each meal for what was successful, how it was eaten, the emotional tenor of the meal and the ultimate outcome in terms of caloric gain and parental success in managing the AN.

Phase 2 (sessions 11-16). This phase begins with a change in the tenor of the treatment: the patient submits to parental re-feeding efforts and conflict around regular nutrition improves, resulting in steady weight gain, as well as a change in the mood of the family (i.e., relief after having taken charge of the eating disorder). Often families make subtle transitions between sessions without realizing that they are taking initial steps toward increasing independence (e.g., patient begins "plating" their food with parental observation rather than parent dictated portions). The therapist shifts task demands to emphasize movement toward independence for the patient. Although symptoms remain a central focus, weight gain with minimum tension is encouraged. Resumption of developmentally appropriate eating behaviors are encouraged throughout the sessions; initially with parental monitoring and, in the face of success, with full independence. Other areas of concern or family functioning (e.g., trust, defining appropriate independence) might be brought forward, although these are selectively addressed in terms of their relationship to maintenance of weight and normalized eating behaviors.

Phase 3 (sessions 17-20). The third phase begins when the patient achieves a stable weight and is generally able to resume normal eating behaviors without undue parental monitoring. In our experience, the entry into this final phase can be distinguished by a distinct lack of concern about or desire to focus on eating symptoms by the family and a sense that there are either more pressing or enjoyable issues presented for discussion. Rather than presenting issues of eating conflict, a conversation may focus on dating, curfew or homework completion and, when eating issues are queried, these are dismissed. At this point, the central focus is on establishing a healthy adolescent or young adult relationship with the parents. This is often a challenge, as for many families the illness has constituted the basis of many interactions. Goals may include working towards increased personal autonomy for the adolescent, re-establishing a stronger marital relationship that does not include the patient or siblings, more appropriate family boundaries and improved familial communication.

Modifications Associated with FBT for BN

Although there is a high degree of symptom overlap between AN and BN in adolescents, several key differences require modifications in the implementation of family-based focus. There are individual and symptomatic differences in BN that bear discussion. First, although AN and BN have high rates of co-morbidity with other mental illnesses, BN can be thought of as having a wider range of co-morbid psychiatric disorders, many of which may be viewed as compelling enough to shift the focus of treatment (e.g., substance abuse) while in AN the consequences and physical response to stark emaciation assist both therapists and the family focused upon the illness. Second, although both AN and BN share a common root in body image disturbance, the focus for those with BN is on an over-valuation of shape and weight which leads to maladaptive compensatory behaviors. This contrast is often less striking than the distortions of AN that clearly highlight the disorder. Thirdly, although it may be premature to discuss "typical" family presentations of these disorders, clinical perceptions suggest that AN families tend toward rigidity, perfectionism and compliance while those with BN may better be characterized as less structured and more disorganized. This may make it challenging initially to engage families as well as for some of these families to provide the structure and monitoring necessary for successful implementation of a family-based approach.

In addition to modifications in the strategic implementation of FBT for BN, psychological aspects or characteristics represent important areas for assessment and may require flexibility implementation. Patients with BN are typically perceived as having a greater level of *independence* than their counterparts with AN, although this is sometimes ambivalent independence. Many parents are often reluctant to intervene or may find resuming control in the area of food or eating more challenging than in patients with AN. Parents may benefit from adopting a "back on track" approach when facing BN, with a push toward normal developmental independence and frequent reminders that their adolescent is, with respect to food, in a regressed state. This is further complicated by the potential for families to see the identified patient as being "beyond guidance" or having a wider range of experiences or challenges than average adolescents. Unlike AN, which is characterized by low levels of insight, levels of *insight* vary in patients with BN. Symptoms of BN are generally ego-dystonic and thus many adolescents can accept that they are ill, although they may not like the nature of parental control. Acknowledgement of illness is an important point upon which the therapist can establish a therapeutic relationship with the identified patient and can assist in the development of a collaborative stance including the parents and the patient. Alternatively, if levels of insight are low, patients with BN may be particularly resistant to parental control over food and eating behaviors. Level of *parental motivation* may be related to the factors above, as well as potential difficulties in recognizing the extent and seriousness of symptoms in the patient. Although many individuals with AN are secretive in their illness, the striking emaciation associated with the disorder often prompts parents to take action. In contrast, patients with BN present at or above normal weight guidelines and often lack the clear medical fragility of their AN counterparts. Parents may also struggle with the secretive nature of BN symptoms and may struggle to separate eating disorder symptoms from more age appropriate adolescent development. This may manifest as more criticism or family hostility directed at the adolescent and/or difficulty identifying and managing eating symptoms.

There are many core tenets of family-based treatment that provide a framework for treatment implementation. First and foremost, the model supports parents as key agents of change in their child's recovery and emphasis on parental knowledge and expertise within the family is reinforced throughout the sessions. In this sense, parents are viewed as experts in their children, while the therapist is an expert in eating disorders. This changes the nature of the relationship, with parents expected to play an active role in identifying ways in which they might modify behavior patterns and the therapist assuming an inquisitive and coaching role, with less emphasis on behavioral directions and interventions. For a relationship of this nature to be truly collaborative, parents must not feel they are being pathologized, stigmatized or responsible for their child's illness, and thus FBT maintains an agnostic stance as to the cause of the illness.

The therapist must also bring a set of skills to the practice of family-based treatment for eating disorders. Critical to success is the therapist's ability to maintain a fairly single-minded focus upon the eating disorder, despite often more enticing and seemingly psychologically fruitful distractions that may arise in family sessions. The focus and entrainment upon eating disorder symptoms in early sessions serves to keep the family's focus on eating pathology and emphasizes the vital importance of parental control over eating and return to nourishment for the identified patient. This can be quite challenging, as a patient's obvious emaciation is replaced by indicators of health, families often wish to shift focus away from the eating disorder to address other, seemingly more pressing issues. Taking ones "eyes off the eating disorder" at too early a stage in treatment can lead to decreased pressure on eating symptoms, failure to make expected weight gains and maintenance at "partial remission" status. It can be all too tempting to address more compelling family dynamics and issues raised, and great skill is essential in refocusing the discussion on eating while validating and tabling these concerns until later in treatment. Preventing complacency and "burnout" in weight restoration efforts requires a mix of humor, compassion and ability to manage both the specific eating disorder symptoms with greater familial dynamics.

In addition to a fairly tenacious focus on eating disorder concerns at the outset of treatment, the therapist must also ground his or her work in a strong developmental framework. Therapists should be knowledgeable of adolescent development and the ways in which eating disordered behavior may interfere with or delay normal development. This is particularly important as self-starvation or highly disorder eating behaviors themselves, assumes a level of developmental regression in independence skills. The therapist must be aware of normal developmental patterns to assist parents in encouraging age appropriate expressions of affect and behaviors, rather than playing out developmental concerns in the realm of food, weight and shape. This knowledge and support of appropriate adolescent development forms the core of the connection that the therapist must develop with the adolescent to sustain rapport and demonstrate respect for the tremendous challenge facing the family. Namely, the removal of otherwise developmentally appropriate independence skills (eating) while actively encouraging strides toward independence in other domains (social).

Case Presentation

To assist clinicians in the implementation of treatment, the following case history outlines implementation of treatment with an adolescent patient with binge-purge subtype anorexia nervosa. This case was chosen to illustrate the ways in which family therapy tackles both severe emaciation as well as binge-purge behaviors.

History taking and first session. K.S., a sixteen year-old female, presented with her family for treatment following several previously unsuccessful therapies to address a three year history of AN. K.S. presented to the outpatient clinic following an extended stay on an inpatient unit, where she was admitted directly from residential treatment. She was accompanied to treatment by her parents, Mrs. C and Mr. S., who had divorced six years prior. Her older sister, age 17 and her younger brother, age 8, were also present for treatment. At the time of the intake session, K.S. and her family reported a three-year history of illness, beginning the summer prior to K.S.'s entry to high school. She began restricting and dropped in weight, which was not seen as alarming to parents, as K.S. had been overweight for much of her childhood and was borderline obese at the time of her weight loss. Weight loss was rapid and significant, falling from 126 pounds at a height of 4 feet, 11 inches to 86 pounds with a concurrent growth spurt that placed her at five feet, three inches in height. At the time of admission to residential treatment, K.S. had a one-year history of binge eating and purging behaviors, which she described as instrumental to keeping her weight low. She had been binge eating once per day, although her binges had decreased in quantity to reflect subjective, rather than objective binge eating amounts. She induced vomiting after most meals and had experimented with laxatives and appetite suppressants. She entered residential treatment after an inpatient hospital stay and was able to increase her weight to 90 pounds, however, she was discharged to the inpatient unit for acute food refusal and violent behavior on the unit.

Her mother reported great guilt around her failure to recognize the severity and significance around this weight loss, while K.S.'s father expressed great hostility toward his ex-wife for allowing their daughter to become ill, while simultaneously questioning the significance of the illness, as he felt it was better to be "too thin than too fat." Parents were alerted to concerns by K.S.'s pediatrician who monitored her low weight for a year. Mother noted the family had been reluctant to seek outpatient care during that time, as they felt this was just a "phase" and a reaction to Mrs. C's recent remarriage. For his part, Mr. S. reported that Mrs. C prevented regular contact with the children and that he had "no idea" about the severity of illness until his daughter was hospitalized. K.S. described her current state as "borderline fat" and reported great distress at the idea of gaining weight. Despite this, she was able to note that her illness had prevented her from leading a "normal" life, having missed a majority of her sophomore and half of her junior year of high school, not being able to drive, and having "never had a boyfriend." Her sister noted that K.S. required a great deal of attention from the family and her frequent hospitalizations or threat of hospitalizations resulted in great disruption and conflict between Mr. S. and Mrs. C. as well as between Mrs. C and her husband. K.S.'s sister reported a great deal of love and concern for her sister and felt AN was a way to "make our parents talk to each other and maybe work together." K.S.'s brother remained silent throughout much of intake session, despite questioning, and he frequently became tearful when asked about his thoughts about his family and his sister's illness.

The therapist discussed the medical consequences and concerns associated with restriction, binge eating and purging. During this conversation, K.S. sat silently and reported that she had "heard all this before." When the therapist confronted her fears of weight gain and concerns that the therapist may try to make her overweight, K.S. stated, "It isn't your job to make me fat, it's your job to make me like it!" Mrs. C wept openly at her concerns regarding her daughter's bone density, cardiac functioning and fears that she was "killing herself." Mr. S. asked many questions about risk and reversibility of risk. At the end of the session, the therapist charged the family with the task of bringing a meal that would be capable of increasing K.S.'s low weight.

The family meal. The family presented with a meal from a local restaurant. As the family unpacked the meal and began eating, the therapist observed, then began asking questions. The family all had similar meals: burritos, tortilla chips and salad, served "family style" apart from the burritos, which were served individually. Mr. S and Mrs. C appeared tense, watching K.S. closely as her siblings divided up the food and served themselves. K.S.'s sister took the lead in serving the family, passing out burritos and placing chips and salad on a plate for each family member. She provided her sister the same portions to each member of her family, serving K.S. last. All other family members ate readily, while watching K.S. surreptitiously. The family ate quietly, although they were able to laugh about the unnatural situation (eating in front of a therapist) and admitted their regular meals were less quiet at home. The therapist discussed who had chosen the food and the parents admitted that Mrs. C. had chosen a meal she felt K.S. was likely to eat and something she had requested, rather than "risk upsetting her." The therapist discussed how this played out at home, with the family allowing K.S. to select meals and what happened when she did not eat the foods offered by the family. Mrs. C. expressed great frustration around this and noted that she felt she was "bending over backwards." K.S.'s siblings reported that this was very unfair, as they were not able to get their parents to purchase their favorite foods on a regular basis. Mr. S. reported that his ex-wife had long "given in" and did not like conflict with K.S. or anyone else. The therapist noted that the family re-feeding approach was one in which conflict and struggles were brought out into the open and faced directly. With that, the therapist provided a paradoxical injunction to K.S. – to eat only as much as she wanted to and not to give in without a challenge.

During the discussion of conflict avoidance, K.S. began crying. The therapist wondered if she was feeling criticized or attacked by her family and she nodded quietly, stating that she didn't "ask" to have her parents treat her in a certain way or "give in" to her. The therapist guided a discussion of the ways in which parent choices for meals and taking the "power of choice away from anorexia" can be challenging in the moment but provide relief from eating disordered choices and ruminations. The therapist also encouraged the family to move away from resentment of K.S. for being ill and to make a separation between K.S. and the illness.

During this discussion, K.S. ate very little and took very prominent bites of food only when watched closely by her family. The therapist noted this and modeled separation of the patient and her illness by suggesting that it was easier for the AN to allow her to eat when observed. She resisted this suggestion, but her parents both eagerly responded that they had noticed exactly this pattern – K.S. would cut her food into "micro-portions" that were then moved about the plate, but eaten only when "fixated with a death stare." The therapist encouraged the parents to move in closer to K.S. to provide support and help her fight her eating disordered thoughts, since her eating improved when she was monitored. At this suggestion she immediately picked up her food and began eating, as though to show she did not need this assistance. Her parents, however, moved to the seats on either side of her and took turns talking to the therapist while the other provided gentle verbal encouragement.

Although she resisted, crying, pushing away her food, the therapist encouraged the parents to remain steadfast in their alliance. Both Mr. S. and Mrs. C. joked that this was the most they had agreed and worked together since their divorce and this statement led to K.S. tearfully crying that she did not want her AN to be the only thing that made them work together. Her siblings agreed vocally and the parents began to discuss this as a family, with the therapist encouraging their return and focus to AN as the most important issue facing the family in the moment. The therapist highlighted for the family the ways in which AN can distract from the task at hand and divert focus and controversy as a means to maintain a grip on the patient. The parents agreed that this occurred frequently in both households: diversions, arguments and provocations all occurred more frequently at mealtimes. The therapist encouraged the parents to maintain a steadfast focus on eating disordered behaviors and to take control, which would strengthen their resolve as well as allow K.S. some relief from her eating disordered symptoms. This also helped the parents in making a separation between their daughter and her illness.

Remainder of Phase 1. At the subsequent sessions, the family explored many issues that prevented the parents from confronting the eating disorder, although they quickly gained skills as evidenced by K.S.'s steady weight gain. Mrs. C. struggled when K.S. would escalate in her upset around food and eating and reported it was a challenge to keep her "eye on the AN." However, she did an excellent job in distinguishing her daughter from "the beast" and took active steps to keep K.S. active between meals. This was particularly useful to prevent purging behaviors, which required monitoring for an hour or more after meals and significantly curtailed K.S.'s independence. Mrs. C. was creative in her distracting techniques and also provided many age-appropriate activities, such as hosting "movie madness" nights with peers, "bake-a-thons" that allowed K.S. to cook and eat a snack with her peers or sister and kept boredom to a minimum. She required repeated reassurance that her confrontation of the eating symptoms would actually relieve anxiety for K.S. and would not be "overly stressful." In session six she proudly stated that she had set a goal for herself to require K.S. to finish all of her portions and realized that this not only did not engender as much conflict as she feared, it resulted in a tremendous feeling of power and satisfaction in her ability handle AN. At that point she was able to provide and monitor sufficient caloric intake at each meal. She also felt empowered to search K.S.'s room to remove all laxatives and created a contract in which K.S. agreed to toxicology screens in exchange for greater privacy.

For his part, Mr. S. struggled to make the distinction between his daughter and AN, often unwittingly making statements about K.S.'s behavior that assumed she was in complete control and directed her symptoms to provoke or express upset. This was more delicate, as K.S. was able to admit that this was sometimes the case when she was alone with the therapist. The therapist worked with the family to distinguish normal adolescent strivings for independence and control and the ways in which the eating disorder had modified this expression. At times Mr. S. was overtly critical of K.S., and the therapist worked directly with this to modify these interactions. As Mr. S. was better able to make a distinction between his daughter and her illness, the entire family began to speak of the illness as "the beast" and K.S. began to be more vocal in expressing other demands, particularly related to independence. Mr. S. often compared K.S. to her sister, much to the chagrin of both girls, who encouraged him to view them as separate and quite unique. This had the effect of unifying the girls against their father and supporting one another.

At the end of phase 1, K.S. had reached approximately 90% of her ideal body weight, had ceased using laxatives and had decreasing self-induced vomiting episodes greatly, with only six purging episodes during the first phase. The family demonstrated many of the skills that are key to success in family re-feeding – they were able to acknowledge that K.S.'s goals were concerning to them, but expressed a belief that she could, in fact, handle independence and set up parameters for maintenance of this. For her part, K.S. had enlisted her sister to support this independence and had been able to find a voice to more easily discuss her desire for the ways in which she wanted her parents to help her. Rather than arguing against the AN, K.S. began to externalize the illness herself and was able to discuss her more shameful and conflict-ridden behaviors more openly. This had a cyclical effect of helping parents find ways to assist her in managing these behaviors. Parental openness and flexibility, as well as a decrease in hostility in communication set the stage for K.S. to assume greater independence.

Phase 2. K.S. had returned to school during phase 1 and had meals monitored by school staff. This was perceived as embarrassing and socially awkward by K.S., who suggested that she move to independent meals at lunch. As noted above, her parents were initially quite concerned but were able to recount her significant progress and identified this as an important area in which K.S. could resume a "normal" life. They agreed on a "partial monitoring" program in which K.S. ate with her friends, then brought her lunch to a school staff member who observed the remainder. K.S. was aware that she could be observed by school staff at any point and that staff would report to her parents if they had concerns. As expected, this transition was difficult for K.S., who was able to note that she had appreciated the structure that observation gave her to remove eating disordered choices. She worked with her family to discuss options that made it less likely that she would limit portions or hide food, including calling her sister or her mother if stressed during lunch, asking for help with friends or going to her guidance counselor. K.S. took the step of recruiting a peer to support her, and this system worked well. However, both parents and K.S. noted on-going concerns related to purging behaviors, with K.S. noting an increasing desire to binge eat. One two occasions the family felt K.S. had hidden or hoarded food and perceived her eating as "out of control" although K.S. denied binge eating. This led to negotiation around trust, independence and ways in which parents could monitor behaviors appropriately.

At home, meals were less structured over time and K.S. was able to serve her own meals. However, the family struggled eating out of the house, as K.S. often expressed great anxiety about portion sizes and calorie counts in restaurants. With parental encouragement, K.S. agreed to take steps toward eating out of the home, with the family agreeing to eat out once per week. This initially caused sibling conflict, as K.S. requested that she choose the restaurant. However, the family compromised, by allowing K.S. to choose two separate restaurants in two weeks (until the next session). At the following session the family negotiated that K.S. would choose one week, but one of her siblings would choose the following week. This worked well and K.S.'s siblings showed great compassion in discussion whether it was better to surprise her with the choice or allow her the opportunity to plan around this "uncontrolled" meal.

K.S. struggled with independence in other domains, however, and as independent eating improved, K.S.'s family expressed concern that she appeared to continue to be "overly dependent" on them and unwilling to go out with peers. Mrs. C. acknowledged her own feeling that this helped K.S.'s recovery – "she won't get into trouble with us watching her" – but also created a significant limitation, as K.S. "needed a life." The therapist worked with the family to notice areas of gains and to continue to modify family criticism toward K.S. The family shifted focus to both encouraging independence, by scheduling previously enjoyable activities, while also managing their anxiety about the way this independence would impact weight and eating.

Phase 3. In this final phase of treatment, K.S. and her family set a goal of encouraging attainment of important milestones of independence – getting a driver's license, visiting colleges for applications and spending the night at a friend's house. She established these goals for herself and recruited her parents in managing her anxiety about engaging in these behaviors. This phase of treatment highlighted the ways in which K.S. responded with great sensitivity to any perceived criticism. She worked with her parents to "check in" with the meaning of their statements and improved her ability to confront and discuss concerns. The family also made a specific behavior plan with "rewards" for K.S. to engage in independence seeking behaviors. As a marker of her new independence, K.S. drove to the final family session.

Conclusion

Although the evidence base for treatment of adolescent eating disorders is remarkably limited, family treatment appears to be a reasonable approach for many. What studies have been conducted, despite their limitations and flaws, suggest is that Gull was mistaken in his observation about parents in most cases. Overall, treatment models of adolescent AN and BN both deserve further study and evaluation. Larger studies that compare family treatment to individual treatment may identify not only if one approach is superior to the other, but may identify for whom which treatment is best suited. In addition, studies that compare types of family treatment are also needed. FBT, with its strong behavioral focus, is the approach that has been systematically examined; however, other family therapy approaches may also be effective for AN. There is also a definite need for more definite studies of family based treatments for BN. A study comparing individual approaches such as cognitive-behavioral therapy to family based treatment would be particularly important to build upon the extremely limited data base for these two approaches in adolescent BN.

References

Bruch H. (1973). *Eating Disorders: Obesity, Anorexia Nervosa, and the Person Within*. New York: Basic Books.

Dare C, Eisler I. (1997). Family therapy for anorexia nervosa. In: *Handbook of Treatment for Eating Disorders*. Garner DM, Garfinkel P, eds. New York: Guilford Press, pp 307-324.

Eisler I, Dare C, Russell GFM, Szmukler GI, Le Grange D, Dodge E. (1997). Family and individual therapy in anorexia nervosa: A five-year follow-up. *Archives of General Psychiatry*, 54, 1025-1030.

Fairburn CG. (1988). The current status of the psychological treatments for bulimia nervosa. *Journal of Psychosomatic Research*, 32, 635-45.

Fairburn CG. (1997). Interpersonal psychotherapy for bulimia nervosa. In: *Handbook of Treatment for Eating Disorders, Second Edition*. Garner DM, Garfinkel P, eds. New York: Guilford Press.

Fairburn CG, Brownell K. (2002). *Eating Disorders and Obesity: A Comprehensive Handbook*. New York: The Guilford Press.

Goldfarb LA, Fuhr R, Tsujimoto RN, Rischman SE. (1987). Systematic desensitization and relaxation as adjuncts in the treatment of anorexia nervosa: A preliminary study. *Psychological Reports*, 60, 511-518.

Gull W. (1874). Anorexia Nervosa (apepsia hysterica, anorexia hysterica). *Transactions of the Clinical Society of London*, 7, 222-228.

Hoek H, Hoeken DV. (2003). Review of prevalence and incidence of eating disorders. *International Journal of Eating Disorders*, 34, 383-396.

Le Grange D, Lock J. (2005). The dearth of psychological treatment studies for anorexia nervosa. *International Journal of Eating Disorders*, 37, 79-81.

Le Grange D, Lock J. (2007). *Treatment Manual for Bulimia Nervosa: A Family-Based Approach*. New York: Guilford Press.

Le Grange D, Lock J, Dymek M. (2003). Family-based therapy for adolescent with bulimia nervosa. *American Journal of Psychotherapy*, 67, 237-251.

Le Grange D, Schmidt U. (2005). The treatment of adolescents with bulimia nervosa. *Journal of Mental Health*, 14, 587-597.

Lock J, Le Grange D, Agras WS, Dare C. (2001). *Treatment manual for anorexia nervosa: A family-based approach*. New York: Guilford Publications, Inc.

Lucas AR, Crowson C, O'Fallon WM, Melton L. (1999). The ups and downs of anorexia nervosa. *International Journal of Eating Disorders*, 26, 397-405.

Minuchin S, Rosman B, Baker I. (1978). *Psychosomatic Families: Anorexia Nervosa in Context*. Cambridge, MA: Harvard University Press.

Mitchell J, Seim HC, Colon E. (1987). Medical complications and medical management of bulimia. *Annals of Internal Medicine*, 107, 71-77.

Palazzoli M. (1974). *Self-starvation: From the intrapsychic to the transpersonal approach to anorexia nervosa*. London: Chaucer Publishing.

Palazzoli M, Boscolo L, Cecchin G, Prata G. (1980). Hypothesizing-circularity-neutrality: three guidelines for the conductor of the session. *Family Process*, 19, 3-12

Pawluck D, Gorey K. (1998). Secular trends in the incidence of anorexia nervosa: integrative review of population-based studies. *International Journal of Eating Disorders*, 23, 347-352.

Robin A, Siegal P, Moye A, Gilroy M, Dennis A, Sikand A. (1999). A controlled comparison of family versus individual therapy for adolescents with anorexia nervosa. *Journal of the American Academy of Child and Adolescent Psychiatry*, 38, 1482-1489.

Russell GF, Szmukler GI, Dare C, Eisler I. (1987). An evaluation of family therapy in anorexia nervosa and bulimia nervosa. *Archives of General Psychiatry*, 44, 1047-56.

Schmidt U, Landau S, Pombo-Carril MG, Bara-Carril N, Reid Y, Murray K, Treasure JL, Katzman M. (2006). Does personalized feedback improve the outcome of cognitive-behavioural guided self-care in bulimia nervosa? A preliminary randomized controlled trial. *British Journal of Clinical* Psychology, 45, 111-121.

Selvini Palazzoli M. (1974). *Self-starvation: From the intrapsychic to the transpersonal approach.* London: Chaucer.

Tierney S, Wyatt K. (2005). What works for adolescents with AN? A systematic review of psychosocial interventions. *Eating and Weight Disorders*, 10, 66-75.

Touyz SW, Williams H, Marden K, Kopec-Schrader E, Beumont P. (1994). Videotape feedback of eating behaviour in patients with anorexia nervosa: Does it normalise eating behavior? *Australian Journal of Nutrition and Dietetics*, 51, 79-82.

In: Evidence-Based Treatments for Eating Disorders
Author: Ida F. Dancyger and Victor M. Fornari

ISBN 978-1-60692-310-8
© 2009 Nova Science Publishers, Inc.

Chapter XVII

Emotion, Eating Disorders, and Integrative Cognitive-Affective Therapy

Scott G. Engel[1], Andrea Wadeson[2], Chad M. Lystad[3],
Heather K. Simonich,[3] and Steve A. Wonderlich[1]
1University of North Dakota, Grand Forks, North Dakota
2North Dakota State University, Fargo, North Dakota
3Neuropsychiatric Research Institute
Fargo, North Dakota, USA

Abstract

Recent clinical reports and empirical findings suggest that emotion is an important factor in the etiology and maintenance of eating disorders. As a result of this, emotion may have an important role in the treatment of eating disorders. In this chapter we briefly review a selected sample of empirical research on emotion and eating disorders. We briefly discuss the role of neurobiology and emotion, emotional processing, and ecologically valid findings in eating disorder research. We then discuss how this research has shaped new treatments of eating disorders. Finally, we describe the key features of a new treatment for bulimia nervosa, called Integrative Cognitive-Affective Therapy (ICAT). ICAT is an emotion-focused treatment that highlights modifying emotion regulation skills in bulimic patients. We discuss core features of the four phases of ICAT and provide prototypical examples of clinical interventions in each phase.

In the past three decades, research on emotion has increased exponentially. Accompanying this dramatic increase in research are new theories of emotion, new research methodologies for studying emotion, and a variety of therapies that incorporate emotion as a core component of treatment (Rottenberg and Johnson, 2007). Emotional processes are often thought to be key constructs in a number of forms of psychopathology, for example, bipolar disorder, alcoholism, anxiety disorders (Johnson, Gruber, and Eisner, 2007; Curtin and Lang, 2007; Farach and Mennin, 2007). In eating disorder (ED) research, scientists have begun to investigate emotion and the role it may play in the etiology and/or maintenance of ED behaviors (e.g., Engel et al., 2007).

The field of emotion is often considered to be "messy", with few areas agreed upon. For example, even the fundamental structure of emotion is debated today (Feldman-Barrett, 2006), with scientists questioning whether we have discrete emotions for example, fear, sadness, anger (Watson and Vaidya, 2003) or whether emotion is best described as a dimensional construct (Russell, 1980). Regardless of the many debates in the area of emotion, we will attempt to provide some definitional information regarding the basics of the affective science field (which, of course, are highly debated!)

In this chapter we use emotion-related terms that are generally consistent with Russell (2003). Emotion is a general term meant to refer to both affect and mood. Mood is thought to be enduring, trait-like experience of core affect. The use of the term affect is meant to convey the momentary experience of state-like emotional experiences. We will most frequently make use of the terms emotion (the more general term) and affect (the more specific term that implies momentary experience), but, admittedly, use them somewhat interchangeably.

Emotion and Models of Eating Disorder Behavior

An increasing amount of research attention has been devoted to studying etiological and maintaining variables in EDs. Much of this research, particularly the initial studies, has focused on dietary restriction as a causal and maintaining factor in EDs. More recently, the research has focused on alternative predictive variables, such as negative affect.

Dietary Restraint Model

According to the dietary restraint model, before individuals engage in bulimic behaviors they experience low self-esteem and appearance concerns. These concerns are defined mainly by an excessive focus on one's weight and shape. In an attempt to improve their self-esteem and reduce these concerns, the individual begins a period of extreme dieting. This severe food restriction leads the individual to be both physiologically and psychologically vulnerable, which then leads to binge eating. In order to compensate for the binge eating, the individual then engages in purging behavior which may take the form of vomiting, excessive exercise or abuse of laxatives. Following this behavior, the original shape and weight concerns often reappear and the individual will return to the original dieting behavior, which begins the cycle again (Fairburn and Cooper, 1989).

While the dietary restraint model has a great deal of empirical support (Steiger, Lehoux, and Gauvin, 1999; Stice, Nemeroff, and Shaw, 1996; Stice, 2001), not all available data are consistent with the model. Stice, Presnell, Groesz and Shaw (2005) recruited 188 adolescent females to test the dietary restraint model. Each participant was randomly assigned to a healthy weight management program or a control group. Stice and colleagues found that those in the experimental condition showed a significant decrease in bulimic symptoms and negative affect, less risk of obesity and weight gain, and better weight management. These findings are contradictory to the dietary restraint model, which would argue that a weight management program, which involves dietary restriction, would increase one's bulimic symptoms. Further, research has shown that not all individuals with bulimia nervosa (BN) engage in dieting prior to engaging in bulimic symptoms; with as many as 9-17 percent of individuals with BN reporting no dieting preceding bulimic symptoms (Mussell et al., 1997; Bulik, Sullivan, Carter, and Joyce, 1997).

Negative Affect Model

Contrary to the focus on dieting in dietary restriction models, negative affect models argue that negative affect is an important predictor in the etiology and maintenance of EDs, particularly BN. Much of the data concerning the negative affect model come from Heatherton and Baumeister's (1991) escape theory. This theory contends that binge eating serves as a way to escape from negative affective states, often related to an awareness that the person is not living up to a standard or expectation. The theory posits that in the face of such negative self awareness, individuals will "cognitively narrow" their thinking style which produces a more concrete and potentially irrational thought process, which is associated with a decreased inhibition of behavior. While the individual is in the "cognitively narrowed" state, binge eating is thought to be more likely because inhibitory restraints are diminished and also such behavior may reduce negative affect.

Stice, Nemeroff, and Shaw (1996) proposed a dual pathway model that states it is both dietary restraint and negative affect that lead to body dissatisfaction, which in turn leads to BN. Extreme dieting is, in part, caused by body dissatisfaction given the belief that it is a valuable method of weight control. Further, dietary restraint has also been shown to lead to negative affect, due to the failures associated with such extreme dieting (Stice, 2001). Furthermore, body dissatisfaction has also been shown to produce negative affect (Stice and Shaw, 1994). The binge-purge behavior characteristic of BN becomes a way to regulate such negative affect, at least temporarily (Heatherton and Baumeister, 1991). It is important to note that it is not necessary for both pathways to be present for BN to develop; rather each of the pathways is considered sufficient to cause the onset of BN (Stice, 2001). In support of this model, it has been found that body dissatisfaction, negative affect, dietary restraint, along with the thin-ideal internalization, are all risk factors for the development of BN (Stice, Nemeroff, and Shaw 1996; Stice, 1998, 2001).

To summarize the negative affect model, those who binge eat tend to have high demands of themselves and a high level of self awareness. Since their expectancies are so high, they become aware of their inadequacies, which results in negative affect. Binge eating allows these individuals to escape from these negative affect states, at least temporarily, and is therefore negatively reinforcing (Heatherton and Baumeister, 1991). Below, we will examine, in a selective and limited review, empirical evidence indicating that emotional variables may have significance in terms of both onset and maintenance of ED behavior.

Research on Emotion and Eating Disorders

While currently, there is little research that specifically investigates emotional processes in patients with EDs, there are a number of studies that are relevant to those interested in emotions and the role they may play in EDs. In an attempt to briefly review some of this literature, we pose three interesting and clinically relevant questions below about emotion and EDs and offer a brief review of the literature that addresses each question.

1) Is there a neurobiological explanation for the emotional problems of ED patients?

A number of studies have examined neurobiological causes and/or correlates of EDs. The work of Kaye and colleagues has suggested that disturbances in serotonin regulation are associated with negative emotions in BN patients (Kaye, Weltzin, and Hsu, 1993). Providing support for their hypothesis, Kaye et al. (2000) showed that BN participants were particularly likely to display negative affect, mood lability and binge urges following tryptophan depletion. Further, research implementing PET scans suggests that such abnormalities persist after patients have recovered from BN (Kaye et al., 2001).

Studies of the neurobiological correlates of emotion function have also been conducted with anorexia nervosa (AN) patients. Similar to BN, AN patients have also been found to have abnormal serotonin functioning (Bailer et al., 2007) and also, several studies have shown that AN patients display serotonin irregularities after they are weight restored and no longer meet diagnostic status for an ED (Bailer et al., 2004; Frank et al., 2002; Kaye et al., 2003; Bailer et al., 2005, 2006). These findings are consistent with the idea that emotion regulation difficulties may represent a predisposing trait for AN. The findings also strongly implicate a neurobiological explanation for the emotion dysregulation seen in ED patients.

2) Is there evidence that ED individuals display Deficits in emotional processes?

As previously mentioned, Stice, Nemeroff and Shaw (1996) found that in addition to dietary restraint, negative affect mediated the relationship between sociocultural pressure for thinness and BN symptoms. Stice (1998) has also found that both dieting and negative affect predict an increase in BN symptoms in a nonclinical sample of girls. Finally, a number of studies have shown that ED patients report a number of emotional abnormalities (compared to controls): difficulty recognizing and verbally expressing emotions (Zonneyvylle-Bender et al., 2004), difficulty recognizing and describing their emotional states (Zonneyvylle-Bender et al., 2005), decreased emotional awareness and deficient emotional control (Gilboa-Schechtman, Avnon, Zubery, and Jaczmein, 2006), and increased suppression of both positive and negative affect (Nandrino et al., 2006). All of these studies suggest that patients with EDs may have difficulty identifying and regulating emotional experiences. These emotional experiences appear to increase their risk of ED behavior, which in turn, may assist these individuals in regulating or controlling negative emotional states.

3) All that research is great, but it is often done in artificial laboratories and I'm not sure how well it generalizes to patients. Has any research been conducted on emotion and eating disorders that is specifically designed to generalize to the lives of patients?

Research employing experience sampling methodology (ESM; Csikszentmihalyi, 1994) or ecological momentary assessment (EMA; Stone and Shiffman, 1994) is specifically designed to maximize the extent to which the research environment parallels the participants' natural environment. Therefore, findings from ESM or EMA research theoretically generalize to the participants' every day lives to the greatest extent possible. Besides conducting research in the participants' natural setting, ESM and EMA research use real-time assessment techniques to reduce memory biases that are problematic with many other forms of assessment (Engel, Wonderlich, and Crosby, 2005). EMA technology has recently been used to clarify the relationship between emotion and ED behavior (Smyth et al., 2001). While EMA and ESM research are technically not the same, they are conceptually very similar and will be referred to as EMA research in the rest of this chapter.

EMA research has been conducted to better understand the role of environmental factors, emotion states and behaviors in AN, BN, and binge eating disorder (BED). Early research suggested that AN participants experience more negative affect than controls (Larson and Johnson, 1991). Two other small EMA studies have suggested that: 1) negative affect is related to AN behaviors (Pieters et al., 2006), but 2) AN patients report considerable variability in mood functioning (Engel et al., 2005). It is worth noting that these findings are somewhat preliminary given that all three of these studies had very small sample size.

Two EMA studies of particular relevance to BED are worth noting. Wegner et al. (2002) found that BED participants reported worse mood on binge days compared to non-binge days. Similarly, Stein et al. (2007) found that negative mood was higher before a binge, but contrary to their expectations, they also found that participants' post-binge negative mood was even higher than pre-binge mood.

The first EMA study of BN patients was conducted in 1982, by Johnson and Larson. They found that BN participants reported significantly more negative affect than control participants. Steiger et al. (1999) expanded on this finding and reported that BN patients and recovered BN patients reported greater levels of negative affect and self-criticism than non-ED participants following a negative social interaction, thus implying that BN subjects may be particularly sensitive to social cues. Several recent studies further clarify the relationship of emotion and bulimic behavior in the natural environment. Smyth et al. (2007) found that significant increases in negative affect precede BN behaviors and, importantly, negative affect markedly drops following a BN behavior. Engel et al. (2007) reported that the relationship between negative emotion and binge eating does not appear to be the same across all individuals with BN: those high in impulsivity displayed a much stronger emotion-behavior relationship than less impulsive subjects. These findings imply that while emotions may predict the likelihood of binge eating in some BN patients, they do not do so for all subgroups of people with BN. In total, the findings from this area of research demonstrate that emotions may be a particularly relevant antecedent to eating disorder behavior, not only in the research laboratory, but also in the natural environments of ED patients.

Summary

Although the evidence presented in this chapter is selective and brief, there is increasing data suggesting that emotional variables have a significant, and potentially clinically important, relationship to ED behaviors. This opens up potential opportunities for new treatments which target emotional correlates of ED behavior. Below, we will provide a brief overview of recent psychological treatments which target emotion related variables and also a small, but developing, literature on emotion focused treatments in the EDs.

Rationale for Focusing on Emotion in the Treatment of Bulimia Nervosa

Currently, cognitive-behavioral therapy (CBT; e.g., Agras et al., 1992; Fairburn et al., 1993; Mitchell et al., 1990) is the most widely tested and effective form of treatment for BN and represents a variation of standard cognitive therapy as defined by Aaron Beck (1967, 1976, 1987). In spite of continued demonstrations of at least moderate effectiveness, cognitive therapy has come under criticism (e.g., Beidel and Turner, 1986; Safran, 1990a, 1990b; Stoppard, 1989; Westen, 2000; Zinbarg, 2000) regarding several issues. Clark (1995) has summarized the criticisms of cognitive therapy and suggested they fall into four categories. These include: 1) a limited view of emotional responding; 2) an inadequate consideration of interpersonal factors; 3) insufficient attention to the therapist-client relationship and 4) overemphasis on conscious controlled cognitive processing. Samoilov and Goldfried (2000) suggest that CBT may be enhanced by eliciting, rather than managing or suppressing emotion in CBT. Zinbarg (2000) suggests that CBT may also be criticized for failing to address issues of resistance, or ambivalence, which may influence compliance with CBT techniques and consequent magnitude of change. Associated with these criticisms of cognitive therapy, there have been numerous efforts to extend or modify traditional cognitive theory and therapy. For example, it has been argued that cognitive therapy should maintain a stronger focus on interpersonal and affective issues (Safran and Segal, 1996; Samoilov and Goldfried, 2000); consider borrowing from constructivist theories to enhance treatment technique (Neimeyer, 1993); include narrative and metaphorical strategies (Meichenbaum, 1993); utilize the therapeutic relationship more thoroughly as a clinical technique (Robbins and Hayes, 1993; Safran and Segal, 1996; Westen, 2000; Zinbarg, 2000); and place greater emphasis on developmental and systemic issues (Guidano, 1986).

At the same time, there have been recent developments in the broader behavior therapy community in which emotion focused models of psychopathology and associated treatments have emerged (Farach and Mennin, 2007). For example, Allen, McHugh, and Barlow, (2007) outline a unified protocol for emotional disorders which highlights identification of typically avoided emotional responses and exposure to such disavowed emotions as a core of treatment. Similarly, Hayes and colleagues (Hayes, Strosahl, and Wilson, 1999) argue that behavioral analysts should carefully consider the functional relationships between emotional states and efforts to manage or cope with such states when deriving their clinical interventions. Their Acceptance and Commitment Therapy (ACT) is another example which attempts to minimize the avoidance of negative emotions and experience as core interventions. Furthermore, the work of Greenberg (2002) depicts an emotion focused treatment which emphasizes identification, experience, expression, and modification of emotional states and structures in the treatment of a variety of forms of psychopathology, including depression and marital dysfunction. All of these approaches highlight an increased emphasis on emotional experience and a new range of interventions which not only modify such emotional responding, but also have been shown to reduce various forms of psychopathology.

Clinical research in EDs has also supported the idea of expanding or extending the range of interventions in CBT for BN. Recently, the original CBT model of BN was tested and found to have more power in predicting bulimic symptomatology when factors such as interpersonal variables and emotional variability were included (von Ranson and Schnitzler, 2007) , thus providing some empirical support for a broader conceptual model. Additionally, Fairburn and colleagues have adapted their original CBT and created a new treatment (i.e., Cognitive Behavior Therapy-Enhanced or CBT-E; Fairburn, Cooper and Safran, 2003) which includes interventions that target perfectionism, low self-esteem, interpersonal factors, and emotional lability. Such adaptations were included because these variables were thought to serve as significant maintenance factors which limited the efficacy of original CBT for BN. Also, recent developments in the application of dialectical behavior therapy (DBT; e.g., Safer et al., 2001) reflect the research community's interest in the potential relevance of this emotionally focused treatment for severe personality disturbances in bulimic individuals. Although modified from its original form, the current DBT treatment for BN retains an emphasis on emotion regulation, distress tolerance, and interpersonal factors and has been shown to be at least somewhat effective in a randomized control trial with CBT as the comparison condition (Safer et al., 2001). These extensions and modifications of the original CBT for BN seem to reflect a growing consensus that a broader model with associated interventions for previously untargeted maintenance factors could provide incremental treatment efficacy.

Thus, CBT-E and DBT are examples of ED treatments which have more fully targeted emotion related variables and processes. Another emotion-focused treatment that not only targets emotion, but other important maintaining variables is integrative cognitive-affective therapy (ICAT) for BN, which is a new emotion focused treatment. We are in the process of finalizing pilot testing with ICAT and have received a federal grant to ultimately conduct a randomized control trial comparing it to the original CBT for BN. Hopefully, this will further clarify the relevance of emotion focused treatments for the treatment of EDs.

Integrative Cognitive – Affective Therapy for BN: A New Emotion-Focused Treatment

The model of etiology and maintenance of BN which underlies ICAT is multifactorial and attempts to integrate a broad array of emotional, interpersonal, cognitive, and biological factors thought to increase the risk of developing, and maintaining behaviors associated with BN. The conceptual model underlying ICAT has been more completely described in several publications (e.g., Wonderlich et al., 2001; Peterson et al., 2004). The model is graphically depicted in Figure 1 and can be summarized in the following manner. Bulimic individuals are thought to display high levels of a harm avoidance trait (e.g., Bulik et al., 1995) and to have experienced significant interpersonal problems and conflicts (Fairburn et al., 1997), which together, result in high levels of self-discrepancy (Higgins, 1987). That is, their actual self does not correspond to standards regarding how they wish they could be ideally or feel they must, or ought to be. Such discrepancy is thought to provoke high levels of negative emotion, which influence the bulimic individual's behavior in a momentary fashion. Furthermore, individuals with such high levels of self-discrepancy who internalize an ideal of thinness (Stice et al., 1994) are likely to display appearance discrepancy which manifests itself as body dissatisfaction.

The right half of Figure 1 depicts the posited behavioral reaction to negative emotions in BN associated with high levels of self discrepancy. Specifically, bulimic individuals are thought to attempt to regulate negative emotion with coping strategies which are defined as self-directed styles and interpersonal patterns. (Wonderlich et al., 2001). Bulimic individuals may also perceive a discrepancy between who they believe they are and who they feel they would like to or must be (self-discrepancy; Higgins, 1987). Further, they may deal with their discrepancy-oriented negative emotion with high levels of self-control (e.g., dietary restriction) or self-attack (e.g., self- disparagement, self-harm behaviors) in an effort to reduce negative affect and underlying self-discrepancies. Alternatively, some bulimic individuals may use a neglect oriented self-directed style (e.g., excessive drinking, numbing out), again in an effort to manage underlying emotional states. Furthermore, bulimic individuals may attempt to regulate emotions through a variety of interpersonal patterns including extreme submissiveness, social withdrawal, or a hostile attack oriented pattern. Each of these interpersonal styles is thought to be a means of trying to regulate emotional states and relationships in a fashion that minimizes the experience of discrepancy.

Finally, in the face of high levels of discrepancy, associated negative emotions, and self-damaging coping styles, bingeing and purging are likely to emerge (Smyth et al., 2007). Such behaviors may serve to block negative emotions or provide a sense of escape from the awareness of such negative feelings. In this regard, bulimic behaviors are considered emotion driven behaviors which are likely to be elicited when emotion states reach exceedingly high levels.

Structure and Format of ICAT

Presently, ICAT is a structured, short term therapy developed explicitly for individuals with normal weight bulimia or subclinical variations of this disorder. It consists of 20 psychotherapeutic sessions distributed over 16 weeks. Patients are seen twice a week during the first four weeks of treatment. Treatment is guided by a clinician manual, patient workbook, and a series of computerized treatment modules on a hand held personal digital assistant.

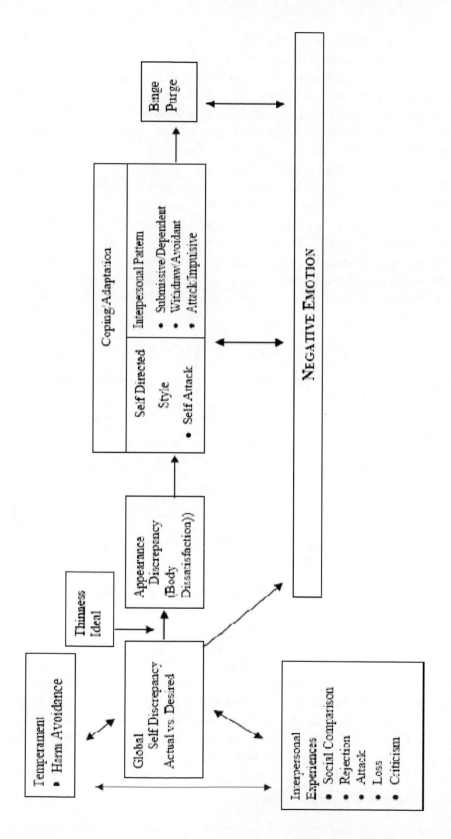

Figure 1. ICAT Model of Bulimia Nervosa.

The treatment is typically administered in a series of four phases which sequentially address motivation and psychoeducation (Phase I), the development of a meal plan and exposure to emotions related to eating (Phase II), modification of self-directed styles and interpersonal patterns associated with emotion regulation (Phase III), and relapse prevention (Phase IV). Furthermore, over the course of treatment five core skills are used to organize the various phases of treatment and focus the clinician and patient on essential processes thought to promote recovery in ICAT. These core skills are outlined in Table 1 and are identified in the treatment by their acronym (second column of Table 1). The FEEL skill is an essential emotion identification skill which is introduced early in Phase I and maintained throughout treatment. The CARE skill is introduced in Phase II and focuses on meal planning and food logging. The SAID and SPA skills refer explicitly to interpersonal patterns and self directed styles, respectively. Finally, the WAIT skill is a generic skill which targets reduction of impulsive or urgent decision making which can result in eating disorder symptomatology. The Patient Workbook complements and extends these skills and they are also included as a series of PDA based modules. Below, we will provide a more detailed description of each of the central phases of ICAT.

Table 1. Core Skills in ICAT

Coping Skill	Acronym for Skill	Elements in Acronym
Emotion Identification	FEEL	Focus, Experience, Examine and Label
Meal Planning	CARE	Carefully Arrange Regular Eating
Assertiveness	SAID	Sensitively Assert Ideas and Desires
Self Regulation	SPA	Self Protect and Accept
Impulse Control	WAIT	Watch All Impulses Today

Phase I: Enhancing Motivation and Psychoeducation - Sessions 1-2

Early sessions of treatment emphasize educating the patient about BN, largely through the patient workbook, and also conducting a collaborative interview with the patient to identify *general* discrepancies between their current behavior and broader life goals (Miller and Rollnick, 1991). This process is typically done by conducting a brief review of the history of their bulimic symptoms and the social and interpersonal context in which they developed. Relying on techniques from Motivational Interviewing (Miller and Rollnick, 1991), these early sessions are utilized to explore and enhance the patient's motivation for treatment. Clearly, the first step in treatment is to attempt to establish a collaborative therapeutic relationship that provides a safe context in which the patient may examine her behavior and consider the implications of change.

In addition, the therapy must remain focused on the patient's *emotional* reaction within each session. This emotion-focused aspect of the treatment is thought to be essential in assisting the patient to cope effectively with fear associated with behavioral change and recovery. The therapist is encouraged to acknowledge and explore patients' feelings as they occur in the session. Therapist interventions may appropriately consist of questions such as "Can you describe what the feeling is like for you as you consider change?" This may then be followed by a series of questions or statements that deepen or clarify the emotional response (e.g., "Is it frightening?" or "It seems hard to even think about it"). By exploring the emotional significance, the therapist clarifies motivational forces that may maintain the ED symptoms.

Another important consideration in Phase I is the introduction of the first core skill, which is the FEEL skill. This skill is essentially an emotion-focused skill designed to assist the patient in the identification and experiencing of emotions. The skill is introduced in the first and second session and the therapist is encouraged to underscore the importance of this skill throughout the treatment. It will be particularly important during Phase II, when meal planning will be introduced and identification and exposure to feelings associated with food, shape, and weight will be emphasized.

In an effort to complement learning of the FEEL skill, patients are asked to carry a Palmtop computer for two days and complete the Positive and Negative Affects Scale (PANAS) on several occasions. Completion of this scale allows the patient to begin to develop a language for identifying feelings in the moment. It is easy to collect the information on Palmtop computers, but this scale could also be delivered through a paper and pencil means if a Palmtop was not available.

Below, we present the case of Ms. S as a demonstration of the importance of emotion avoidance. Ms. S is a 28 year old, divorced, female who had a long standing history of BN and significant abuse of alcohol. Ms. S displayed a significant difficultly tolerating and managing negative emotional states. Although many interpersonal and work related situations posed significant difficulties for her, she had a fundamental inability to identify her emotional experience and, in ICAT terminology, demonstrated an emotional avoidance through eating disorder behavior and alcohol use which became a target in treatment. The transcript clarifies such emotional avoidance.

> Therapist: Now, what are we doing here? What I'm noticing is I'm hammering away at this with you and you are holding firm and steady with a hint of curiosity.
>
> Patient: Well right, I mean how have I done it up until this time in my life…with alcohol and throwing up. That's where my serenity, if I'm going to have any comes from. Just numb me up which means I'm not actually having any serenity in the first place. I'm just numbing the rest of my world out.
>
> Therapist: Right, and if you begin to tune into instead of numbing out, so if you use the Palm Pilot to begin to tune into what's going on inside of you…
>
> Patient: That's going to suck.
>
> Therapist: Because?
>
> Patient: Because it's going to be work and who knows what I'm going to see.
>
> Therapist: What are you going to see?
>
> Patient: I mean, I don't know.
>
> Therapist: I think you have a clue otherwise you wouldn't be so afraid.
>
> Patient: Well probably a lot of things I don't like.

Therapist: Like?

Patient: I don't know.

Therapist: Take a minute.

Patient: I really - I don't know, I mean probably—

Therapist: Slow down,

Patient: I thought I was going too slow.

Therapist: Slow down and think about it. What are you so afraid of?

Patient: I guess probably seeing what's in there and we're both pretty certain there is pain in there and probably seeing that. Not only seeing it but having it come out and deal with it. No, no, not only deal with it, but having it come out.

Therapist: And what will happen if it comes out?

Patient: It will be painful. Pain is uncomfortable and there is no room.

Therapist: It would swamp what you do. There would be no room for it.

Patient: Nope. Well there is no room because I've not ever allowed there to be room because the feeling of pain is not something like the feeling of wanting to cry or crying, or if like I'm going to be angry. I just don't like that feeling. I don't like the feeling of being hurt. I just don't and so…and if you are hurt and allow yourself to be hurt that infects the rest of your world.

Patient: A perfect example is the phone call that I had where I hung up the phone and I was almost immediately in tears because I had felt like such a failure I took everything told to me by the other teacher so personally that it just overwhelmed me to the point I lost all of my business-like composure and I became emotional - like creeped in without me realizing it was going to. I don't like that feeling because it a) hurts and b) there is no control.

Therapist: So it's just better to just block it out than try to figure out what it is, try and respond to it?

Patient: That's all I've ever known

Much of the early phase of treatment with Ms. S was focused on trying to identify her emotional experiences and states. This was a difficult procedure for Ms. S and she frequently denied the importance of her feelings and attempted to engage the therapist in a process which identified her as hopeless and untreatable. Although it took considerable time, Ms. S ultimately did benefit from continued psychotherapy and an intensive inpatient stay which gave her some control over her eating and drinking behavior and appeared to substantially improve her ability to process her emotional responding.

Phase II: Normalization of Eating and Associated Coping Skills – Sessions 3-8

Phase II, which generally runs from Session 3 through Session 8, relies on the direct encouragement of behavioral change in the area of eating and meal planning. Similar to other treatments for BN (e.g., CBT), patients are encouraged to eat three meals a day along with several snacks by prescribing a formal meal plan. Eating a variety of foods is encouraged and introducing feared foods is also part of this intervention. The treatment assumes that much of the reluctance that patients exhibit when asked to increase food intake is based on fear and

Goals of Phase I

1) Establish a treatment relationship which clearly includes the patient as a significant collaborator in her treatment.
2) Enhance motivation by noting discrepancies between the effects of the eating disorder symptoms and broader life goals.
3) "Side with the disorder" in terms of acknowledging possible benefits of the symptoms.
4) Remain sensitive to patients' emotional state and make efforts to identify emotional reactions. This will serve as a basic strategy that will be employed throughout the therapy.
5) Introduce FEEL skill and PDA methods.
6) Begin self-monitoring of food intake.

anxiety rather than oppositional defiance or characterologic resistance. Consistent with this perspective, the introduction of the meal plan is considered not only a nutritionally oriented exercise, but an emotion specific exercise. That is, while the therapist will assist the patient in incorporating food related issues, there will be a thorough and committed effort to understand emotions with the patient as they approach the meal plan, change their eating patterns, and particularly when they continue to have difficulty with eating regular meals and engage in binge eating.

An important element of Phase II is to emphasize continuation of the FEEL skill while the new core skill entitled CARE is introduced. The CARE skill is considered a very significant companion to the FEEL skill during this early phase of treatment. Using a variety of formats (e.g., PDA's, index cards, and their workbook), the therapist and patient together will attempt to increase the direct practicing of these skills in therapy sessions and outside of sessions. The acronyms for the core skills will be used to facilitate a language which emphasizes these skills. For example, the therapist may say to the patient "While you are working on your CARE skill tonight, it might be important to leave yourself time to practice FEEL again as well." This combination of identifying emotions while in the process of arranging meals and eating is a critical component of the therapy at this point in time.

Goals of Phase II

1) Continue self-monitoring food intake.
2) Implement formal meal planning with an emphasis on nutritionally adequate meals and snacks.
3) Introduce the CARE skill while continuing to practice the FEEL skill in and outside of sessions.

Phase III: Interpersonal Patterns, Self-Directed Styles, and Cognitive

Processes Sessions 9-18

In Phase III of treatment, there is a clear shift in therapeutic focus from nutritional rehabilitation to the interpersonal patterns, self-directed styles, and cognitive processes that are considered coping strategies in ICAT. Of particular interest is how these factors may serve to manage negative emotions, potentially related to self discrepancy, and may ultimately lead to emotion driven bulimic behaviors. These concepts are outlined in Figure 2, which is included in the Patient Workbook.

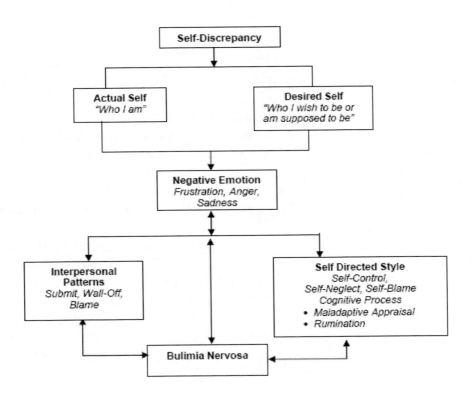

Figure 2. Phase III Treatment Components.

A major task in Phase III of treatment is for the therapist to work with the patient to clarify the patient's interpersonal patterns and self-directed styles developed to cope with negative moods. Also, the negative emotions should be elicited and experienced thoroughly by the patient. Through careful listening to the patient's descriptions of their interpersonal transactions, the therapist hypothesizes about the interpersonal rules, or "scripts" (Leahy, 1991), which seem to guide the patient's interpersonal patterns and self-directed styles (Benjamin, 1996, 2003). Thus, the patient gains an understanding of their interpersonal and self-directed behavior in "if-then" terms (e.g., "if others do x, I do y"). For example, a patient may have an interpersonal pattern which incorporates the if-then statement "If I submit to others, then others will love me." Alternatively, a patient may have developed a self directed style which relies on the "if-then" statement "If I can control myself perfectly, I will be O.K."

The therapist's focusing on the elements of the interpersonal patterns and self-directed styles must continue to be *emotion-focused*. That is, if the patient is only able to describe such interpersonal patterns or self-directed styles in a sterile and intellectualized manner, it is unlikely to be optimally effective in terms of behavioral change. Thus, the therapist must remain attentive to the emotional quality of the patient's descriptions of their interpersonal encounters and their self-views.

Below, we provide a transcript from Ms. M., a patient with AN-binge purge type. This section of a therapy session highlights the efforts to identify the interpersonal patterns and self directed styles that this patient frequently experienced and figured prominently in her ED behaviors.

Therapist: O.K., so something happened last night when you were talking to your boyfriend on the phone.

Patient: Yeah.

Therapist: Can you tell me about what took place last night, all of what happened with him?

Patient: Well, it was a bad night. I got home from work and called him and I just got the feeling he was preoccupied. Some of the guys from his softball team wanted him to go out later and I had thought we were going to do something. (She sees him as SEPARATE)

Therapist: Can you say what it was like, that is what you were feeling, when he was talking about going out with his friends on the phone.

Patient: I was mad! He always does this. He has got softball games all summer and every time he has a softball game, he has to be with his friends. But then when he has got time free, he expects me to be available. ("mad" is obviously an emotion word and explored further below)

Therapist: So you saw him as sort of doing his own thing and not being very available to you and you noticed that you were angry? Can you describe more completely what that was like for you when you were angry? (Further effort to clarify feelings)

Patient: I don't know, I just get mad.

Therapist: Yes, I understand that, but what happens when you get mad? What does it feel like internally and what do you do? (continued emotion exploration)

Patient: I just get crazy. I feel like I want to cry and scream. I pace and I don't seem to be able to sit still. That's when I do my (bulimic) behaviors. (beginning to see the action tendency)

Therapist: Did you in this case?

Patient: Yeah.

Therapist: Did those behaviors help you?

Patient: For a little while, but I was still freaking out.

Therapist: Can you tell me what you wound up doing then, after your behaviors, when you were feeling so upset and your boyfriend was not going to be available to you?

Patient: Well, I talked to him later and screamed at him and told him what a jerk I thought he was. I told him that he was insensitive and spoiled and that I was sick of being treated like dirt. (therapist is beginning to identify a possible ATTACK pattern)

Therapist: So you really sort of let him have it?

Patient: Yeah, I did and he really deserved it.

Therapist: And what happened then? (looking for consequences of behavior)

Patient: Well, then he got really quiet. He wouldn't talk to me and I got sort of nervous. I kept asking him to talk to me and he told me that he thought that maybe we needed a break from each other and that he was sick of dealing with my tantrums. (Boyfriend appears to be WALLING-OFF)

Therapist: So he was sort of pulled back. Sounds like he was threatening to leave.

Patient: Yeah, that freaked me out. ("freaked-out" is an emotion word)

Therapist: Freaked you out? What did you do? (identifying the action tendency)

Patient: Well, I did what I always do. I told him I was sorry and I would never do it again. That I was out of line. That I was acting like a bitch and I would try and do better next time. (possible evidence of reaction of SUBMIT and self-directed behavior of SELF-BLAME)

Therapist: Do you remember what you were feeling once you started to take the blame?

Patient: I am not sure. I know I get really nervous when he threatens to leave me. I think that I just keep telling him I'll be better and kind of begging him to stay. I don't know what I feel. Probably something like scared.

Therapist: There is one more thing I want to clarify. Earlier you told me that when you were angry at your boyfriend because he was not going to be able to see you, you were pretty mad. As I understood it, you called him some names and kind of put him down (ATTACK). I was wondering what you were hoping he might do when you got down on him. Any thoughts?

Patient: I don't know. I wanted him to know that he was a jerk and he was hurting me and I didn't like it.

Therapist: What did you hope he would do?

Patient: Well, I suppose I wanted him to say that he wouldn't go with his friends and that he would be with me. I wanted him to change his mind. (Wants CONTROL and wishes for boyfriend to SUBMIT)

Therapist: I see. You wanted to have some influence on him. I never did understand if it worked. Did he spend the night with you or did he go with his friends?

Patient: He went with his friends. (He WALLED-OFF)

Finally, during Phase III three additional core skills are introduced. Each of these focuses on a particular aspect of interpersonal or self directed behavior or action tendencies. For example, the SAID skill focuses on expression of feelings, desires, and ideas to other people assertively. The SPA skill emphasizes the development of self protecting and self accepting self directed styles. Finally, the WAIT skill targets impulsive behaviors and encourages a careful reflection on feelings and needs before acting (see Table 1). Each of these skills is again included in the PDA, on index cards, and in the workbook.

Phase IV: Relapse Prevention and Lifestyle Management - Sessions 19-20

The final phase of treatment focuses on consolidating improvements and preventing relapse. This process requires the therapist and patient to review progress in treatment, especially identifying interventions that were particularly helpful and effective. Final sessions should also include discussions of the patient's feelings and thoughts about ending treatment.

Goals of Phase III

1) Identify and modify maladaptive self-directed styles.
2) Identify and modify maladaptive interpersonal patterns.
3) Identify the connection between emotion and interpersonal patterns and self-directed styles and how these relate to bulimic symptoms.
4) Continue to modify extreme discrepancies between actual self and evaluative standards for the patient.
5) Implement SPA, SAID, and WAIT core skills.

An essential component of Phase IV is to educate the patient about the nature of relapse in order to prevent its occurrence. Specifically, the therapist should emphasize the distinction between a "lapse" compared to a "relapse" in order to prevent the patient from overgeneralizing the importance of a minor slip, a process that can lead to symptomatic deterioration. In addition, the patient is asked to consider various relapse scenarios, and to formulate coping strategies using skills developed in treatment. The patient also identifies her own potential cognitive, interpersonal, and behavioral triggers of lapses and relapses, and develops plans to get back on track should these occur.

Finally, the patient and therapist review the changes made in treatment and develop a maintenance plan to facilitate continued improvement. As part of the maintenance plan, components of a healthy life style are identified and implemented. In addition, the therapist should focus on emotions related to ending the treatment.

Goals of Phase IV

1) Review coping strategies that can be used to prevent relapse from occurring and learn about the nature of relapse. Include an emphasis on 3-D coping.
2) Identify risk factors of relapse and plan specific strategies for getting back on track if symptoms worsen.
3) Review progress in treatment.
4) Develop a maintenance plan for continued improvement and healthy lifestyle.
5) Focus on emotions related to termination.

An increasing amount of research suggests that emotion may be particularly relevant to a number of forms of psychopathology (Rottenberg and Johnson, 2007). In particular, research shows that emotional processes may be particularly important to eating disorders. Accordingly, new therapies for eating disorders have attempted to better incorporate emotional processes into treatment. In particular, the present chapter provides a brief overview of integrative affective therapy, which is a new emotion- focused therapy for BN. This treatment integrates the direct modification of meal planning and eating behavior with emotion-oriented interventions which address identification of feelings states and also adaptive emotion regulation strategies. Given the apparent strong association between emotional experience and eating disorder behaviors, new treatments which attempt to modify the experience of emotions and eating disordered individuals strategies for managing such emotions may provide an important step in the next generation of ED treatments.

References

Agras, W.S., Rossiter, E.M., Arnow, B., Schneider, J.A., Telch, C.F., Raeburn, S.D., Bruce, B., Perl, M., and Koran L.M. (1992). Pharmacologic and cognitive-behavioral treatment for bulimia nervosa: a controlled comparison. *American Journal of Psychiatry, 149,* 82-87.

Allen, L.B., McHugh, R.K., and Barlow, D.H. (2007). Emotional disorders: A unified protocol. In D.H. Barlow (Ed.), *Clinical handbook of psychological disorders* (4th ed.). New York: Guilford Press.

Bailer, U. F., Frank, G. K., Henry, S. E., Price, J. C., Meltzer, C. C., Mathis, C. A., Wagner, A., Thornton, L., Hoge, J., Ziolko, S. K., Becker, C. R., McConaha, C. W., and Kaye, W.H. (2007). Exaggerated 5-HT1A but normal 5-HT2A receptor activity in individuals ill with anorexia nervosa. *Biological Psychiatry, 61,* 1090-1099.

Bailer, U. F., Frank, G. K., Henry, S. E., Price, J. C., Meltzer, C. C., Weissfeld, L, Mathis, C. A., Drevets, W. C., Wagner, A., Hoge, J., Ziolko, S. K., McConaha, C. W., Kaye, W. H. (2005). Altered brain serotonin 5-HT1A receptor binding after recovery from anorexia nervosa measured by positron emission tomography and [carbonyl^{11}c]way-100635. *Archives of General Psychiatry, 62,* 1032-1041.

Bailer, U. F., Price, J. C., Meltzer, C. C., Mathis, C. A., Frank, G. K., Weissfeld, L., McConaha, C. W., Henry, S. E., Brooks-Achenbach, S., Barbarich, N. C., and Kaye, W. H. (2004). Altered 5-HT2A receptor binding after recovery from bulimia-type anorexia nervosa: Relationships to harm avoidance and drive for thinness. *Neuropsychopharmacology, 29,* 1143-1155.

Beck, A. T. (1967). *Depression: Clinical, experimental, and theoretical aspects.* New York: Harper and Row.

Beck, A. T. (1976). *Cognitive therapy and the emotional disorders.* New York: International Universities Press.

Beck, A. T. (1987). Cognitive models of depression. *Journal of Cognitive Psychotherapy, 1,* 5-37.

Beidel, D. C. and Turner, S. M. (1986). A critique of the theoretical bases of cognitive-behavioral theories and therapy. *Clinical Psychology Review, 6,* 177-197.

Benjamin, L. S. (1996). *Interpersonal diagnosis and treatment of personality disorders.* (2nd ed.). New York: Guilford Press.

Benjamin, L. S. (2003). *Interpersonal reconstructive therapy: Promoting change in nonresponders.* New York: Guilford Press.

Bulik, C. M., Sullivan, P. F., Carter, F. A., and Joyce, P. R. (1997). Initial manifestations of disordered eating behavior: Dieting vs. binging. *International Journal of Eating Disorders, 22,* 195-201.

Bulik, C. M., Sullivan, P. F., Weltzin, T. E., and Kaye, W. (1995). Temperament in eating disorders. *International Journal of Eating Disorders, 17*, 251-261.

Clark, D. A. (1995). Perceived limitations of standard cognitive therapy: A consideration of efforts to revise Beck's theory and therapy. *Journal of Cognitive Psychotherapy: An International Quarterly, 9*, 153-172.

Clore, G. L., Schwarz, N., and Conway, M. (1994). Affective causes and consequences of social information processing. In R. S. Wyer and T. K. Srull (Eds.), *Handbook of social cognition* (pp. 121-144). Mahwah, NJ: Lawrence Erlbaum Associates, Inc.

Csikszentmihalyi, M. (1994). *Flow: The psychology of optimal experience.* New York, NY: Harper Collins.

Curtin, J.J. and Lang, A.R. (2007). Affective processes in psychopathology. In J. Rottenberg and S.L. Johnson (Eds.), *Emotion and psychopathology: Bridging affective and clinical science* (pp. 215-240). Washington, D.C.: American Psychological Association.

Engel, S. G., Boseck, J. J., Crosby, R. D., Wonderlich, S. A., Mitchell, J. E., Smyth, J., Miltenberger, R., and Steiger, H. (2007). The relationship of momentary anger and impulsivity to bulimic behavior. *Behaviour Research and Therapy, 45*, 437-447.

Engel, S. G., Wonderlich, S. A., Crosby, R. D. (2005). Ecological momentary assessment. In J. E. Mitchell and C. Peterson (Eds.), *The assessment of patients with eating disorders* (pp. 203-220). New York, NY: Guilford Publications.

Engel, S. G., Wonderlich, S. A., Crosby, R. D., Wright, T. L., Mitchell, J. E., Crow, S. J., Venegoni, E. E. (2005). A study of patients with anorexia nervosa using ecological momentary assessment. *International Journal of Eating Disorders, 38*, 335-339.

Fairburn, C. G., and Cooper, P. J. (1989). Eating disorders. In K. Hawton, P. M. Salkovskis, J. Kirk, and D. M. Clark (Eds.), *Cognitive behaviour therapy for psychiatric problems: A practical guide* (pp. 277-314). New York, NY: Oxford University Press.

Fairburn, C. G., Cooper, Z., and Safran, R. (2003). Cognitive behaviour therapy for eating disorders: A "transdiagnostic" theory and treatment. *Behaviour Research and Therapy, 41*, 509-528.

Fairburn, C.G., Jones, R., Peveler, R.C., Hope, R.A., and O'Connor, M. (1993). Psychotherapy and bulimia nervosa. Longer-term effects of interpersonal psychotherapy, behavior therapy and cognitive behavior therapy. *Archives of General Psychiatry, 50*, 419-428.

Fairburn, C.G., Welch, S. L. and Doll, H. (1997). Risk factors for bulimia nervosa: A community-based case-control study. *Archives of General Psychiatry, 54*, 509-517.

Farach, F.J. and Mennin, D.S. (2007). Emotion-based approaches to the anxiety disorders. In J. Rottenberg and S.L. Johnson (Eds.), *Emotion and psychopathology: Bridging affective and clinical science* (pp. 243-262). Washington, D.C.: American Psychological Association.

Feldman-Barrett, L. (2006). Are emotions natural kinds? *Association for Psychological Science, 1*, 28-58.

Frank, G. K., Kaye, W. H., Meltzer, C. C., Price, J. C., Greer, P., McConaha, C., and Skovira, K. (2002). Reduced 5-HT2A receptor binding after recovery from anorexia nervosa. *Biological Psychiatry, 52*, 896-906.

Greenberg, L.S. (2002). *Emotion-focused therapy: Coaching clients to work through their feelings.* Washington, DC: American Psychological Association.

Guidano, V. F. (1986). The self as mediator of cognitive change in psychotherapy. In L. M. Hartman and K. R. Blankstein (Eds.), *Perception of self in emotional disorder and psychotherapy* (pp. 305-330). New York: Plenum Press.

Hayes, S. C., Strosahl, K. D. and Wilson, K. G. (2002). Acceptance and commitment therapy: An experiential approach to behavior change. *Cognitive and Behavioral Practice, 9,* 164-166.

Heatherton, T. F., and Baumeister, R. F. (1991). Binge eating as escape from self-awareness. *Psychological Bullletin, 110,* 86-108.

Higgins, E. T. (1987). Self-discrepancy: A theory relating self and affect. *Psychological Review, 94,* 319-340.

Johnson, S.L., Gruber, J., and Eisner, L.R. (2007). Emotion and bipolar disorder. In J. Rottenberg and S.L Johnson (Eds.), *Emotion and psychopathology: Bridging affective and clinical science* (pp. 123-150). Washington, D.C.: American Psychological Association.

Johnson, C., and Larson, R. (1982). Bulimia: An analysis of moods and behavior. *Psychosomatic Medicine, 44,* 341-351.

Kaye, W. H., Barbarich, N. C., Putnam, K., Gendall, K. A., Fernstrom, J., Fernstrom, M., McConaha, C. W., Kishore, A. (2003). Anxiolytic effects of acute tryptophan depletion in anorexia nervosa. *International Journal of Eating Disorders, 33,* 257-267.

Kaye, W. H., Frank, G. K., Meltzer, C. C., Price, J. C., McConaha, C. W., Crossan, P. J., Klump, K. L., and Rhodes, L. (2001). Altered serotonin 2A receptor activity in women who have recovered from bulimia nervosa. *American Journal of Psychiatry, 158,* 1152-1155.

Kaye, W. H., Weltzin, T. E., and Hsu, L. K. G. (1993). Serotonin and norepinephrine activity in anorexia and bulimia nervosa: Relationship to nutrition, feeding, and mood. In J. J. Mann and D. J. Kupfer (Eds.), *Biology of depressive disorders, part b: Subtypes of depression and comorbid disorders* (pp. 127-149). New York, NY: Plenum Press.

Larson, R., and Johnson, C. (1981). Anorexia nervosa in the context of daily experience. *Journal of Youth and Adolescence, 10,* 455-471.

Leahy, R. L. (1991). Scripts in cognitive therapy: The systemic perspective. *Journal of Cognitive Psychotherapy, 5: Special issue: Narrative,* 91-304.

Meichenbaum, D. (1993). Changing conceptions of cognitive behavior modification: Retrospect and prospect. *Journal of Consulting and Clinical Psychology, 61,* 202-204.

Miller, W. R., and Rollnick, S. (1991). *Motivational interviewing: Preparing people to change addictive behavior.* New York: Guilford Press.

Mitchell, J.E., Pyle, R.L., Eckert, E.D., Hatsukami, D., Pomeroy, C., and Zimmerman, R. (1990). A comparison study of antidepressants and structured intensive group therapy in the treatment of bulimia nervosa. *Archives of General Psychiatry, 47,* 149-157.

Mussell, M. P., Mitchell, J. E., Fenna, C. J., Crosby, R. D., Miller, J. P., and Hoberman, H. M. (1997). *International Journal of Eating Disorders, 21,* 353-360.

Nandrino, J. L., Doba, K., Lesne, A., Christophe, V., and Pezard, L. (2006). Autobiographical memory deficit in anorexia nervosa: Emotion regulation and effect of duration of illness. *Journal of Psychosomatic Research, 61*, 537-543.

Neimeyer, R. A. (1993). An appraisal of constructivist psychotherapies. *Journal of Consulting and Clinical Psychology, 61*, 221-234.

Peterson, C.B., Wimmer, S., Ackard, D.M., Crosby, R., Cavanagh, L.C., Engbloom, S., and Mitchell, J.E. (2004). Changes in body image during cognitive-behavioral treatment in women with bulimia nervosa. *Body Image, 1*, 139-153.

Pieters, G., Vansteelandt, K., Claes, L., Probst, M., Van Mechelen, I., and Vandereycken, W. (2006). The usefulness of experience sampling in understanding the urge to move in anorexia nervosa. *Acta Neuropsychiatrica, 18*, 30-37.

Rottenberg, J. and Johnson, S.L. (Eds.). (2007). *Emotion and psychopathology: Bridging affective and clinical science.* Washington, D.C.: American Psychological Association.

Russell, J.A., (1980). A circumplex model of affect. *Journal of Personality and Social Psychology, 39*, 1161-1178.

Russell, J. A. (2003). Core affect and the psychological construction of emotion. *Psychological Review, 110*, 145-172.

Safer, D.L., Telch, C.F., and Agras, W.S. (2001). Dialectical behavior therapy adapted for bulimia: A case report. *International Journal of Eating Disorders, 30*, 101-106.

Safran, J. D. (1990a). Towards a refinement of cognitive therapy in light of interpersonal theory: I. theory. *Clinical Psychology Review, 10*, 87-105.

Safran, J. D. (1990b). Towards a refinement of cognitive therapy in light of interpersonal theory: II. practice. *Clinical Psychology Review, 10*, 107-121.

Safran, J. D. and Segal, Z. V. (1996). *Interpersonal process in cognitive therapy.* Northvale, NJ: Aronson.

Samoilov, A. and Goldfried, M. R. (2000). Role of emotion in cognitive-behavior therapy. *Clinical Psychology: Science and Practice, 7*, 373-385.

Smyth, J., Wonderlich, S., Crosby, R., Miltenberger, R., Mitchell, J., and Rorty, M. (2001). The use of ecological momentary assessment approaches in eating disorder research. *International Journal of Eating Disorders, 30*, 83-95.

Smyth, J., Wonderlich, S., Heron, K., Sliwinski, M., Crosby, R., Mitchell, J., and Engel, S. (2007). Daily and momentary mood and stress are associated with binge eating and vomiting in bulimia nervosa patients in the natural environment. *Journal of Consulting and Clinical Psychology, 75*, 629-638.

Steiger, H., Gauvin, L., Engelberg, M. J., Ying Kin, N. M. K., Israel, M., Wonderlich, S. A., Richardson, J. (2005). Mood- and restrain-based antecedents to binge episodes in bulimia nervosa: Possible influences of the serotonin system. *Psychological Medicine, 35*, 1553-1562.

Steiger, H., Gauvin, L., Jabalpurwala, S., Seguin, J. R., and Stotland, S. (1999). Hypersensitivity to social interactions in bulimic syndromes: Relationship to binge eating. *Journal of Consulting and Clinical Psychology, 67*, 765-775.

Steiger, H., Lehoux, P. M., and Gauvin, L. (1999) Impulsivity, dietary control and the urge to binge in bulimic syndromes. *International Journal of Eating Disorders, 26*, 261-274.

Stein, R. I., Kenardy, J. K., Wiseman, C. V., Zoler Dounchis, J., Arnow, B. A., and Wilfley, D. E. (2007). What's driving the binge in binge eating disorder?: A prospective examination of precursors and consequences. *International Journal of Eating Disorders, 40*, 195-203.

Stice, E. (1998). Relations of restraint and negative affect to bulimic pathology: A longitudinal test of three competing models. *International Journal of Eating Disorders, 23*, 243-260.

Stice, E. (2001). A prospective test of the dual-pathway model of bulimic pathology: Mediating effects of dieting and negative affect. *Journal of Abnormal Psychology, 110*, 124-135.

Stice, E., Nemeroff, C., and Shaw, H. E. (1996). Test of the dual pathway model of bulimia nervosa: Evidence for dietary restraint and affect regulation mechanisms. *Journal of Social and Clinical Psychology, 15*, 340-363.

Stice, E., Presnell, K., Groesz, L., and Shaw, H. (2005). Effects of a weight maintenance diet on bulimic symptoms in adolescent girls: An experimental test of the dietary restraint theory. *Health Psychology, 24*, 402-412.

Stice, E., Schupak-Neuberg, E., Shaw, H. E., and Stein, R. I. (1994). Relation of media exposure to eating disorder symptomatology: An examination of mediating mechanisms. *Journal of Abnormal Psychology, 103*, 836-840.

Stice, E., and Shaw, H. E. (1994). Adverse effects of the media portrayed thin-ideal on women and linkages to bulimic symptomology. *Journal of Social and Clinical Pscyhology, 13*, 288-308.

Stone, A., and Shiffman, S. (1994). Ecological momentary assessment (EMA) in behavioral medicine. *Annals of Behavioral Medicine, 16*, 199-202.

Stoppard, J. M. (1989). An evaluation of the adequacy of cognitive/behavioural theories for understanding depression in women. *Canadian Psychology, 30*, 39-47.

von Ranson, K. and Schnitzler, C. (2007, October). Adding impulsivity and thin-ideal internalization to the cognitive-behavioral model of bulimic symptoms. Poster session presented at the annual Eating Disorder Research Conference, Pittsburgh, PA.

Watson, D. (2002). *Mood and temperament.* New York, NY: Guilford Press.

Watson, D., Clark, L. A., and Tellegen, A. (1988). Development and validation of brief measures of positive and negative affect: The PANAS scales. *Journal of Personality and Social Psychology, 54*, 1063-1070.

Wegner, K. E., Smyth, J. M., Crosby, R. D., Wittrock, D., Wonderlich, S. A., and Mitchell, J. E. (2002). An evaluation of the relationship between mood and binge eating in the natural environment using ecological momentary assessment. *International Journal of Eating Disorders, 32*, 352-361.

Westen, D. (2000). Commentary: Implicit and emotional processes in cognitive-behavioral therapy. *Clinical Psychology: Science and Practice, 7*, 386-390.

Wonderlich, S. A., Mitchell, J. E., Peterson, C. B., and Crow, S. (2001). Integrative cognitive therapy for bulimic behavior. In R. H. Striegel-Moore and L. Smolak (Eds.), *Eating disorders: Innovative directions in research and practice* (pp. 173-195). Washington, DC: American Psychological Association.

Zinbarg, R. E. (2000). Comment on "Role of emotion in cognitive behavior therapy": Some quibbles, a call for greater attention to patient motivation for change, and implications of adopting a hierarchical model of emotion. *Clinical Psychology: Science and Practice, 7*, 394-399.

Zonnevylle-Bender, M. J. S., van Goozen, S. H. M., Cohen-Kettenis, P. T., van Elburg, A., and van Engeland, H. (2004). Emotional functioning in adolescent anorexia nervosa patients. *European Child and Adolescent Psychiatry, 13*, 28-34.

Zonnevylle-Bender, M. J. S., van Goozen, S. H. M., Cohen-Kettenis, P. T., Jansen, L. M. C., van Elburg, A., and van Engeland, H. (2005). *Psychiatry Research, 135*, 45-52.

In: Evidence-Based Treatments for Eating Disorders
Author: Ida F. Dancyger and Victor M. Fornari

ISBN 978-1-60692-310-8
© 2009 Nova Science Publishers, Inc.

Chapter XVIII

Pharmacological Therapies for Anorexia Nervosa

James L. Roerig[1,2], Kristine J. Steffen[2], James E. Mitchell[1,2], and Scott J. Crow[3]

1.University of North Dakota School of Medicine and Health Sciences
Fargo, North Dakota, USA
2.Neuropsychiatric Research Institute, Fargo, North Dakota, USA
3.University of Minnesota Medical School
Minneapolis, Minnesota, USA

Abstract

This chapter will review the evidence surrounding the use of pharmacotherapy in the treatment of anorexia nervosa [AN]. Medications are divided into three classes; antidepressants, atypical antipsychotics and miscellaneous agents. Randomized, double blind, placebo controlled trials will be emphasized. In the absence of controlled trials uncontrolled data is presented. Lastly, suggestions for future studies will be presented.

Introduction

In recent years, substantial advances in pharmacological treatment approaches have been realized in many psychiatric conditions, including schizophrenia, bipolar disorder, and major depressive disorder. This progress has not been paralleled in AN, and definitive data to support the routine use of any pharmacotherapy in this disorder remains lacking. Historically, pharmacological agents have been chosen based on their ability to cause weight gain or to improve mood rather than their efficacy on other core AN symptoms. This may have contributed to the current state of affairs, in which the number of controlled pharmacological trials in the field has been modest and the few studies that have been completed have generally yielded negative or inconclusive results.

This chapter will review the state of the art, as it is somewhat shy of science, in terms of pharmacotherapy approaches. Discussion of the use of antidepressants, second generation antipsychotics and miscellaneous agents will serve to inform the current practice of pharmacotherapy. Lastly, a discussion of future treatment approaches and areas of inquiry will be presented.

The treatment course of AN is generally regarded as being biphasic; the initial focus of treatment is on promoting medical stability and encouraging weight restoration whereas the goal later shifts toward facilitating weight maintenance which requires a focus on the psychopathological symptoms of the illness. Currently, this treatment includes psychotherapy, education and nutritional rehabilitation, with pharmacotherapy in an adjunctive role.

As will be discussed below, there is little data on which to base treatment decisions. However, that may not reflect current clinical practice. As with any difficult to treat illness, clinicians will attempt to treat symptoms that the patient presents even in the absence of clear data supporting efficacy. In some cases the patient will benefit from this practice. However, many patients also experience complex therapies and are at times exposed to the risk of medication side effects, drug interactions and finally, high costs.

In exploring the "core" AN symptoms, a possibility exists to discover clues to aid in the development of more effective drug treatment. Some of the AN symptoms are illustrated in the following case:

Denise was a 20-year old female with a diagnosis of AN binge/purge subtype. She had developed AN about one year previously and had been quite resistant to outpatient treatment when she presented at 92 pounds and 5'5" tall. She was admitted to the partial hospital program and managed to gain weight to 98 pounds; but in general she continued to be quite resistant to weight gain. She was then placed in twice a week in outpatient psychotherapy and was seen by a family physician every other week to monitor her weight and laboratory work. However, she continued to do poorly and lost to 90 pounds at which time she was hospitalized as an outpatient treatment failure.

In the hospital she was quite depressed, and in general, not cooperative with treatment. She was quite obsessed with body image concerns and spent much of the day attempting to measure body parts with her hands or by checking in the mirror. She was very moody, but generally down, and she was also very obsessional and perfectionistic. She attempted to do all her assignments "perfectly", and repeatedly complained about having to eat all her meals. She had slept poorly and had a great deal of difficulty relating to staff or other patients. Because of this the decision was made to try her on the atypical antipsychotic olanzapine in addition to the therapeutic milieu on the inpatient unit and the behavioral contingencies for weight gain. She was started at a dose of 2.5 mg. which was increased five days later to 5 mg., and five days subsequent to that to 7.5 mg. The effect was dramatic. She reported, and the staff observed, decreased symptoms of anxiety and depression, and in particular less obsessionality about weight and shape issues. She reported that she was finding it somewhat easier to eat and began a steady pattern of weight gain. Her mood continued to improve and she became much more amenable to psychotherapy, and developed a good working relationship with her inpatient therapist. She was discharged several weeks later at a target weight of 110 pounds and was transferred back to fairly intensive outpatient treatment. The medication was continued for the next two months while her weight gain continued and then stabilized, as she progressed in psychotherapy.

Treatment

Antidepressants

The antidepressant class of medications has received the most extensive study among psychotropic agents in the treatment of AN. Although this research is arguably not yet exhaustive, the majority of antidepressant trials conducted to date have yielded negative findings. As reflected in the preceding case, patients with AN frequently have comorbid psychopathology which in itself might be an indication for the use of an antidepressant medication, including major depressive disorder, anxiety symptoms, and obsessive-compulsive disorder symptoms

Early controlled trials failed to demonstrate the superiority of tricyclic antidepressants [TCAs] over placebo [Lacey and Crisp, 1980; Biederman et al., 1985; Halmi et al., 1986]. Tricyclic antidepressants work by inhibiting reuptake of norepinephrine and/or serotonin, and also act as antagonists at a variety of receptors including alpha-1 adrenergic, muscarinic acetylcholine [M1], and histamine-1 [H1] receptors [Feighner, 1999]. It is the H1 antagonism of these drugs that is thought to lead to sedation as well as weight gain [Richelson, 2003]. Depression treatment research has shown that TCA use leads to a continuous, dose-dependent weight gain of 0.57-1.37 kg/month [Garland, Remick and Zis, 1988]. Although the H1 antagonism of the TCAs may therefore be of theoretical benefit in AN, their antagonism of alpha-1 and M1 receptors can lead to adverse effects such as orthostatic hypotension and anticholinergic effects, respectively.

Lacey [1980] compared clomipramine, 50 mg/day, to placebo in 16 hospitalized patients with AN. In this study, there were no significant differences in weight gain or the time that elapsed prior to achieving target weight between groups. Clomipramine appeared to increase hunger ratings during the first two months of treatment, but was equal to placebo during the final three weeks of the study. Participants in this trial received concomitant psychotherapy and a 2600 kcal/day nutritional rehabilitation program. In addition to the potential confounding effects of these multiple interventions, the clomipramine dose used in this study was likely subtherapeutic. Currently, therapeutic antidepressant clomipramine doses are generally regarded to be above 100 mg/day.

Similarly, Biederman [1985] studied a mixture of 38 inpatients and outpatients with AN. In a five week trial, amitriptyline [mean dose 115 ± 31 mg/day, maximum dose 175 mg/day] was compared to a placebo group and a control group. The control group was comprised of drug-refusers who received psychosocial treatment only. Across the three groups, weight gain was similar and no greater decrease in depressive symptoms occurred in the amitriptyline group. The amitriptyline group did, however, experience side effects that included diaphoresis, drowsiness, dry mouth and hypotension.

Finally, Halmi [1986] studied 72 inpatients for four weeks, comparing amitriptyline [maximum of 160 mg/day], cyproheptadine [maximum of 32 mg/day], and placebo. Cyproheptadine is a histamine, acetylcholine, and serotonin antagonist. This study was conducted in two locations, with differing findings in each. There were 15/46 treatment failures in one location versus 4/26 at the other location. Patient's pretreatment weight status appeared to influence outcome. Cyproheptadine increased what was termed treatment efficiency in the non-bulimic subgroup and decreased efficiency in the bulimic subgroup. There was an antidepressant effect in the bulimic subgroup with cyproheptadine.

By virtue of their improved adverse effect profile, the SSRIs have largely supplanted TCA use in the field of psychiatry. In patients with AN, there are additional issues related to TCA use that should be considered. First, it has been reported that underweight patients are at higher risk of developing an arrhythmia with TCA use [Kotler and Walsh, 2000]. Secondly, many patients with AN are adolescent and TCA's have been associated with sudden death in children. A series of eight cases of sudden death are described in a 2001 review in which child or adolescent patients were treated with either imipramine or desipramine [Varley, 2001]. This author postulates that this risk extends to all TCA's, not just imipramine and desipramine. Finally, all antidepressant medications now contain a Black Box warning regarding an increased risk of suicidal thinking and behavior in children, adolescents, and most recently also in young adults between the ages of 18 and 24. This warning has been instituted in response to a request from the U.S. Food and Drug Administration [FDA]. This risk appears to be highest within the first two months after initiating treatment with an antidepressant (FDA U.S. Food and Drug Administration, 2007). The FDA does make it clear that patients under age 24 can still receive antidepressants and treatment should be based on an assessment of the risk-benefit ratio in each patient. These warnings, however, do necessitate educating patients and caregivers about this risk.

SSRI's have been studied in the treatment of AN. There are essentially two types of trials with SSRIs; acute treatment trials and maintenance trials. Acute treatment typically occurs in patients who are often severely underweight and are hospitalized, and the primary treatment goal is weight gain. Maintenance treatment occurs after weight restoration has occurred, and the primary goal of treatment becomes relapse prevention. There are currently controlled data with fluoxetine both in acute treatment and as maintenance treatment. There are also uncontrolled data with a variety of other SSRIs.

Controlled data includes a study by Attia [1990], who showed that in low-weight AN inpatients, seven weeks of fluoxetine at a maximum daily dose of 60 mg failed to improve weight gain or mood over placebo. Several explanations may exist to account for this finding. Tryptophan, the amino acid precursor required for serotonin synthesis, decreases following acute dieting [Anderson et al., 1990; Wolfe, Metzger and Stollar, 1997]. Therefore, underweight patients may be unable to synthesize sufficient serotonin for the SSRIs to be effective. However, findings regarding plasma tryptophan levels have been inconsistent in AN. Some data have suggested lower concentrations of tryptophan in AN versus matched control subjects [Askenazy et al., 1998] and other data showed no difference between underweight AN patients and controls [Goodwin et al., 1989]. A "ceiling effect" may also be operative, in which the unique contribution of a drug would be statistically indiscernible over and above the array of simultaneous andgenerally to some degree effective, interventions these patients already receive.

Controlled relapse-prevention trials have also been performed with SSRIs in weight-restored patients. While an earlier controlled trial demonstrated improved weight maintenance and decreased core symptoms with fluoxetine over placebo at one year [Kay et al., 2001], a subsequent, more rigorously controlled, larger trial failed to substantiate these findings [Walsh et al., 2006]. The latter trial enrolled 93 AN outpatients and demonstrated that similar percentages of patients remained in the trial at 52 weeks and maintained a BMI of at least 18.5 [fluoxetine, 26.5%; placebo, 31.5%; p=0.57].

Table 1. Controlled Antidepressant Trials in Anorexia Nervosa

Reference	Drug and Dose (mg/day)	Duration	N	Inpatient or Outpatient	Outcome
Lacey and Crisp, 1980	Clomipramine 50mg Versus Placebo	Variable Length Study	16 females	Inpatient	Trial continued until patients met target weight. Concomitant psychotherapy and nutritional program. No significant difference in amount or rate of weight gain between groups.
Biederman et al., 1985	Amitriptyline Max 175mg Mean 115mg ($\pm$ 31) mg Versus Placebo Versus Control	5 Weeks	38 (sex not reported)	Inpatient and Outpatient	Control group comprised of patients who refused drug and were given psychosocial treatment. No difference on weight gain or depression measures between groups. There were adverse effects in the amitriptyline group, including diaphoresis, dry mouth, and hypotension.
Halmi et al., 1986	Amitriptyline Max 160mg Versus Cyproheptadine Max 32mg versus Placebo	4 Weeks	72 females	Inpatient	Cyproheptadine increased treatment efficiency in the non-bulimic subgroup. Cyproheptadine group also had an antidepressant effect.
Attia et al., 1998	Fluoxetine Max 60mg Mean 56mg	7 weeks	33 females	Inpatient	Participants also involved in nutritional and cognitive behavioral therapy program. Groups did not differ on weight gain or mood symptoms. Fluoxetine was tolerated well.
Kaye et al., 2001	Fluoxetine range of doses; 20mg every other day to 60mg/day	52 weeks	39 females	Outpatients	Higher number of fluoxetine treated patients remained on drug at one year (10/16) versus placebo (3/19). Fluoxetine group increased weight and decreased core eating disorder symptoms at 52 weeks. Participation in psychotherapy was optional in this study.
Walsh, et al., 2006	Fluoxetine mean: 63.5 ($\pm$ 15.8) mg/day versus Placebo	52 weeks	93 females	Outpatients	No difference between groups in time to relapse. 26.5% of the fluoxetine group and 31.5% of the placebo group maintained a BMI of 18.5 and remained in the study for 52 weeks.
Abbreviations: BMI=body mass index					

Atypical Antipsychotics

The second class of compounds that are clinically used in AN treatment are antipsychotic agents. While traditional [1st generation] antipsychotics have not been shown to be of benefit relative to placebo [Vandereycken and Pierloot, 1982; Vandereycken, 1984], atypical [2nd generation] antipsychotics have recently demonstrated some promise in uncontrolled reports and modest trials. As with antidepressants, the weight gain liability of some of the 2nd generation agents contributed to interest in these agents. Also, it has been suggested that patients with AN have distorted perceptions of body shape and/or weight, which have a delusion-like quality [Jones and Watson, 1997]. Symptoms of anxiety surrounding meals, obsessive features and sleep disruption have been reported to improve with atypical antipsychotic use. While they are not devoid of side effects, the atypical agents are generally less likely to cause extrapyramidal side effects [EPSE] including pseudoparkinsonism, dystonias, and akathisia as well as being less likely to cause tardive dyskinesia [TD], a condition for which adequate treatment does not exist [Umbricht and Kane, 1996]. Unfortunately, only three small controlled trials have been presented as posters/oral presentation at several meetings [Bissada et al., 2007; Kafantaris et al., 2007, Attia et al. 2008]. The Bissada trial has now been published [Bissada et al. 2008]. However, several uncontrolled studies and case series have suggested benefit of using these drugs in AN [See Table 2].

In reviewing these data, an effect on core AN symptoms has been described. Areas such as anxiety, depression and obsessive compulsive symptoms as well as thought disturbance are frequently improved with the atypical agents [Powers et al., 2007; Mondraty et al., 2005; Malina et al., 2003; Mehler, et al., 2001]. In addition, rating scales have demonstrated significant improvement including the Positive and Negative Symptom Scale [PANSS] total score and subscales of general psychopathology, anxiety and depression, the Brief Psychiatric Rating Scale [BPRS] total score, the Eating Disorder Inventory- 2 [EDI-2] total score and the subscales drive for thinness, perfectionism, impulse regulation, social insecurity, bulimia subscale, body dissatisfaction, ineffectiveness, interoceptive awareness and maturity fears [Powers et al., 2007; Powers, Santana and Bannon, 2002]; and the Yale Brown Cornell Scale for Eating Disorders [YBC-EDs] [Barbarich et al., 2004].

One consideration is that weight gain, rather than the drug therapy, may be responsible for these improvements. However, a difference in the comparison group's weight gain was not consistently shown. Thus, while weight gain is associated with improvement of symptoms, it may be that the drug's effect in reducing the core symptoms of the illness allow the patient to return to healthful eating and a better quality of life. These speculations must be demonstrated however, in larger, randomized, double blind, placebo controlled trials. These studies will have to address relevant questions including choice of agent, dosage and side effect liability.

Table 2. Antipsychotic Trials in Anorexia Nervosa

Reference	Drug and Dose [mg/day]	Study Design	N	Inpt/ Outpt	Outcome
Gaskill et al., 2001	Olanzapine Range: 1.25-15 mg	Open-label [non-randomized]	46 (sex not reported)	Inpt	Study enrolled inpatients. Weight gain was not different between olanzapine and non-treated group.
Mehler et al., 2001	Olanzapine Range: 5-12.5 mg	Case Report 6 – 8 weeks	5 females	---	Age range of 12-17. Olanzapine failed to increase weekly average weight gain. Decreased delusional thinking and improved social interaction observed in 5 patients.
Ruggiero et al., 2001	Fluoxetine 28 [$\pm$10.32] Clomipramine 57.69 [$\pm$25.79] Amisulpride 50 [$\pm$0]	Single-blind 3 months	35 females	Inpt	Patients were treated during the beginning of refeeding phase. Exclusion of subjects with clear depression, anxiety, obsessive compulsive disorder, and delusional body image thinking. Weight increase was not significantly different between groups.
Carver et al., 2002	Risperidone Range: 0.5-1.5 mg	Retro-spective Chart Review	30 females	----	Study enrolled refractory inpatients with AN. Risperidone treated patients demonstrated slightly higher weight gain [3.6 vs. 3.4 kg] and caloric intake [1017 vs 943 kcal].
Powers et al., 2002	Olanzapine 10 mg	Open-label 10 weeks	18 (16 female, 2 male)	Outpt	10 of 14 completers gained average of 8.75 lb. 4 drop-outs gained an average of 3.25 lbs. 4 completers lost an average of 2.25 lb but 3 of the 4 had low OLZ plasma levels. Patients who gained weight had significant improvement on psychiatric rating scales by week 10
Barbarich, et al., 2004	Olanzapine Mean: 4.7 [$\pm$1.6 mg] Range: 2.5-7.5 mg	Open-label 6 weeks	17 (sex not reported)	Inpt	Depression, anxiety, and core eating disorder symptoms improved. Weight increased significantly, from entrance weight of 69 [$\pm$ 10] % IBW to final weight of 81 [$\pm$9] % IBW [p=0.000]. Some subjects were also taking SSRIs.
Mondraty, et al., 2005	Olanzapine Range: 5-15 mg [mean: 10 mg]. Chlorpromazine Range: 25-100 mg [mean: 50 mg]	Randomized open-label. Up to 79 days	15 (sex not reported)	Inpt	Duration of the trial was 46 $\pm$ 31 days for olanzapine and 53 $\pm$ 26 days for chlorpromazine. Patients were hospitalized. The reduction in ruminative thinking on the Padua Inventory was significantly greater in the olanzapine group [54% decrease] vs. the chlorpromazine group [9% decrease] [p=<0.01]. Average weight gain was 5.5 kg, with no significant differences between groups. Participants also received standard inpatient care, consisting of psychiatric, nutritional, and medications.

Table 2. (Continued)

Reference	Drug and Dose [mg/day]	Study Design	N	Inpt/ Outpt	Outcome
Powers, et al., 2007	Quetiapine 150-300 mg	Open-label 10 week	19 (18 females, 1 male)	Outpt	Study enrolled outpatients. 10-wk study. LOCF analysis performed. 14 participants completed the study. Total scores on the PANSS as well as on the psychopathology and depression scales decreased significantly [p=0.024, 0.10, 0.0005, respectively]. Improvements were seen in anxiety, depression, and obsessive-compulsive symptoms. Mean weight gain was 0.73 kg. No participants withdrew due to adverse effects.
Bosanac et al., 2007	Quetiapine 50 – 800 mg/d 8 wk =mean dose 520mg, SD 277.49	Open-label 8 week	8 females	Inpt	7 completed 4 weeks 5 completed 8 weeks 4 weeks significant difference in the EDE-12 restraint score 8 weeks significant differences on BMI and EDE-12 restraint subscale scores SE of initial mild sedation
Bissada et al., 2007	Olanzapine 2,5 – 10mg/d	Double blind, placebo controlled 13 week	14 each group (sex not reported)	Outpt. 4 day/w k DH	Olan. + DH gained weight at a faster rate than plac. + DH. [p=.04 intent to treat]. Of completers 100% of Olan group was weight restored [BMI > 18.5] vs. 71.4% of the placebo group [p=.03]. No evidence of adverse side effects among any patients. Depression, anxiety, OC symptoms significantly improved in both groups.
Kafantaris et al., 2007	Olanzapine (dose unknown)	Double blind, placebo controlled 10 week	20 subjects total (sex not reported)	9 hospit al- ized, 11 in day progr am	No difference in weight gain. Significant improvement in total BPRS (p<.004) and Ham-D (p<.014) scores and significantly less depressed affect [p<.003], insomnia [p<.005] and increase in appetite [p<.039] in Olan group.
Attia et al., 2008	Olanzapine	Double blind, placebo controlled, 8 week	23 subject s	Outpt.	Olan. associated with statistically significant higher rate of weekly weight gain (0.9 ± 0.94 vs. -0.15 ± 1.07, p = 0.043). No significant difference between groups on multiple psychological symptoms

Abbreviations: BMI =Body Mass Index; BPRS =Brief Psychiatric Rating Scale; DH = Day Hospital; EDE-12=Eating Disorder Examination-12th Edition; Ham-D =Hamilton Depression rating scale; IBW=Ideal Body Weight; Inpt=Inpatient; OC=Obsessive Compulsive; Olan.=Olanzapine; Outpt.=Outpatient; PANSS=Positive and Negative Syndrome Scale; SE=Side Effects; wk=week

As can be seen in Table 2, olanzapine, quetiapine and risperidone are frequently used agents. All of these agents can cause weight gain with olanzapine having the greatest effect, quetiapine somewhat less [Allison et al., 1999] and risperidone's effect being approximately half of olanzapine [Roerig et al., 2005]. Is the weight gain liability of the atypicals necessary for a positive effect? No data currently address this question. The weight liability may cause non-compliance with the drug treatment in AN patients due to their fear of gaining weight. Also the weight liability may not have any role to play in response to the agent. Studies with weight neutral agents are needed to explore this question. Currently there are two weight neutral atypical agents marketed in the U.S., aripiprazole and ziprasidone. As discussed below, ziprasidone has the liability of affecting cardiac conduction and would not be recommended in this population.

Dosages of these agents have run from low to moderate levels [see Table 2]. Usually the dosage of the selected agents is initiated at a low level and gradually titrated to effect or mid dosing range. However, controlled data will have to guide these selections in the future, as it is always best to utilize the minimum effective dose to avoid side effect burden.

In general, these agents are well tolerated and the various reports listed above confirm this. However, the agents do differ somewhat in adverse reaction liability. As mentioned, olanzapine has the greatest effect on weight and in the population of patients with schizophrenia also has the greatest effect on serum lipids and glucose control [Lieberman et al., 2005]. Both olanzapine and quetiapine are sedating, although this effect usually decreases in the first week of treatment. Lastly, risperidone represents the agent with the greatest dopamine-2 receptor blocking affinity which results in elevated prolactin and dose related EPSE particularly as the dose approaches and exceeds 4 mg/day [Lieberman et al., 2005; Hamner, 2002]. Another concern in underweight AN patients is cardiac conduction. Many agents can lengthen the QTc interval and result in a higher risk for cardiac arrhythmias such as Torsade De Pointes. Of the atypicals, olanzapine has the least effect on the QTc interval and ziprasidone the greatest [Harrigan et al., 2004]. For this reason we would recommend against using ziprasidone in this population.

Finally, if data support the efficacy and effectiveness of selected atypical agents in the acute treatment of AN, the question of maintenance treatment becomes important. Currently there are no data addressing the duration of treatment. Various case reports and series have patients continuing on the atypical for weeks to months. As with the data reported by Walsh et al [2006] concerning fluoxetine maintenance therapy, it will be important to design rigorous trials to determine if there is any benefit to continuing atypical agents and if so, how long.

Miscellaneous Agents

Medications other than antidepressants and antipsychotics have also been tried in a handful of controlled trials in AN. Owing either to unfavorable adverse effect profiles or to a lack of demonstrated efficacy, these medications have not earned a place in the clinical management of AN. Medications in this category include tetrahydrocanabinol [Gross et al., 1983], naltrexone [Marrazzi et al., 1995], clonidine [Casper, Schlemmer and Javaid, 1987], recombinant human growth hormone [Hill, Bucuvalas and McClain, 2000], and the prokinetic agents metoclopramide, domperidone, and cisapride [Stacher et al., 1986; Saleh and Lebwohl, 1980; Szmukler, Yound and Miller, 1995]. Trials are summarized in Table 3.

In contrast to the preceding list of medications, zinc supplementation has also been studied [summarized in Table 3. and may have some role in the management of AN [Birmingham, Goldner and Bakan, 1994; Katz and Keen, 1987]. Although the results of the studies with zinc showed benefits on some outcome measures and not on others, the risk of side effects with zinc is low, potentially creating a favorable risk-benefit ratio and warranting consideration of its use.

Table 3. Miscellaneous Agents in Anorexia Nervosa

Author Year	Intervention	Proposed Mechanism	N Inpt/Outpt	Study Duration, Design	Outcome	Comments
Gross et al., 1981	Lithium carbonate (dosed to achieve serum concentration between 0.9-1.4 mEq/liter) versus Placebo	Weight gain, Improvement in affective state	16 female Inpt	Four-week, Double-Blind, Parallel Group	Significant group x time interaction occurred for weight gain. No difference between groups at weeks 1 and 2. At weeks 3 ($p=0.04$) and 4 ($p=0.03$), lithium group gained significantly more weight. Overall, weight gain in lithium group was 6.8 ± 0.4 kg (baseline weight 35.7 ± 1.1 kg) versus 5.2 ± 0.1 kg (baseline weight 32.7 ± 1.9 kg) in the placebo group.	All patients received a behavior modification treatment program and tube feedings as needed. Three of eight lithium treated patients had minor tremor and dizziness. No electrolyte abnormalities in either group. Thyroid assessments did not differ between groups.
Gross et al., 1983	Delta-9-tetrahydrocannabinol 30 mg/day versus diazepam 15 mg/day	Appetite Stimulation Improvement in affective state	11 female Inpt	4week Crossover, Double-Blind, Randomized	3 patients had dysphoric reactions (paranoid ideation and feeling of loss of control) on THC and withdrew (ITT analysis performed). No difference in weight gain or caloric intake between treatments.	Concomitant behavior modification, occasional tube feedings. After two weeks, participants crossed over to opposite treatment. No washout period between treatments.

Table 3. (Continued)

Author Year	Intervention	Proposed Mechanism	N Inpt/Outpt	Study Duration, Design	Outcome	Comments
Casper et al., 1987	Clonidine 500-700 mcg/day versus Placebo	Stimulation of eating. Clonidine is an alpha-2 adrenergic agonist.	4 female Inpt	8 week, Randomized, Placebo-Controlled Crossover. Multiple trials per participant.	Significant reductions in blood pressure on clonidine vs. placebo. No significant differences in weight change, hunger, or satiety during clonidine versus placebo administration.	Patients were selected due to failure to improve during hospitalization. No washout period. Concomitant psychotherapy, nutritional program. All patients considered clonidine an "unpleasant drug." Side effects included sedation, lightheadedness, one patient had severe bradycardia with a Wolf-Parkinson-White syndrome.
Katz et al., 1987	Elemental zinc 50 mg/day versus Placebo	Correct zinc depletion (patients found to have low zinc intake and urinary zinc excretion)	14 females	6 months, double-blind, placebo-controlled	Decreased depression ($p<0.05$) and anxiety ($p<0.05$) in the zinc group. Weight gain not statistically different between groups.	Patients also received psychotherapy and nutritional treatment
Stacher et al., 1993	Cisapride 10 mg tid versus placebo	Acceleration of gastric emptying	12 Outpt (sex not reported)	6 week double-blind, then 6-week open label	Acceleration of gastric emptying of a semisolid meal occurred in all 6 patients on cisapride. Weight gain in 5/6 cisapride patients versus 4/6 on placebo.	During the open –label phase, 4/6 of the patients originally treated with placebo had gastric emptying acceleration when switched to cisapride

Table 3. (Continued)

Author Year	Intervention	Proposed Mechanism	N Inpt/Outpt	Study Duration, Design	Outcome	Comments
Birmingham et al., 1994	Elemental zinc 14 mg/day versus Placebo	Weight gain	35 females	Randomized, double-blind, placebo-controlled	Rate of increase in BMI in zinc group was 0.079 (± 0.07)/day, versus 0.039 (± 0.06)/day in the placebo group (p=0.03). Number of days in the study did not differ between groups.	Patients received standard inpatient treatment, including nutritional, psychological, and concomitant medication therapy
Marrazzi et al., 1995	Naltrexone 100 mg bid versus placebo	Narcotic antagonism to block the endogenous opioids and interrupt the addictive cycle of dieting	19 female Outpt Sample included both AN (N=6) and BN	6 weeks per treatment period. Crossover, Randomized, Double-Blind	Significant differences between groups on binges, purges, urges to binge, urges to purge, daily food intake, and binge food ratio (p<0.05). Some patients with AN gained weight while others did not achieve weight restoration.	Population was both AN and BN patients. Patients drug-free except for hormone preparations and prn use of antihistamines and antibiotics. 1 month antidepressant washout before trial. Weekly psychotherapy. No washout between treatment periods.
Szmukler et al., 1980	Cisapride 10 mg tid before meals versus Placebo	Promote gastric emptying	29 Inpt (sex not reported)	8 week Randomized, Double-Blind, Placebo-Controlled	No difference on gastric emptying time between groups or on weight gain. Cisapride group showed greater improvement on ratings of hunger versus placebo (p<0.02), although prior to trial commencement they were significantly less hungry than placebo patients. Cisapride treated patients also	Patients also undergoing refeeding program with psychological support. No side effects that warranted participant withdrawal from the trial.

Table 3. (Continued)

Author Year	Intervention	Proposed Mechanism	N Inpt/Outpt	Study Duration, Design	Outcome	Comments
					rated themselves better on the global rating of improvement in symptoms associated with eating (p<0.03).	
Hill et al., 2000	Recombinant Human Growth Hormone 0.05 mg/kg/day SQ versus Placebo	Promotion of nitrogen retention, increase in serum IGF-1 levels, enhancement of fluid retention, improve dehydration, improve CV instability	15 Inpt (14 females, 1 male)	28-day, Randomized, Double-Blind	rhGH treated patients reached medical/CV stability sooner than the placebo patients (median 17 vs. 37 days, p=0.02). Median length of hospitalization decreased for rhGH group vs. placebo (32 days vs. 39 days, NS). Difference in rate of weight gain NS between groups.	All patients received a standard refeeding protocol.

Abbreviations: AN=Anorexia Nervosa; BN=Bulimia Nervosa; bid=twice daily; BMI=body mass index; CV=cardiovascular; Inpt=inpatient; NS=nonsignificant; Oupt=outpatient; SQ=subcutaneous; tid=three times daily

Pathophysiology

The current state of pharmacotherapy for AN leaves much to be desired. The matching of drugs to symptoms thus far has not produced strong therapeutic effects. SSRIs appear ineffective for mood and OC symptoms. Traditional antipsychotics appear to add nothing to treatment. The use of atypical antipsychotic agents is providing some hint of potential utility.

Rather than matching traditional symptoms to drug entities a better approach may be to explore what is known about the pathophysiology of AN and seek out agents that can modify the pathology. Dopamine, serotonin and norepinephrine have been associated with novelty seeking, harm avoidance and reward dependence respectively [Gerra et al., 2000; Hennig et al., 2000]. In addition, these transmitters have effects on eating. Thus, these neurotransmitters provide a starting point to explore possible drug targets. In exploring the function of these systems the binding affinity at receptor sites can be determined as well as binding affinity at the 5-HT transporter [5-HTT]. Also, regional blood flow can be explored through the use of functional Magnetic Resonance Imaging [fMRI].. Selected studies exploring these questions are listed in Table 4.

Table 4. Neurotransmitter and Receptor Studies in Anorexia Nervosa

Parameter	Method	Subjects	Result	Effect	Reference
5HIAA	CSF analysis	AN-R Ill	Significantly reduced	Reduced 5-HT in brain	Kaye et al.2005Kaye et al. 1991
5HIAA	CSF analysis	AN-R Recovered	Significantly elevated	Increased 5-HT in brain	Kaye et al. 1991
HVA	CSF analysis	AN-R Recovered	Decreased compared to recovered AN-BP or BN women	Decreased dopamine in brain	Kaye et al. 1999
5-HT1A	PET	AN-R Ill	30%–70% increase in binding potential	Reduced firing of 5-HT neurons	Bailer et al. 2007
5-HT1A	PET	AN-R Recovered	30 to 60% increase	Correlated with trait anxiety and harm avoidance	Bailer et al. 2005
5-HT2A	PET	AN-ill	Normal binding potential	Positive correlation to harm avoidance	Bailer et al. 2007
5-HT2A	PET	AN-R Recovered	Activity reduced		Bailer et al. 2004; Frank et al. 2002; Kaye et al. 2001
5-HT2A	SPECT	AN-BP	Reduced in the parietal cortex in AN-BP in comparison with AN-R	Positive correlation between reward dependence and parietal 5-HT2A binding index	Goethals et al. 2007
5-HTT Binding	PET	Bulimic ED	Reduced binding		Kuikka et al. 2001; Tauscher et al. 2001
5-HTT Binding	PET	AN-R Recovered	Increased compared to REC AN-BP	Increased 5-HTT activity may respond to higher SSRI doses	Bailer et al. 2007
rCBF	fMRI Studies of the insula	AN-R Recovered	Significantly reduced fMRI signal response	Insular neural activity did not correlate with pleasantness ratings for sucrose in AN women but did for the control women	Wagner et al. 2007
Dopamine D2/D3	PET	AN-R Recovered	Significantly higher [11C]raclopride binding potential in the antero-ventral striatum than CW.	Binding potential was positively related to harm avoidance.	Frank et al. 2005

5HIAA= 5-hydroxyindolacetic acid; 5-HT Transporter=5-HTT; AN-R Ill =Anorexia nervosa-restrictor ill; AN-BP=Anorexia nervosa-binge/purge; Control Women= CW; HVA=Homovanillic acid; Positron emission tomography=PET; rCBF=regional cerebral blood flow; Single photon emission computed tomography=SPECT

Future Directions

As listed above, in acutely ill AN patients, the 5-HT1A receptor has been shown to be up-regulated. This activity may give rise to anxiety, dysphoria and rigid behavior. The 5-HT2A activity is normal to down-regulated. Recovered AN patients also have an increase in activity of the 5-HT transporter. It also appears that the insula activity is reduced which could give rise to the distorted body image, diminished motivation to change, lack of recognition of the symptoms of malnutrition, and failure to appropriately respond to hunger. This recent literature provides interesting findings regarding the pathophysiology of AN. However, further work will be needed before this data can guide our drug selection.

At this point an immediate need in the pharmacotherapy of AN is to conduct placebo controlled, randomized, double blind trials utilizing selected atypical antipsychotics. Repeatedly, drugs that have looked beneficial in case reports or uncontrolled studies have been proven to have no effect when subjected to the more rigorous study design. The large number of reports of possible benefit in selected patients is very interesting. However, atypical antipsychotics have significant side effects that could be detrimental to the therapy of AN patients. Thus, it is necessary to definitively answer the question of their efficacy.

In light of the data that indicates heightened 5-HT1A receptor activity, a treatment that affects this system may prove to be beneficial. Also, recent evidence that glutamate antagonists possess antidepressant effects would indicate another avenue of exploration [Zarate et al., 2006].

Multiple problems present themselves in this type of research. AN is a very difficult disorder in which to study treatment interventions, given that many of these patients are not motivated for treatment, that many of them require a multiplicity of interventions simultaneously, and that AN is a relatively rare condition compared to many psychiatric disorders. In addition, randomized, controlled trials investigating new treatments are methodologically very complex and expensive to conduct. The development of a short-term method of screening pharmacological agents for possible efficacy in treating core symptoms associated with AN would aid in identifying potentially efficacious agents. Such paradigms could be utilized in searching for and evaluating the potential of new drug moieties for further study. The identified agents could then be tested in full, placebo controlled, randomized clinical trials; allowing these more complicated and expensive assessments to be carried out on the most likely agents to show a benefit in the treatment of AN.

Conclusion

In summary, much work has to be done to determine the role, if any, of pharmacotherapy in AN. It seems reasonable to search for compounds to target the core symptoms of the illness rather than just agents that cause weight gain as a side effect. With lessening or elimination of at least some of the core symptoms, individuals with AN may be able to return to healthful eating and a better quality of life. In the absence of such agents, aggressive nutritional rehabilitation remains critical, however, difficult in the face of the core symptomatology of AN.

References

Allison DB, Mentore JL, Heo M, Chandler LP, Cappelleri JC, Infante MC, et al. (1999). Antipsychotic-induced weight gain: a comprehensive research synthesis. *American Journal of Psychiatry*, 156, 1686–96.

Anderson IM, Parry-Billings M, Newsholme EA, Fairburn CG, Cowen PJ. (1990). Dieting reduces plasma tryptophan and alters brain 5-HT function in women. *Psychological Medicine*, 20, 785-91.

Askenazy F, Candito M, Caci H, Myquel M, Chambon P, Darcourt G, et al. (1998). Whole blood serotonin content, tryptophan concentrations, and impulsivity in anorexia nervosa. *Biological Psychiatry*, 43, 188-95.

Attia E, Haiman C, Walsh BT, Flater SR. (1998). Does fluoxetine augment the inpatient treatment of anorexia nervosa? *American Journal of Psychiatry*, 155, 548-51.

Attia E, Kaplan AS, Haynos A, Yilmaz Z, Musante D. (2008) Olanzapine vs. placebo for outpatients with anorexia nervosa: a pilot study. Presented at Eating Disorders Research Society's Annual meeting, September, Montreal Quebec, Canada.

Bailer UF, Price JC, Meltzer CC, Mathis CA, Frank GK, Weissfeld L, et al. (2004). Altered 5-HT2A receptor binding after recovery from bulimia-type anorexia nervosa: relationships to harm avoidance and drive for thinness. *Neuropsychopharmacology*, 29, 1143–55.

Bailer UF, Frank GK, Henry SE, Price JC, Meltzer CC, Weissfeld L, et al. (2005). Altered brain serotonin 5-HT1A receptor binding after recovery from anorexia nervosa measured by positron emission tomography and [11C]WAY100635. *Archives of General Psychiatry*, 62, 032-41.

Bailer UF, Frank G, Henry S, Price J, Meltzer C, Mathis C, et al. (2007). Exaggerated 5-HT1A but normal 5-HT2A receptor activity in individuals ill with anorexia nervosa. *Biological Psychiatry*, 61, 1090–99.

Bailer UF, Frank GK, Henry SE, Price JC, Meltzer CC, Becker C, et al. (2007). Serotonin transporter binding after recovery from eating disorders. *Psychopharmacology (Berl)*, Aug 11; [Epub ahead of print].

Barbarich NC, McConaha CW, Gaskill J, La Via M, Frank GK, Achenbach S, et al. (2004). An open trial of olanzapine in anorexia nervosa. *Journal of Clinical Psychiatry*, 65, 1480-82.

Biederman J, Herzog DB, Rivinus TM, Harper GP, Ferber RA, Rosenbaum JF, et al. (1985). Amitriptyline in the treatment of anorexia nervosa: A double-blind, placebo-controlled study. *Journal of Clinical Psychopharmacology*, 5,10-16.

Birmingham CL, Goldner EM, Bakan R. (1994). Controlled trial of zinc supplementation in anorexia nervosa. *International Journal of Eating Disorders*, 15, 251-55.

Bissada H, Tasca G, Barber A, Jacques B. (2007). A randomized controlled trial of olanzapine in the treatment of anorexia nervosa. Presented at the International Conference on Eating Disorders. May; Baltimore, MD.

Bissada H, Tasca GA, Barber AM, Bradwejn J. (2008) Olanzapine in the treatment of low body weight and obsessive thinking in women with anorexia nervosa: a randomized, double-blind, placebo-controlled trial.

Am J Psychiatry. 165:1281-8.

Bosanac P, Kurlender S, Norman T, Hallam K, Wesnes K, Manktelow T, et al. (2007). An open-label study of quetiapine in anorexia nervosa. *Human Psychopharmacology*, 22, 223-30.

Carver A.E., Miller S., Hagman J., Sigel E. (2002). The use of risperidone for the treatment of anorexia nervosa. Presented at the Academy of Eating Disorders Annual Meeting. April; Boston MA.

Casper RC, Schlemmer RF, Javaid JI. (1987). A placebo-controlled crossover study of oral clonidine in acute anorexia nervosa. *Psychiatry Research*, 20, 249-60.

FDA U.S. Food and Drug Administration. (2007). Antidepressant Use in Children, Adolescents, and Adults. Available from: http://www.fda.gov/cder/ drug /antidepressants /default.htm

Feighner JP. (1999). Mechanism of action of antidepressant medications. *Journal of Clinical Psychiatry*, 60(Suppl 4), 4-11.

Frank GK, Kaye WH, Meltzer CC, Price JC, Greer P, McConaha C, et al. (2002). Reduced 5-HT2A receptor binding after recovery from anorexia nervosa. *Biological Psychiatry*, 52, 896–906.

Frank GK, Bailer UF, Henry SE, Drevets W, Meltzer CC, Price JC, et al. (2005). Increased dopamine D2/D3 receptor binding after recovery from anorexia nervosa measured by positron emission tomography and [11c]raclopride. *Biological Psychiatry*, 58, 908-12. Epub Jun 29.

Garland EJ, Remick RA, Zis AP. (1988). Weight gain with antidepressants and lithium. *Journal of Clinical Psychopharmacology*, 8, 323-30.

Gaskill JA, Treat TA, McCabe EB, Marcus MD. (2001). Does olanzapine affect the rate of weight gain among inpatients with eating disorders? *European Eating Disorders Review*, 12, 1-2.

Gerra G, Zaimovic A, Timpano M, Zambelli U, Delsignore R, Brambilla F. (2000). Neuroendocrine correlates of temperamental traits in humans. *Psychoneuroendocrinology*, 25, 479-96.

Goethals I, Vervaet M, Audenaert K, Jacobs F, Ham H, Van de Wiele C, et al. (2007). Differences of cortical 5-HT2A receptor binding index with SPECT in subtypes of anorexia nervosa: relationship with personality traits? *Journal of Psychiatric Research*, 41, 455-8.

Goodwin GM, Shapiro CM, Bennie J, Dick H, Carroll S, Fink G. (1989). The neuroendocrine responses and psychological effects of infusion of L-tryptophan in anorexia nervosa. *Psychological Medicine*, 19, 857-64.

Gross H, Evert MH, Faden VB, et al. (1983). A double-blind trial of Δ^9 Tetrahydrocannabinol in primary anorexia nervosa. *Journal of Clinical Psychopharmacology*, 3, 165-71.

Gross HA, Ebert MH, Faden VB, Goldberg SC, Nee LE, Kaye WH. (1981). A double-blind controlled trial of lithium carbonate primary anorexia nervosa. *Journal of Clinical Psychopharmacology*, 1, 376-81.

Halmi KA, Eckert E, LaDu TJ, Cohen J. (1986). Anorexia nervosa: Treatment efficacy of cyproheptadine and amitriptyline. *Archives of General Psychiatry*, 43, 177-81.

Hamner M. (2002). The effects of atypical antipsychotics on serum prolactin levels. *Annals of Clinical Psychiatry*, 14, 163-73.

Harrigan EP, Miceli JJ, Anziano R, Watsky E, Reeves KR, Cutler NR, et al. (2004). A randomized evaluation of the effects of six antipsychotic agents on QTc, in the absence and presence of metabolic inhibition. *Journal of Clinical Psychopharmacology*, 2, 62–9.

Hennig J, Toll C, Schonlau P, Rohrmann S, Netter P. (2000). Endocrine responses after d-fenfluramine and ipsapirone challenge: further support for Cloninger's tridimensional model of personality. *Neuropsychobiology*, 41, 38-47.

Hill K, Bucuvalas J, McClain C. (2000). Pilot study of growth hormone administration during the refeeding of malnourished anorexia nervosa patients. *Journal of Child and Adolescent Psychopharmacology*, 10, 3-8.

Jones E, Watson JP. (1997). Delusion, the over valued idea and religious beliefs: A comparative analysis of their characteristics. *British Journal of Psychiatry*, 170, 381–386.

Kafantaris V, Leigh E, Berest A, Hertz S, Meyer-Sterling W, Schehendach J, et al. (2007). Pilot study of olanzapine in the treatment of anorexia nervosa. Presented at the American Association of Child and Adolescent Psychiatry. October; Boston, MA.

Katz RL, Keen CL, Litt IF, et al. (1987). Zinc deficiency in anorexia nervosa. *Journal of Adolescent Health*, 8, 400-6.

Kaye WH, Gwirtsman HE, George DT, Ebert MH. (1991). Altered serotonin activity in anorexia nervosa after long-term weight restoration. Does elevated cerebrospinal fluid 5-hydroxyindoleacetic acid level correlate with rigid and obsessive behavior? *Archives of General Psychiatry*, 48, 556–562.

Kaye, W.H.; Frank, G.K.; McConaha, C. (1999). Altered dopamine activity after recovery from restricting-type anorexia nervosa. *Neuropsychopharmacology*, 21, 503-6.

Kaye WH, Nagata T, Weltzin TE, Hsu LK, Sokol MS, McConaha C, et al. (2001). Double-blind placebo-controlled administration of fluoxetine in restricting and purging type anorexia nervosa. *Biological Psychiatry*, 49, 644-52.

Kaye WH, Frank GK, Meltzer CC, Price JC, McConaha CW, Crossan PJ et al. (2001). Altered serotonin 2A receptor activity in women who have recovered from bulimia nervosa. *American Journal of Psychiatry*, 158, 1152–1155.

Kaye WH, Frank GK, Bailer UF, Henry SE. (2005). Neurobiology of anorexia nervosa: clinical implications of alterations of the function of serotonin and other neuronal systems. *International Journal of Eating Disorders*, 37, S15–S19.

Kotler LA, Walsh BT. (2000). Eating disorders in children and adolescents: Pharmacological therapies. *European Child and Adolescent Psychiatry*, 9(Suppl 1), 108-16.

Kuikka JT, Tammela L, Karhunen L, Rissanen A, Bergstrom KA, Naukkarinen H, et al. (2001). Reduced serotonin transporter binding in binge eating women. *Psychopharmacology (Berl)*, 155, 310–14.

Lacey JH, Crisp AH. (1980). Hunger, food intake and weight: The impact of clomipramine on a refeeding anorexia nervosa population. *Postgraduate Medical Journal*, 56(Suppl 1), 79-85.

Lieberman JA, Stroup TS, McEvoy JP, Swartz MS, Rosenheck RA, Perkins DO, et al. (2005). Effectiveness of antipsychotic drugs in patients with chronic schizophrenia. *New England Journal of Medicine*, 353, 1209–23.

Malina A, Gaskill J, McConaha C, Frank GK, LaVia M, Scholar L, et al. (2003). Olanzapine treatment of anorexia nervosa: a retrospective study. *International Journal of Eating Disorders*, 33, 234-7.

Marrazzi MA, Bacon JP, Kinzie J, Luby ED. (1995). Naltrexone use in the treatment of anorexia nervosa and bulimia nervosa. *International Clinical Psychopharmacology*, 10, 163-72.

Mehler C, Wewetzer C, Schulze U, Warnke A, Theisen F, Dittmann RW. (2001). Olanzapine in children and adolescents with chronic anorexia nervosa. A study of five cases. *European Child and Adolescent Psychiatry*, 10, 151-7.

Mondraty N, Birmingham CL, Touyz S, Sundakov V, Chapman L, Beumont P. (2005). Randomized controlled trial of olanzapine in the treatment of cognitions in anorexia nervosa. *Australasian Psychiatry*, 13, 72-5.

Powers, P.S., Santana, C.A., Bannon, Y.S. (2002). Olanzapine in the treatment of anorexia nervosa: an open label trial. *International Journal of Eating Disorders*, 32,146-54.

Powers PS, Bannon Y, Eubanks R, McCormick T. (2007). Quetiapine in anorexia nervosa patients: an open label outpatient pilot study. *International Journal of Eating Disorders*, 40, 21-6.

Richelson E. (2003). Interactions of antidepressants with neurotransmitter transporters and receptors and their clinical relevance. *Journal of Clinical Psychiatry*, 64(Suppl 13), 5-12.

Roerig JL, Mitchell JE, de Zwaan M, Crosby RD, Gosnell BA, Steffen KJ, et al. (2005). A Comparison of the Effects of Olanzapine and Risperidone versus Placebo on Eating Behaviors. *Journal of Clinical Psychopharmacology*, 25, 413–18.

Ruggiero G.M., Laini V., Mauri M.C., Ferrari V., Clemente A., Lugo F., et al. (2001). A single blind comparison of amisulpride, fluoxetine and clomipramine in the treatment of restricting anorectics. *Progress In Neuro-psychopharmacology and Biological Psychiatry*, 25, 1049-59.

Saleh JW, Lebwohl P. M. (1980). etoclopramide-induced gastric emptying in patients with anorexia nervosa. *American Journal of Gastroenterology*, 74, 127-32.

Stacher G, Kiss A, Wiesnagrotzki S, Bergmann H, HobartJ, Schneider C. (1986). Oesophageal and gastric motility disorders in patients categorized as having primary anorexia nervosa. *Gut,* 27, 1120-1126.

Stacher G, Abatzi-Wenzel TA, Wiesnagrotzki S, Bergmann H, Schneider C et al. (1993). Gastric emptying, body weight and symptoms in primary anorexia nervosa. Long-term effects of cisapride. *British Journal of Psychiatry*, 162, 398-402

Szmukler GI, Young GP, Miller G, Lichtenstein M, Binns DS. (1995). A controlled trial of cisapride in anorexia nervosa. *International Journal of Eating Disorders*, 17, 347-57.

Tauscher J, Pirker W, Willeit M, de Zwaan M, Bailer U, Neumeister A, et al. (2001). [123I]beta-CIT and single photon emission computed tomography reveal reduced brain serotonin transporter availability in bulimia nervosa. *Biological Psychiatry*, 49, 326–32.

Umbricht D, Kane JM. (1996). Medical complications of new antipsychotic drugs. *Schizophrenia Bulletin*, 22, 475-83.

Vandereycken W, Pierloot R. (1982). Pimozide combined with behavior therapy in the short-term treatment of anorexia nervosa. *Acta Psychiatrica Scandinavica*, 66, 445-50.

Vandereycken W. (1984). Neuroleptics in the short term treatment of anorexia nervosa; a double-blind placebo controlled study with sulpiride. *British Journal of Psychiatry*, 144, 288-92.

Varley, CK. (2001). Sudden death related to selected tricyclic antidepressants in children: epidemiology, mechanisms, and clinical implications. *Paediatric Drugs*, 3, 613-27.

Wagner A, Aizenstein H, Mazurkewicz L, Fudge J, Frank GK, Putnam K, et al. (2007 May 9). Altered insula response to taste stimuli in individuals recovered from restricting-type anorexia nervosa. *Neuropsychopharmacology*, [Epub ahead of print].

Walsh BT, Kaplan AS, Attia E, Olmsted M, Parides M, Carter JC, et al. (2006). Fluoxetine after weight restoration in anorexia nervosa: a randomized controlled trial. *JAMA*, 295, 2605-12. Erratum in: *Jourral of the American Medical Association,* 2605-12.

Wolfe BE, Metzger ED, Stollar C. (1997). The effects of dieting on plasma tryptophan concentration and food intake in healthy women. *Physiology and Behavior*, 61, 537-41.

Zarate CA Jr, Singh JB, Carlson PJ, Brutsche NE, Ameli R, Luckenbaugh DA, Charney DS, Manji HK. (2006). A randomized trial of an N-methyl-D-aspartate antagonist in treatment-resistant major depression. *Archives of General Psychiatry*, 63, 856-64.

In: Evidence-Based Treatments for Eating Disorders
Author: Ida F. Dancyger and Victor M. Fornari

ISBN 978-1-60692-310-8
© 2009 Nova Science Publishers, Inc.

Chapter XIX

Pharmacological Therapies for Bulimia Nervosa

Amanda Joelle Brown[1], Lisa A. Kotler[2] and B. Timothy Walsh[2]
1. The New York State Psychiatric Institute
New York, New York, USA
2. Columbia University College of Physicians and Surgeons
New York, New York, USA

Abstract

There are a number of established pharmacologic therapies for the treatment of bulimia nervosa (BN). In response to clinical observations suggesting a link between BN and mood disorders, the majority of double-blind, placebo-controlled trials have tested the safety and efficacy of antidepressant medications for the treatment of BN. Positive outcomes in early trials using tricyclic antidepressants (TCAs) and monoamine oxidase inhibitors (MAOIs) suggested that antidepressants were indeed effective treatments for BN, although they were often associated with various side effects. Newer antidepressant agents, particularly selective serotonin reuptake inhibitors (SSRIs) such as fluoxetine, proved to be as effective as earlier classes of medications while causing fewer side effects, and this combination of safety and efficacy prompted the FDA's approval of fluoxetine for the treatment of BN in 1994. This chapter summarizes the evidence-based literature on medication trials in BN and concludes with a case example illustrating the application of evidence-based pharmacological treatments for BN.

Introduction

Since bulimia nervosa (BN) was first described in print (Russell, 1979), more than 20 clinical trials have been conducted to assess the safety and efficacy of various pharmacological agents for reducing the behavioral and psychological symptoms of BN (see Shapiro et al., 2007; Zhu and Walsh, 2002 for reviews). Early trials were brief (i.e. six to eight weeks) and mainly focused on testing the efficacy of antidepressant agents such as tricyclic antidepressants (TCAs), monoamine oxidase inhibitors (MAOIs), and atypical antidepressants, as it was commonly noted that many patients with BN presented for treatment with co-morbid depressive symptoms that had historically responded well to treatment with these medications. The majority of these early studies showed that almost all of the then-available classes of antidepressant medication were significantly more effective than placebo in reducing the symptoms of BN, including the frequency of binge eating and purging. As new classes of antidepressants have become available, particularly selective serotonin reuptake inhibitors (SSRIs), research groups have conducted double-blind, placebo-controlled trials in BN using these agents. More recent clinical trials have focused on novel pharmacological interventions such as the anticonvulsant topiramate and serotonin receptor agonist ondansetron, and many of these trials have produced promising data, opening up new avenues for future research.

Many clinical trials of pharmacological therapies in BN have focused exclusively on the effectiveness of a single medication, while others have compared more than one pharmacological agent, and still others have looked at the effectiveness of medication in conjunction with psychological treatments such as self-help, cognitive-behavioral therapy (CBT), and interpersonal therapy (IPT). Overall, clinical trials of pharmacological interventions for BN have had varying degrees of success in treating the symptoms of the disorder, and many of the pharmacological interventions have both costs and benefits that must be considered before making a recommendation for any individual patient. This chapter summarizes the available evidence-based literature on randomized, double-blind, placebo-controlled trials of pharmacological therapies for children, adolescents, and adults with BN. It will then apply the relevant data to a clinical case example provided at the end of the chapter.

Early Clinical Trials of Pharmacological Therapies for BN

In response to a growing awareness of the frequent co-morbidity of BN and affective disorders, particularly major depression (Pope and Hudson, 1982; Stewart et al., 1984), the first placebo-controlled medication trials in patients with BN examined the efficacy of both short-term and longer-term treatment with antidepressant medications. The most commonly studied classes of antidepressants were the TCAs and MAOIs, but other atypical antidepressants also received some attention in early clinical trials.

TCAs

Six clinical trials have investigated the safety and efficacy of TCAs for the treatment of BN. Pope and colleagues (1983) found that six weeks of treatment with imipramine (200 mg/day) was associated with a mean 70% decrease in binge frequency and 50% reduction in Hamilton Depression Scale (HAM-D) scores, while placebo treatment had no effect on eating or mood symptoms. Agras et al. (1987) reported comparable decreases in the behavioral and psychological symptoms of BN following a 16-week course of treatment with imipramine (average dose: 167 mg/day), suggesting that this medication may be efficacious for the treatment of BN over various lengths of time. Hughes et al. (1986) reported that desipramine (200 mg/day) was not only superior to placebo in reducing binge frequency, but also effective in completely eliminating behavioral symptoms in nearly 50% of participants by the end of the six-week trial. Walsh et al. (1991) replicated Hughes' findings in an eight-week, randomized, double-blind trial of desipramine (200-300 mg/day) versus placebo, and then openly treated those who had achieved at least a 50% reduction in binge frequency with desipramine for 16 more weeks. Participants who sustained their initial improvement during the open trial then entered a 24-week double-blind "discontinuation trial." While desipramine was superior to placebo in the short-term treatment of BN, longer-term treatment was neither well-tolerated nor effective; in fact, only five of the original 78 participants completed all 48 weeks of the study, as many discontinued treatment due to lack of efficacy or on account of side effects associated with desipramine use such as sedation, dizziness, and tremulousness.

Two trials investigated the efficacy of TCAs in combination with a behavioral intervention for the treatment of adults with BN. Mitchell and Groat (1984) studied the effects of amitriptyline (150 mg/day) in the context of a treatment program that incorporated elements of CBT and found that both active drug and placebo groups improved significantly from baseline but did not differ from each other on any behavioral measures. This negative finding may be due to a "ceiling effect" resulting from the overall benefit of the behavioral intervention. In another study investigating the efficacy of a combined treatment approach, Agras and colleagues (1992, 1994) randomly assigned women with BN to receive either 16 weeks of desipramine alone (average dosage: 168 mg/day), 16 weeks of desipramine combined with CBT, CBT alone for 16 weeks, desipramine alone for 24 weeks, or 24 weeks of desipramine combined with CBT. The 24-week combined treatment proved superior to 16 weeks of medication alone in terms of reducing binge eating and vomiting frequency, both at the end of the trial and at a one-year follow-up assessment point. The results of these studies indicate that combining TCAs with behavioral interventions may be an effective method for treating adults with BN.

MAOIs

As trials of TCAs were underway, another class of antidepressants, MAOIs, also began to receive attention from clinicians and researchers working in the field of eating disorders. MAOIs were thought to be potentially effective in patients with BN because these patients frequently presented for treatment with atypical depressive symptoms such as mood reactivity and anxiety, symptoms that generally responded well to MAOIs in patients with mood and anxiety disorders. Walsh and colleagues (1988) found that eight weeks of treatment with phenelzine (60-90 mg/day) reduced binge frequency and scores on several measures of psychological functioning to a significantly greater degree than did placebo treatment. Kennedy et al. (1988) found that iscarboxazid (60 mg/day) was associated with greater improvement in the frequency of vomiting, but not binge eating, episodes compared with placebo. After the isocarboxazid trial, Kennedy's group (Kennedy et al., 1993) found similar results in a trial of brofaromine (average dose 175 mg/day). Brofaromine-treated patients reported significantly fewer vomiting, but not binge eating episodes compared with the placebo group at the end of the trial. More recently, Carruba and colleagues (2001) found no difference in outcome between adult female outpatients treated with moclobemide (600 mg/day), a selective and reversible MAOI, and those treated with placebo over the course of a six-week trial. Overall, the results of clinical trials using MAOIs indicated that this class of medications may be helpful for treating symptoms of BN, but a number of side effects including orthostatic hypotension, sleep disturbance, dizziness, constipation, and sedation have been associated with members of this class of medications, and the emergence of newer agents limit the use of MAOIs in this population.

Other Early Clinical Trials

While TCAs and MAOIs received the most attention in early clinical trials of treatments for BN, other medications known to affect the psychological and behavioral symptoms of BN were also being tested. The atypical antidepressant mianserin (Sabine et al., 1983) and mood stabilizer lithium (Hsu et al., 1987) were not found to be more effective than placebo in reducing binge eating and vomiting frequency in adults with BN. Pope et al. (1989) found that the antidepressant trazodone (400 mg/day) was superior to placebo in reducing binge eating and vomiting frequencies over the course of their six-week trial. Horne and colleagues (1988) found that eight weeks of treatment with bupropion (300-450 mg/day) resulted in significantly greater improvement in patients with BN compared with placebo treatment. Unfortunately, four patients assigned to treatment with bupropion reported grand mal seizures during the trial, and this 5.8% prevalence of seizures could not be accounted for by commonalities in the medical history, laboratory findings, concurrent medication use, or other clinical characteristics of the four affected patients. The study was prematurely terminated, and the investigators concluded that bupropion should not be prescribed as a first-line treatment for BN. Based on the above findings, bupropion is now contraindicated by the FDA for the treatment of patients with a prior or current diagnosis of BN. The extended release version of the medication also carries this contraindication, although studies assessing the safety and efficacy of this newer agent have not been conducted.

Based on an earlier open trial (Jonas and Gold, 1988) in which naltrexone (200-300 mg/day) was found to be associated with significant reductions in binge eating and purging, Mitchell et al. (1989) conducted a randomized double-blind trial of naltrexone (50 mg/day) versus placebo and found that this low dose of the opioid antagonist was not superior to placebo in reducing bingeing and purging frequency or HAM-D scores. Likewise, Alger et al. (1991) found that treatment with naltrexone (100 mg/day) did not reduce binge frequency significantly more than did treatment with placebo. However, the lower doses of naltrexone used in these studies may not have been sufficient to cause a significant decrease in BN symptom severity, and future research with naltrexone may benefit from an investigation of the safety and efficacy of higher doses. In light of research demonstrating the efficacy of naltrexone in the treatment of alcohol dependence (see Assanangkornchai and Srisurapanont, 2007 for review), future clinical trials in BN may be warranted both to investigate the benefit conferred by naltrexone and to better understand links between the neurobiological underpinnings of eating and substance use disorder.

Summary

The early years of clinical research assessing the safety and efficacy of various pharmacological therapies were rich with evidence to suggest that many patients respond well to treatment with medications such as TCAs, MAOIs, and atypical antidepressants. However, the introduction of newer agents, particularly SSRIs, has relegated these older agents to second or third-line treatment status.

More Recent Clinical Trials: The Advent of SSRIs and Beyond

SSRIs

In 1987, the antidepressant medication fluoxetine was approved by the FDA for the treatment of mood disorders. Fluoxetine specifically targets the intercellular transmission of serotonin, a neurotransmitter implicated in the etiology of mood disorders and in the control of eating behavior. As the efficacy of antidepressant medications for the treatment of BN had been supported by much of the early clinical trials, fluoxetine soon received the attention of clinicians and researchers in the field of eating disorders because of its improved safety and tolerability compared to TCAs and MAOIs. After open-label trials produced encouraging results (Freeman and Hampson, 1987; Mitchell et al., 1989), double-blind, placebo-controlled clinical trials of fluoxetine for the treatment of BN were initiated. Two large multisite trials have investigated the efficacy of fluoxetine in reducing the symptoms of BN in nearly 400 outpatients, and the significant benefit conferred by fluoxetine treatment in these trials led the FDA to approve a specific indication for BN in 1994. To date, fluoxetine is the only medication approved by the FDA for the treatment of BN, although newer SSRIs such as fluvoxamine and sertraline have also received research support in small controlled trials. Many studies have focused exclusively on medication management with fluoxetine while others have investigated the synergistic and comparative effects of fluoxetine and behavioral interventions such as CBT or supportive psychotherapy. The promising results from these trials have led to the widespread use of fluoxetine in the treatment of BN.

Fluoxetine without Behavioral Intervention

Freeman and colleagues (1988) reported significant improvements in binge eating and vomiting frequency, Eating Disorder Inventory (EDI), and Eating Attitudes Test (EAT) scores among those subjects assigned to fluoxetine (60-80 mg/day) but not those assigned to placebo in their six-week double-blind trial. They also noted that six of the 20 fluoxetine-treated patients achieved abstinence from binge eating and vomiting by the end of the trial, whereas no patients assigned to placebo experienced complete symptom remission. Shortly thereafter, the Fluoxetine BN Collaborative Study Group (1992) conducted a randomized, eight-week, double-blind, multisite trial comparing the efficacy of fluoxetine (20 mg/day or 60 mg/day) versus placebo in 382 female outpatients. The results of this Eli Lilly-sponsored trial indicated that fluoxetine (both 20 mg/day and 60 mg/day) was associated with greater reductions in binge eating, vomiting, weight, body dissatisfaction, and food/diet preoccupation compared with placebo. Furthermore, a fluoxetine dose of 60 mg/day was superior to 20 mg/day in reducing binge eating and vomiting frequency. Side effects were relatively rare and the dropout rate due to adverse events was not significantly different between the fluoxetine and placebo groups (8.5% and 6.2%, respectively).

As a follow-up to these encouraging findings, Goldstein et al. (1995) conducted a second large Lilly-sponsored multisite trial aiming to assess the safety and effectiveness of treatment with fluoxetine (60 mg/day) over a 16-week period in 398 male and female late adolescent and adult outpatients. On the primary efficacy measure, change in the number of vomiting episodes per week over the course of the treatment period, fluoxetine-treated patients experienced significantly greater improvement than the placebo-treated group. Fluoxetine was also associated with greater improvement on the EDI, Clinical Global Impression (CGI) scale, and Patient's Global Impression (PGI) scale over the course of the trial. The rate of discontinuation due to an adverse event did not significantly differ between the two treatment groups. The results of this trial supported the longer-term use of fluoxetine in the treatment of BN.

In an even longer-term trial, sponsored by Lilly after fluoxetine had received FDA approval for BN, Romano and colleagues (2002), randomized 150 adult patients with BN to receive fluoxetine (60 mg/day) or placebo in a double-blind fashion for up to 52 weeks following response to an eight-week single-blind trial of fluoxetine (response was defined as reporting at least a 50% decrease from baseline in vomiting frequency for at least one of the final two weeks of the single-blind phase). Although the dropout rate was substantial in both groups in the double-blind treatment phase (83% for the fluoxetine group and 92% for the placebo group), fluoxetine treatment significantly prolonged the time to relapse and was correlated with a significantly lower rate of relapse (33% versus 51%) compared to treatment with placebo. Fluoxetine was also associated with smaller mean increases in vomiting, binge eating, and symptom severity as assessed by the CGI Improvement and Severity scales during the relapse prevention phase. Side effects and adverse events were similar in the two treatment groups, with rhinitis being the only side effect that was reported with significantly higher frequency in the fluoxetine group. The results of this trial offer support for the use of fluoxetine for relapse prevention following acute pharmacological treatment for BN, although the significant benefit conferred by fluoxetine must be interpreted in the context of an extremely high rate of dropout from both arms of the study. In summary, the evidence from the four studies described above demonstrates the efficacy of fluoxetine as a treatment for adults with BN, both in the short term and over longer periods of time.

Fluoxetine in Younger Populations

While nearly all clinical trials of fluoxetine have enrolled adult patients with BN, recent evidence from a small, eight-week open trial of fluoxetine (60 mg/day) for the treatment of BN in adolescent females (Kotler et al., 2003) suggests that fluoxetine may also be efficacious in younger populations. All ten subjects showed improvement on the CGI Improvement scale at the end of the trial. Overall, patients experienced significant decreases in the average number of weekly binge eating and purging episodes over the course of the treatment. Scores on the EAT, EDI, and Self-Report for Childhood Anxiety Related Disorders (SCARED) scales also declined significantly from baseline to week eight of the trial. Furthermore, no patient discontinued fluoxetine because of side effects from the medication. These results indicate that fluoxetine may be useful for treating the symptoms of BN in adolescent populations, although future placebo-controlled trials must be conducted before the safety and efficacy of fluoxetine for a younger population can be considered clearly established.

Additionally, in response to recent concerns about a potential link between increased risk of suicidal thoughts and behaviors and antidepressant medication treatment in adolescents and young adults, the FDA has recommended that antidepressant medications such as fluoxetine carry a black box warning against their use in patients under the age of 25. Certainly, adolescents and young adults undergoing treatment with an antidepressant for BN should be carefully monitored for clinical worsening. Families should also be advised to closely observe younger patients and to communicate frequently and openly with their child or adolescent's treatment provider to ensure the continued monitoring of these at-risk patients.

Fluoxetine Following Inadequate Response to Psychotherapy

Walsh and colleagues (2000) conducted an eight-week double-blind trial of fluoxetine (60 mg/day) versus placebo for patients who had not responded during or had relapsed following a 20-week course of either CBT or IPT (patients were randomly assigned to either treatment condition). Lack of response and relapse were defined as binge eating and vomiting at least once weekly over a one-month period. This research team found that treatment with fluoxetine was associated with decreased frequency of binge eating and purging episodes compared with placebo treatment; in fact, patients on placebo tended to increase the frequency of these behaviors. Furthermore, five of the 13 fluoxetine-treated participants reported abstinence from binge eating and purging during the last 28 days of the study, while no participants receiving placebo reported complete symptom remission at the end of the trial. The results of this study suggest that pharmacotherapy with fluoxetine may benefit patients with BN who do not respond to a course of a psychological treatment such as CBT and IPT.

In another study of fluoxetine treatment after failure to respond to a psychotherapeutic intervention, Mitchell et al. (2002) randomized 62 adult patients with BN who remained symptomatic after completing 20 sessions of CBT (defined more strictly than in Walsh et al.'s study as exhibiting any remaining purging behavior) to receive either 20 sessions of IPT or medication management beginning with fluoxetine (60 mg/day) and switching to desipramine (maximum 300 mg/day) if abstinence from bingeing and purging was not achieved within eight weeks of treatment with fluoxetine. Symptoms were reassessed at the end of the trial (week 33) and again at a week 60 follow-up point. Only 37 of the 62 randomized patients completed the full course of treatment, and no differences were found between the IPT and medication-only groups on measures of eating behavior, rates of abstinence from bingeing and purging, or any psychological measures. Data from the week 60 follow-up assessment indicated that those patients who were abstinent at the end of the trial remained so at week 60, and none of the 26 subjects who failed to achieve abstinence in the trial became abstinent in the post-treatment period. The lack of a placebo control group and the high dropout rate makes the value of a sequential treatment approach in BN difficult to interpret from this study.

Fluoxetine in the Context of Inpatient Treatment

In one of the earliest double-blind, placebo-controlled trials of fluoxetine, Fichter et al. (1991) randomized 40 patients with BN who were participating in an intensive inpatient program to five weeks of treatment with fluoxetine (60 mg/day) or matched placebo. Both groups significantly improved on the Symptom Checklist-90-Revised (SCL-90R), EDI, HAM-D, and CGI over the course of the study, but there were no significant differences on any outcome measure in those treated with fluoxetine compared to those treated with placebo. However, the clear therapeutic benefit of the intensive inpatient program may have overshadowed any additional effects of the medication, and therefore no firm conclusions can be reached about the relative efficacy of fluoxetine and placebo during inpatient treatment for BN based on this study.

Fluoxetine with Nutritional Counseling

Beaumont and colleagues (1997) enrolled 67 adult outpatients with BN in an eight-week, double-blind trial of fluoxetine (60 mg/day) versus placebo accompanied by individual nutritional counseling with a dietitian. As in Fichter et al. (1991), Beaumont et al. (1997) reported that both groups showed similar decreases in the frequency of binge eating and vomiting episodes over the course of the trial. Furthermore, while the fluoxetine-treated patients showed greater improvement on some subscales of the Eating Disorder Examination (EDE) during the active phase of the treatment compared with those taking placebo, the group assigned to active medication experienced a higher rate of relapse during the three-month follow-up period. Again, these results must be interpreted cautiously, as no waitlist control group was used, and the lack of significant difference between the groups may be indicative of a "ceiling effect" whereby the benefits of nutritional counseling limit the measurement of further clinical improvement with either fluoxetine or placebo.

Fluoxetine with CBT

In response to clinical trials supporting the efficacy of CBT for the treatment of BN (see Wilson, 2005 for review), Goldbloom et al. (1997) compared the efficacy of fluoxetine (60 mg/day) alone, CBT alone, and combined treatment over the course of 16 weeks. Seventy-six adult women with BN were enrolled into the study, but only 43 (57%) completed the minimum number of weeks of treatment to be considered "treatment completers" (14 weeks). This high dropout rate was mainly due to side effects from fluoxetine and noncompliance with session attendance. A completer analysis found that treatment with fluoxetine alone was significantly inferior to both CBT alone and combined treatment in decreasing frequency of binge eating and vomiting. There was no difference between CBT alone and combined treatment on these measures, and no differences were found between any of the three conditions in terms of EDE and BDI scores. Again, limitations with the study's design including a high dropout rate, lack of placebo and waitlist control groups, and variable amounts of time participants in each group spent with a treatment provider (fluoxetine alone: 10 sessions each lasting approximately 10 minutes, CBT alone: 16 weekly sessions each lasting one hour, combined: 10 10-minute medication sessions plus 16 one-hour CBT sessions) limit the interpretation of these results. The authors' main conclusion from the results of this trial was that fluoxetine alone appears to be less effective than a treatment combining fluoxetine and CBT for reducing the behavioral symptoms of BN.

In another study looking at the relative efficacy of medication, psychotherapy, and combined treatment, Walsh and colleagues (1997) randomly assigned patients with BN to one of five treatment groups: CBT plus medication, CBT plus placebo, supportive psychotherapy (SP) plus medication, SP plus placebo, or medication alone. Patients first received desipramine (200 mg/day) or matched placebo, and after eight weeks had passed, non-responders (those whose binge frequency remained above 25% of their baseline frequency) and those experiencing intolerable side effects on desipramine were tapered off and started on fluoxetine (60 mg/day) or matched placebo for the remainder of the trial. Overall, patients receiving the combined treatment showed more significant reductions in binge eating frequency, EAT scores, BDI scores, and SCL-90 depression scores compared with those who received placebo with psychological treatment. CBT proved to be superior to SP in reducing behavioral symptoms of BN, and no significant differences were found between the outcomes of patients who received SP plus medication and those who received medication alone. Taken in sum, the results of Walsh et al.'s (1997) study suggest that CBT is more effective than SP in adults with BN, whether used in combination with active drug treatment or with placebo; antidepressant medication is superior to placebo in reducing binge eating and purging frequency and improving mood; and the combination of antidepressant medication and psychological treatment is modestly more effective than either CBT or SP combined with placebo. Since this study did not include a psychotherapy-only group, no conclusions can be drawn about the relative efficacy of psychological treatment without medication management and a treatment combining psychotherapy and medication.

Fluoxetine with Self-Help

Increased demand for more affordable treatment options for patients with eating disorders and concerns about the accessibility of specialized eating disorder treatments have led researchers to examine the effectiveness of self-help manuals for treating patients with BN. In 2001, Mitchell and colleagues conducted a trial comparing the effects of fluoxetine (60 mg/day) alone, placebo alone, combined fluoxetine and self-help, and combined placebo and self-help in 91 adult outpatients with BN. At the end of the 16-week trial, those patients who had received fluoxetine reported reduced vomiting frequency compared with placebo. Access to the self-help manual magnified this differential reduction in vomiting frequency. CGI and PGI scores differed significantly from baseline for the groups receiving fluoxetine but not placebo, with no evidence of additional benefit from the self-help manual. There were no significant differences in outcome on any secondary measures, and remission rates did not differ between the three treatment cells. These results suggest that self-help manuals only modestly augment the benefits of fluoxetine in the treatment of adults with BN.

In another self-help trial, Walsh et al. (2004) randomized participants to either fluoxetine (60 mg/day) alone, placebo alone, guided self-help and fluoxetine, or guided self-help and placebo. Treatment took place in a primary care setting. All patients met with an internist once a month for medication management, and those who received the self-help manual also met with a nurse six to eight times throughout the duration of the study. 91 women entered the study, but nearly 70% dropped out of the trial before the scheduled point of termination. Compared with placebo treatment alone, treatment with fluoxetine alone was associated with decreased frequency of binge eating and vomiting, depressed mood as indicated by the BDI, and lower general symptom index as assessed by the SCL-53. The self-help manual had no independent effect on treatment outcome, and there were no significant interactions between the medication and self-help conditions. At the end of the trial, only eight of the 91 randomized patients had achieved abstinence from binge eating and purging. Although limited by the low rate of treatment completion, which decreased the statistical power to detect differences between combined treatment and medication-only conditions, the available data suggest that a guided self-help manual does not significantly enhance treatment of BN with fluoxetine in a primary care setting.

Other SSRIs

Although fluoxetine is currently the only medication approved by the FDA with an indication for the treatment of BN, other SSRIs have been studied and found useful for reducing symptoms of BN and for preventing relapse following inpatient hospitalization. Milano et al. (2004) conducted a 12-week trial of sertraline (100 mg/day) and found that it reduced binge eating and purging frequency to a significantly greater degree than did placebo treatment. Furthermore, patients reported no serious side effects from the medication. Fichter et al. (1996, 1997) conducted a placebo-controlled trial of fluvoxamine (average dose 182 mg/day) for relapse prevention following intensive inpatient treatment and found that the fluvoxamine group showed significantly less deterioration on behavioral measures compared with the placebo group during the 12 weeks following hospitalization. However, more recent evidence from a double-blind trial (Schmidt et al., 2004) suggests that fluvoxamine (50-300 mg/day), combined with a "stepped care" psychotherapy intervention, may not be more effective than placebo in the short-term or long-term treatment of BN. Fluvoxamine treatment was also associated with severe side effects such as seizures and impaired liver function in this study.

New Research and Future Directions

With the support of the data described above and an FDA approval for the treatment of indication of BN, fluoxetine (60 mg/day) is currently considered the "gold standard" of pharmacological therapies for the disorder, especially when combined with a psychotherapy like CBT. However, while fluoxetine is typically the pharmacological treatment of choice for BN, other medications may be equally or more safe or effective for any given patient, and further research is required to investigate the efficacy of new pharmacological agents. Recent clinical trials have highlighted the potential efficacy of topiramate (100-250 mg/day), an anticonvulsant and mood stabilizer, in the treatment of BN. In two 10-week, randomized, double-blind, placebo-controled trials (Hoopes et al., 2003, Hedges et al., 2003, Nickel et al., 2005), topiramate was associated with significant reductions in binge eating and vomiting frequency, and no patients in either study reported serious side effects resulting from topiramate treatment. These encouraging results point to topiramate as a pharmacological therapy for BN that warrants further investigation in larger randomized clinical trials.

Other medications that may hold promise for the future are ondansetron, a 5-HT3 antagonist typically prescribed to alleviate nausea associated with chemotherapy (Faris et al., 2002); flutamide, an androgen receptor antagonist (Sundblad et al., 2005); and baclofen, a GABA-B agonist used to treat alcohol and drug dependence (Broft et al., 2007). Each of these pharmacological agents has shown at least some evidence of utility in reducing symptoms of BN in double-blind or open trials. Faris et al. (2002) found that patients who took four milligrams of ondansetron when feeling an urge to binge eat or vomit significantly reduced the frequency of binge eating and purging and increased consumption of normal meals compared with those assigned to placebo treatment. Sundblad et al. (2005) conducted a randomized 12-week trial comparing treatment with flutamide (500 mg/day) to treatment with citalopram, an SSRI (40 mg/day) and found that patients treated with flutamide reported significantly greater global improvement than those taking citalopram. Most recently, Broft and colleagues (2007) reported that, in an open trial, baclofen (60 mg/day) was associated with a greater than 50% decrease in binge eating frequency in two of three patients with BN, and one of these achieved complete symptom remission by the end of the trial. These results suggest that GABA-B receptors may be implicated in controlling aspects of binge eating, and the utility of future clinical trials of baclofen for the treatment of BN lies not only in examining its efficacy in reducing symptoms, but also in learning more about the underlying neurobiology of the disorder.

One innovative trial has investigated the effectiveness of a non-medication biological intervention; evidence suggesting that patients with BN may have neurochemical disturbances similar to those of patients with seasonal affective disorder led Braun et al. (1999) to conduct a randomized, double-blind, controlled trial of bright light therapy for the treatment of BN. Patients who received the active treatment (10,000 lux bright white light) showed significantly greater improvement in binge frequency during the treatment phase compared with those participants who were given the "placebo" treatment (50 lux dim red light). However, there were no significant differences between the groups during the two-week post-treatment phase, nor were changes in BDI, HAM-D, or HAM-SAD significantly different between the groups at any time point. No subjects withdrew from the study due to side effects. A strong placebo response was observed in this study, which is possibly explained by the fact that every patient guessed at the end of the trial that she had been randomized to receive the active treatment. The findings from this small and short-term study suggest that bright light therapy may be a treatment option for BN, but further study is needed.

The majority of studies that have investigated sequencing pharmacological and psychological interventions have studied the efficacy of medication after insufficient response to psychotherapy (Walsh et al., 2000; Mitchell et al., 2002). Two psychotherapy treatment studies have produced data on outcome predictors in BN, and both have found that early behavioral change in psychotherapy predicts overall outcome (Fairburn et al., 2004; Agras et al., 2000). More specifically, a greater than 70% reduction in purging frequency by the sixth session of CBT is the best predictor of treatment response. Thus, an interesting area of future clinical research might be to examine the benefit of adding a medication at the sixth psychotherapy session if purging frequency has not yet been reduced by 70% or more. In a similar vein, Walsh and colleagues (2006) recently reported evidence that patients with BN who ultimately fail to respond to treatment with an antidepressant medication can be reliably identified by their response during the first two weeks of treatment with that medication. Future research aimed at determining the most appropriate length of time to allow before trying a different medication or recommending a supplemental psychotherapy intervention would be of significant clinical relevance.

Conclusion

BN is a psychiatric disorder that is often characterized by distressing physical and psychological sequelae and affects approximately 1% of women and 0.1% of men (Hoek and van Hoeken, 2003). On average, patients seeking treatment for BN have been ill for 5-9 years (Reas et al., 2001), and as many as 50% may relapse within the first six months after attaining full symptom remission in treatment (Fairburn et al., 1993; Halmi et al., 2002). Fortunately, there are data demonstrating that several pharmacological treatments benefit adults with BN. There is solid evidence indicating that the FDA-approved antidepressant fluoxetine, especially when combined with CBT, aids in the reduction of the behavioral and psychological symptoms of BN. In the case of inadequate response to fluoxetine, a variety of second- and third-line treatment options are available that have received at least some support from clinical studies. Additional controlled trials are needed to refine existing treatment methods to assist an even greater number of patients with BN to achieve complete symptom remission and to protect against relapse.

Clinical Case Example

Melissa is a 26 year-old graduate student with a three-year history of BN who lives alone in an apartment in a large U.S. city. She started dieting three and a half years ago after gaining five pounds while on vacation in the Caribbean. She began cutting out carbohydrates from her meals and was soon skipping breakfast and sometimes lunch. She found it increasingly difficult to sustain this level of restriction and began to have binge eating episodes once or twice a week. She felt excessively guilty after these episodes and began to self-induce vomiting in hopes of counteracting the effects of these binges. The frequency of these binge eating and vomiting episodes has increased steadily over the past three years, and she is currently experiencing daily episodes. She severely restricts her food intake during the day in an attempt to control her body weight and shape, but then typically loses control over her eating during dinner, the one meal she allows herself each day. She is often preoccupied with thoughts about food, and is therefore having a difficult time concentrating in class and completing her assignments on time. She feels sad and down on herself, has little energy, and is experiencing insomnia despite feeling a constant profound tiredness. Formerly a stellar student and devoted friend, Melissa is finding that her academic performance and interpersonal relationships are slowly deteriorating as a result of her impaired concentration, dwindling motivation, and increased social isolation.

After years of avoiding treatment out of feelings of shame and guilt, Melissa finally contacts Dr. X hoping that the psychiatrist will be able to help her break the cycle that is "controlling her life." She is relieved to find Dr. X reassuring and knowledgeable about treatment approaches for BN. Dr. X initiates CBT, as she knows that this type of psychotherapy has received significant research support as a treatment for BN. After six treatment sessions, the frequency of Melissa's binge eating and purging episodes has dropped to four times per week, but she continues to eat restrictively and erratically, and remains preoccupied with thoughts of food, eating, body shape, and weight.

Encouraged by the reduction in Melissa's disordered eating behaviors but concerned about the persistence of her symptoms, Dr. X decides that Melissa, not having been prescribed pharmacological agents in the past, may be a good candidate for treatment with fluoxetine. She chooses this SSRI based on its success in randomized clinical trials and the relatively low rate of side effects associated with its use compared with older agents such as MAOIs and TCAs. Dr. X recommends that Melissa begin with a dose of 20 mg/day and titrates the dose up to 60 mg over the course of a week, as she knows that patients with BN are more likely to respond to this higher dose. She chooses to continue seeing her for weekly CBT sessions, as a number of studies she reads suggest that a combination of psychotherapy and medication is superior to medication treatment alone for BN. After three weeks on 60 mg/day of fluoxetine, the frequency of Melissa's binge eating and purging episodes has decreased to two to three times per week, but she reports experiencing increased anxiety and difficulty sleeping, so Dr. X lowers the dose to 20 mg/day. At this dose, Melissa's binge eating and purging behaviors increase in frequency and her side effects do not abate. She and Dr. X together decide to discontinue the fluoxetine treatment.

Dr. X is encouraged by the improvement in Melissa's eating disorder symptoms while on fluoxetine and suggests that she try a different SSRI. She prescribes sertraline and titrates up to a dose of 100 mg/day. Unfortunately, Melissa's anxiety and insomnia persist on sertraline, although she also does note a slight decrease in her urges to binge and purge. Melissa decides that her side effects are too uncomfortable and requests a change in medication. Dr. X and Melissa decide to try topiramate, a mood stabilizer that she knows has received recent research support for treating BN, and slowly titrates the dose to 250 mg/day. Melissa adjusts well to this medication without experiencing significant side effects. Her positive response to topiramate allows her to better utilize the tools of CBT, and through continued therapy and medication treatment, the frequency of her bingeing and purging episodes continues to decrease. By the end of her second month of combined psychological and pharmacological therapy with Dr. X, Melissa achieves full symptom remission and reports improvements in her mood, physical health, concentration, and overall quality of life. She remains concerned that she may fall back into her old habits of binge eating and purging, but she feels confident that she has gained essential tools to control these symptoms.

References

(No authors listed). (1992). Fluoxetine Bulimia Nervosa Collaborative Study Group. Fluoxetine in the treatment of bulimia nervosa. A multicenter, placebo-controlled, double-blind trial. *Archives of General Psychiatry*, 49(2):139-47.

Agras WS, Dorian, B., Kirkley, B.G., Arnow, B., Bachman, J. (1987). Imipramine in the treatment of bulimia: A double-blind controlled study. *International Journal of Eating Disorders*, 6(1):29-38.

Agras WS, Rossiter EM, Arnow B, Schneider JA, Telch CF, Raeburn SD, et al. (1992). Pharmacologic and cognitive-behavioral treatment for bulimia nervosa: a controlled comparison. *American Journal of Psychiatry*, 149(1):82-7.

Agras WS, Rossiter EM, Arnow B, Telch CF, Raeburn SD, Bruce B, et al. (1994). One-year follow-up of psychosocial and pharmacologic treatments for bulimia nervosa. *Journal of Clinical Psychiatry*, 55(5):179-83.

Alger SA, Schwalberg MD, Bigaouette JM, Michalek AV, Howard LJ. (1991). Effect of a tricyclic antidepressant and opiate antagonist on binge-eating behavior in normoweight bulimic and obese, binge-eating subjects. *American Journal of Clinical Nutrition*, 53(4):865-71.

Assanangkornchai S, Srisurapanont M. (2007). The treatment of alcohol dependence. *Current Opinions in Psychiatry*, 20(3):222-7.

Beaumont PJ, Russell, J.D., Touyz, S.W., Buckley, C., Lowinger, K., Talbot, P. Johnson, G.F. (1997). Intensive nutritional counseling in bulimia nervosa: a role for supplementation with fluoxetine? *Australian and New Zealand Journal of Psychiatry*, 31(4):514-24.

Braun DL, Sunday SR, Fornari VM, Halmi KA. (1999). Bright light therapy decreases winter binge frequency in women with bulimia nervosa: a double-blind, placebo-controlled study. *Comprehensive Psychiatry*, 40(6):442-8.

Broft AI, Spanos A, Corwin RL, Mayer L, Steinglass J, Devlin MJ, et al. (2007). Baclofen for binge eating: An open-label trial. *International Journal of Eating Disorders*, 23.

Carruba MO, Cuzzolaro M, Riva L, Bosello O, Liberti S, Castra R, et al. (2001). Efficacy and tolerability of moclobemide in bulimia nervosa: a placebo-controlled trial. *International Clinical Psychopharmacology*, 6(1):27-32.

Fairburn CG, Peveler RC, Jones R, Hope RA, Doll HA. (1993). Predictors of 12-month outcome in bulimia nervosa and the influence of attitudes to shape and weight. *Journal of Consulting and Clinical Psychology*, 61(4):696-8.

Faris PL, Kim SW, Meller WH, Goodale RL, Oakman SA, Hofbauer RD, et al. (2000). Effect of decreasing afferent vagal activity with ondansetron on symptoms of bulimia nervosa: a randomised, double-blind trial. *Lancet*, 4;355(9206):792-7.

Fichter MM, Kruger R, Rief W, Holland R, Dohne J. (1996). Fluvoxamine in prevention of relapse in bulimia nervosa: effects on eating-specific psychopathology. *Journal of Clinical Psychopharmacology*, 16(1):9-18.

Fichter MM, Leibl C, Kruger R, Rief W. (1997). Effects of fluvoxamine on depression, anxiety, and other areas of general psychopathology in bulimia nervosa. *Pharmacopsychiatry*, 30(3):85-92.

Fichter MM, Leibl K, Rief W, Brunner E, Schmidt-Auberger S, Engel RR. (1991). Fluoxetine versus placebo: a double-blind study with bulimic inpatients undergoing intensive psychotherapy. *Pharmacopsychiatry*, 24(1):1-7.

Freeman CP, Morris, J.E., Cheshire, K.E., Davies, F., Hampson, M. A double-blind controlled trial of fluoxetine versus placebo for bulimia nervosa. Third International Conference on Eating Disorders; 1988; New York, NY; 1988.

Freeman CP, Hampson M. (1987). Fluoxetine as a treatment for bulimia nervosa. *International Journal of Obesity*, 11 Suppl 3:171-7.

Goldbloom DS, Olmsted M, Davis R, Clewes J, Heinmaa M, Rockert W, et al. (1997). A randomized controlled trial of fluoxetine and cognitive behavioral therapy for bulimia nervosa: short-term outcome. *Behavioral Research Therapy*, 35(9):803-11.

Goldstein DJ, Wilson MG, Thompson VL, Potvin JH, Rampey AH, Jr. (1995). Long-term fluoxetine treatment of bulimia nervosa. Fluoxetine Bulimia Nervosa Research Group. *British Journal of Psychiatry*, 166(5):660-6.

Halmi KA, Agras WS, Mitchell J, Wilson GT, Crow S, Bryson SW, et al. (2002). Relapse predictors of patients with bulimia nervosa who achieved abstinence through cognitive behavioral therapy. *Archives of General Psychiatry*, 59(12):1105-9.

Hedges DW, Reimherr FW, Hoopes SP, Rosenthal NR, Kamin M, Karim R, et al. (2003). Treatment of bulimia nervosa with topiramate in a randomized, double-blind, placebo-controlled trial, part 2: improvement in psychiatric measures. *Journal of Clinical Psychiatry*, 64(12):1449-54.

Herzog DB, Keller MB, Sacks NR, Yeh CJ, Lavori PW. (1992). Psychiatric comorbidity in treatment-seeking anorexics and bulimics. *Journal of the American Academy of Child and Adolescent Psychiatry*, 31(5):810-8.

Hoek HW, van Hoeken D. (2003). Review of the prevalence and incidence of eating disorders. *International Journal of Eating Disorders*, 34(4):383-96.

Hoopes SP, Reimherr FW, Hedges DW, Rosenthal NR, Kamin M, Karim R, et al. (2003). Treatment of bulimia nervosa with topiramate in a randomized, double-blind, placebo-controlled trial, part 1: improvement in binge and purge measures. *Journal of Clinical Psychiatry*, 64(11):1335-41.

Horne RL, Ferguson JM, Pope HG, Jr., Hudson JI, Lineberry CG, Ascher J, et al. (1988). Treatment of bulimia with bupropion: a multicenter controlled trial. *Journal of Clinical Psychiatry*, 49(7):262-6.

Hsu LK, Clement L, Santhouse R. (1987).Treatment of bulimia with lithium: a preliminary study. *Psychopharmacology Bulletin,* 23(1):45-8.

Hsu LK, Clement L, Santhouse R, Ju ES. (1991). Treatment of bulimia nervosa with lithium carbonate. A controlled study. *Journal of Nervous and Mental Disorders*, 179(6):351-5.

Hughes PL, Wells LA, Cunningham CJ, Ilstrup DM. (1986). Treating bulimia with desipramine. A double-blind, placebo-controlled study. *Archives of General Psychiatry*, 43(2):182-6.

Kennedy SH, Goldbloom DS, Ralevski E, Davis C, D'Souza JD, Lofchy J. (1993). Is there a role for selective monoamine oxidase inhibitor therapy in bulimia nervosa? A placebo-controlled trial of brofaromine. *Journal of Clinical Psychopharmacology,* 13(6):415-22.

Kennedy SH, Piran N, Warsh JJ, Prendergast P, Mainprize E, Whynot C, et al. (1988). A trial of isocarboxazid in the treatment of bulimia nervosa. *Journal of Clinical Psychopharmacology*, 8(6):391-6.

Kotler LA, Devlin MJ, Davies M, Walsh BT. (2003). An open trial of fluoxetine for adolescents with bulimia nervosa. *Journal of Child and Adolescent Psychopharmacology,* 13(3):329-35.

Milano W, Petrella C, Sabatino C, Capasso A. (2004). Treatment of bulimia nervosa with sertraline: a randomized controlled trial. *Advance Therapy*, 21(4):232-7.

Mitchell JE, Christenson G, Jennings J, Huber M, Thomas B, Pomeroy C, et al. (1989). A placebo-controlled, double-blind crossover study of naltrexone hydrochloride in outpatients with normal weight bulimia. *Journal of Clinical Psychopharmacology,* 9(2):94-7.

Mitchell JE, Fletcher L, Hanson K, Mussell MP, Seim H, Crosby R, et al. (2001). The relative efficacy of fluoxetine and manual-based self-help in the treatment of outpatients with bulimia nervosa. *Journal of Clinical Psychopharmacology,* 21(3):298-304.

Mitchell JE, Groat R. (1984). A placebo-controlled, double-blind trial of amitriptyline in bulimia. *Journal of Clinical Psychopharmacology,* 4(4):186-93.

Mitchell JE, Halmi K, Wilson GT, Agras WS, Kraemer H, Crow S. (2002). A randomized secondary treatment study of women with bulimia nervosa who fail to respond to CBT. *International Journal of Eating Disorders,* 32(3):271-81.

Mitchell JE, Pyle RL, Eckert ED, Hatsukami D, Pomeroy C, Zimmerman R. (1989). Response to alternative antidepressants in imipramine nonresponders with bulimia nervosa. *Journal of Clinical Psychopharmacology*, 9(4):291-3.

Nickel C, Tritt K, Muehlbacher M, Pedrosa Gil F, Mitterlehner FO, Kaplan P, et al. (2005). Topiramate treatment in bulimia nervosa patients: a randomized, double-blind, placebo-controlled trial. *International Journal of Eating Disorders*, 38(4):295-300.

Pope HG, Jr., Hudson JI. (1982). Treatment of bulimia with antidepressants. *Psychopharmacology (Berl)*,78(2):176-9.

Pope HG, Jr., Hudson JI, Jonas JM, Yurgelun-Todd D. (1983). Bulimia treated with imipramine: a placebo-controlled, double-blind study. *American Journal of Psychiatry*, 140(5):554-8.

Pope HG, Jr., Keck PE, Jr., McElroy SL, Hudson JI. (1989). A placebo-controlled study of trazodone in bulimia nervosa. *Journal of Clinical Psychopharmacology*, 9(4):254-9.

Reas DL, Schoemaker C, Zipfel S, Williamson DA. (2001). Prognostic value of duration of illness and early intervention in bulimia nervosa: a systematic review of the outcome literature. *International Journal of Eating Disorders*, 30(1):1-10.

Romano SJ, Halmi KA, Sarkar NP, Koke SC, Lee JS. (2002). A placebo-controlled study of fluoxetine in continued treatment of bulimia nervosa after successful acute fluoxetine treatment. *American Journal of Psychiatry*, 159(1):96-102.

Russell G. (1979). Bulimia nervosa: an ominous variant of anorexia nervosa. *Psychological Medicine,* 9(3):429-48.

Sabine EJ, Yonace A, Farrington AJ, Barratt KH, Wakeling A. (1983). Bulimia nervosa: a placebo controlled double-blind therapeutic trial of mianserin. *British Journal of Clinical Pharmacology*, 15 Suppl 2:195S-202S.

Shapiro JR, Berkman ND, Brownley KA, Sedway JA, Lohr KN, Bulik CM. (2007). Bulimia nervosa treatment: a systematic review of randomized controlled trials. *International Journal of Eating Disorders*, 40(4):321-36.

Stewart JW, Walsh BT, Wright L, Roose SP, Glassman AH. (1984). An open trial of MAO inhibitors in bulimia. *Journal of Clinical Psychiatry*, 45(5):217-9.

Sundblad C, Landen M, Eriksson T, Bergman L, Eriksson E. (2005). Effects of the androgen antagonist flutamide and the serotonin reuptake inhibitor citalopram in bulimia nervosa: a placebo-controlled pilot study. *Journal of Clinical Psychopharmacology*, 25(1):85-8.

Walsh BT, Agras WS, Devlin MJ, Fairburn CG, Wilson GT, Kahn C, et al. (2000). Fluoxetine for bulimia nervosa following poor response to psychotherapy. *American Journal of Psychiatry*, 157(8):1332-4.

Walsh BT, Fairburn CG, Mickley D, Sysko R, Parides MK. (2004). Treatment of bulimia nervosa in a primary care setting. *American Journal of Psychiatry*, 161(3):556-61.

Walsh BT, Gladis M, Roose SP, Stewart JW, Stetner F, Glassman AH. (1988). Phenelzine vs placebo in 50 patients with bulimia. *Archives of General Psychiatry*, 45(5):471-5.

Walsh BT, Hadigan CM, Devlin MJ, Gladis M, Roose SP. (1991). Long-term outcome of antidepressant treatment for bulimia nervosa. *American Journal of Psychiatry*, 148(9):1206-12.

Walsh BT, Stewart JW, Roose SP, Gladis M, Glassman AH. (1985). A double-blind trial of phenelzine in bulimia. *Journal of Psychiatric Research*, 19(2-3):485-9.

Walsh BT, Wilson GT, Loeb KL, Devlin MJ, Pike KM, Roose SP, et al. (1997). Medication and psychotherapy in the treatment of bulimia nervosa. *American Journal of Psychiatry*, 154(4):523-31.

Wilson GT. (2005). Psychological treatment of eating disorders. *Annual Review of Clinical Psychology,* 1:439-65.

Zhu AJ, Walsh BT. (2002). Pharmacologic treatment of eating disorders. *Canadian Journal of Psychiatry*, 47(3):227-34.

Index

C

D

E

I

M

S

T

U

V